Comparative Effectiveness Review
Number 95

Interventions To Modify Health Care Provider Adherence to Asthma Guidelines

Prepared for:
Agency for Healthcare Research and Quality
U.S. Department of Health and Human Services
540 Gaither Road
Rockville, MD 20850
www.ahrq.gov

Contract No. 290-2007-10061-I

Prepared by:
Johns Hopkins University Evidence-based Practice Center
Baltimore, MD

Investigators:
Sande O. Okelo, M.D., Ph.D.
Arlene M. Butz, Sc.D., R.N., C.R.N.P.
Ritu Sharma, B.Sc.
Gregory B. Diette, M.D., M.H.S.
Samantha I. Pitts, M.D., M.P.H.
Tracy M. King, M.D., M.P.H.
Shauna T. Linn, B.A.
Manisha Reuben, B.S.
Yohalakshmi Chelladurai M.B.B.S., M.P.H.
Karen A. Robinson, Ph.D.

AHRQ Publication No. 13-EHC022-EF
May 2013

This report is based on research conducted by the Johns Hopkins University Evidence-based Practice Center (EPC) under contract to the Agency for Healthcare Research and Quality (AHRQ), Rockville, MD (Contract No. 290-2007-10061-I). The findings and conclusions in this document are those of the authors, who are responsible for its contents; the findings and conclusions do not necessarily represent the views of AHRQ. Therefore, no statement in this report should be construed as an official position of AHRQ or of the U.S. Department of Health and Human Services.

The information in this report is intended to help health care decisionmakers—patients and clinicians, health system leaders, and policymakers, among others—make well-informed decisions and thereby improve the quality of health care services. This report is not intended to be a substitute for the application of clinical judgment. Anyone who makes decisions concerning the provision of clinical care should consider this report in the same way as any medical reference and in conjunction with all other pertinent information, i.e., in the context of available resources and circumstances presented by individual patients.

This report may be used, in whole or in part, as the basis for development of clinical practice guidelines and other quality enhancement tools, or as a basis for reimbursement and coverage policies. AHRQ or U.S. Department of Health and Human Services endorsement of such derivative products may not be stated or implied.

Persons using assistive technology may not be able to fully access information in this report. For assistance contact EffectiveHealthcare@ahrq.hhs.gov.

None of the investigators have any affiliations or financial involvement that conflicts with the material presented in this report.

Suggested citation: Okelo SO, Butz AM, Sharma R, Diette GB, Pitts SI, King TM, Linn ST, Reuben M, Chelladurai Y, Robinson KA. Interventions To Modify Health Care Provider Adherence to Asthma Guidelines. Comparative Effectiveness Review No. 95. (Prepared by Johns Hopkins University Evidence-based Practice Center under Contract No. 290-2007-10061-I.) AHRQ Publication No. 13-EHC022-EF. Rockville, MD. Agency for Healthcare Research and Quality. www.effectivehealthcare.ahrq.gov/reports/final.cfm. May 2013.

Preface

The Agency for Healthcare Research and Quality (AHRQ), through its Evidence-based Practice Centers (EPCs), sponsors the development of systematic reviews to assist public- and private-sector organizations in their efforts to improve the quality of health care in the United States. These reviews provide comprehensive, science-based information on common, costly medical conditions, and new health care technologies and strategies.

Systematic reviews are the building blocks underlying evidence-based practice; they focus attention on the strength and limits of evidence from research studies about the effectiveness and safety of a clinical intervention. In the context of developing recommendations for practice, systematic reviews can help clarify whether assertions about the value of the intervention are based on strong evidence from clinical studies. For more information about AHRQ EPC systematic reviews, see www.effectivehealthcare.ahrq.gov/reference/purpose.cfm.

AHRQ expects that these systematic reviews will be helpful to health plans, providers, purchasers, government programs, and the health care system as a whole. Transparency and stakeholder input are essential to the Effective Health Care Program. Please visit the Web site (www.effectivehealthcare.ahrq.gov) to see draft research questions and reports or to join an email list to learn about new program products and opportunities for input.

We welcome comments on this systematic review. They may be sent by mail to the Task Order Officer named below at: Agency for Healthcare Research and Quality, 540 Gaither Road, Rockville, MD 20850, or by email to epc@ahrq.hhs.gov.

Carolyn M. Clancy, M.D.
Director
Agency for Healthcare Research and Quality

Jean Slutsky, P.A., M.S.P.H.
Director, Center for Outcomes and Evidence
Agency for Healthcare Research and Quality

Stephanie Chang, M.D., M.P.H.
Director,
Evidence-based Practice Program
Center for Outcomes and Evidence
Agency for Healthcare Research and Quality

Christine Chang, M.D., M.P.H.
Task Order Officer
Center for Outcomes and Evidence
Agency for Healthcare Research and Quality

Acknowledgments

The authors gratefully acknowledge the continuing support of our AHRQ Task Order Officer, Christine Chang, M.D., M.P.H. We extend our appreciation to our Key Informants and members of our Technical Expert Panel (listed below), all of whom provided thoughtful advice and input during our research process.

The Evidence-based Practice Center thanks Oluwatosin Ikotun, Nelson Biodun Olagbuji, and Oluwaseun Omole for their assistance with reviewing articles and data abstraction.

Key Informants

Michael Cabana, M.D., M.P.H.
University of California, San Francisco
San Francisco, CA

Lisa Cicutto, Ph.D., R.N.
National Jewish Health & University of
    Colorado, Denver
Denver, CO

Cheryl De Pinto, M.D.
Maryland Asthma Control Program
Maryland Department of Health and Mental
    Hygiene
Baltimore, MD

Arethusa Kirk, M.D., FAAP
Total Health Care, Inc.
Baltimore, MD

Margret Schnitzer, M.S.M.
Greater Baltimore Asthma Alliance
Baltimore, MD

Kate Scott, R.N., M.P.H.
Baltimore City Health Department
Healthy Homes and Communities Division
Baltimore, MD

Technical Expert Panel

Michael Cabana, M.D., M.P.H.
University of California, San Francisco
San Francisco, CA

Rey Panettieri, M.D.
University of Pennsylvania
Philadelphia, PA

Frederic Wolf, Ph.D., M.Ed.
University of Washington
Seattle, WA

Barbara Yawn, M.D., M.Sc., FAAFP
Olmsted Medical Center
Rochester, MN

Jessica Zar
American Academy of Pediatrics
Elk Grove Village, IL

Ilene Zuckerman, Pharm.D, Ph.D.
University of Maryland
Baltimore, MD

Interventions To Modify Health Care Provider Adherence to Asthma Guidelines

Structured Abstract

Objective. To synthesize the published literature on the effect of interventions designed to improve health care providers' adherence to asthma guidelines on: (1) health care process outcomes (Key Question 1); (2) clinical outcomes (Key Question 2); (3) health care processes that subsequently impact clinical outcomes (Key Question 3).

Data sources. Reports of studies from MEDLINE®, Embase®, Cochrane Central Register of Controlled Trials (CENTRAL), Cumulative Index to Nursing and Allied Health Literature (CINAHL®), Educational Resources Information Center (ERIC^sm), PsycINFO®, and Research and Development Resource Base in Continuing Medical Education (RDRB/CME), up to July 2012.

Review methods. Paired investigators independently reviewed each title, abstract, and full-text article to assess eligibility. Only comparative studies were eligible. Investigators abstracted data sequentially and independently graded the evidence.

Results. A total of 73 studies were eligible for review. A slight majority of studies were conducted in the U.S. (n=38). We classified studies as assessing eight types of interventions: decision support, organizational change, feedback and audit, clinical pharmacy support, education only, quality improvement (QI)/pay-for-performance, multicomponent, and information only. Half of the studies were randomized trials (n=34), 29 were pre-post, and the remaining 10 were a variety of nonrandomized study designs. The studies took place exclusively in primary care settings. The most frequently cited health care process outcome was prescription of asthma controller medication (n=41), followed by provision of an asthma action plan (n=18), prescription of a peak flow meter (n=17), and self-management education (n=12). Common clinical outcomes included emergency department (ED) visits (n=30) and hospitalizations (n=27), followed by use of short-acting β2 agonists (n=9), missed school days (n=8), lung function tests (n=6), symptom days (n=6), quality of life (n=5), and urgent doctor visits (n=5). We identified 4 critical outcomes for which 68 studies provided information. There was moderate evidence for increased prescriptions of asthma controller medications using decision support, feedback and audit, and clinical pharmacy support interventions and low grade evidence for organizational change, multicomponent interventions. Moderate evidence supports the use of decision support and clinical pharmacy interventions to increase provision of patient self-education/asthma action plans; for the same outcome, low grade evidence supports the use of organizational change, feedback and audit, education only, quality improvement, and multicomponent interventions. Moderate grade evidence supports use of decision support tools to reduce ED visits/hospitalizations while low grade evidence suggests there is no benefit associated with organizational change, education only, and QI/pay-for-performance. Organizational change interventions provided no benefit for lost days of work/school. The evidence for the remainder of interventions was insufficient or low in strength.

Conclusions. There is low to moderate evidence to support the use of decision support tools, feedback and audit, and clinical pharmacy support to improve the adherence of health care providers to asthma guidelines, as measured through health care process outcomes, and to improve clinical outcomes. There is a need to further evaluate health care provider-targeted interventions with a focus on standardized measures of outcomes and more rigorous study designs.

Contents

Tables

Figures

Appendixes

Appendix A. Acronyms and Abbreviations
Appendix B. Detailed Search Strategies
Appendix C. Screening and Data Abstraction Forms
Appendix D. Excluded Studies
Appendix E. Evidence Tables

Executive Summary

Background

Asthma is a respiratory disease characterized by variable and recurring symptoms, airflow obstruction, bronchial hyper-responsiveness, and inflammation of the airways. In the U.S., an estimated 24.6 million people (8.2 percent) currently have asthma.[1] Students with asthma miss more than 14 million school days every year due to illness. In 2005, there were approximately 679,000 emergency room visits in the U.S. due to asthma in children under 15 years of age.[2] Currently, asthma is the third leading cause of hospitalization among children in this age group.[2] Furthermore, certain U.S. population subgroups have higher prevalence rates of asthma in comparison with the national average: children (9.6 percent), poor children (13.5 percent), non-Hispanic African American children (17.0 percent), women (9.7 percent), and poor adults (10.6 percent).[1]

A number of asthma guidelines have been published internationally (e.g., the National Asthma Education and Prevention Program "Expert Panel Report 3: Guidelines for the Diagnosis and Management of Asthma" is also known as EPR-3,[3] a guideline based on a systematic review of published evidence and expert opinion). Following asthma guideline treatment recommendations improves clinical outcomes in a variety of pediatric populations, including high-risk populations, such as inner-city, poor, and/or African American populations.[4-6] The available evidence suggests that most people with asthma can be symptom-free if they receive appropriate medical care, use inhaled corticosteroids when prescribed, and modify their environment to reduce or eliminate exposure to allergens and irritants.

Despite the evidence of improved outcomes associated with adherence to guidelines, their long-term existence (>20 years) and widespread availability, health care providers do not routinely follow asthma guideline recommendations.[7,8] In one study, only 34.2 percent of patients reported receiving a written asthma action plan, while only 68.1 percent had been taught the appropriate response to symptoms of an asthma attack.[8] In the same study, only about one-third of children or adults were using long-term asthma controller medicine such as inhaled corticosteroids. Health care providers do not appropriately assess asthma control in most children,[9-12] resulting in substandard care. Minority children are up to half as likely as Caucasian children to receive inhaled steroids.[13] The significance of these studies is that suboptimal outcomes persist, such as twofold higher rates of emergency room visits for African American children compared with their Caucasian counterparts.[14]

With the lack of adherence to guideline recommendations, attention has been focused on why best practices are not followed (i.e., adhered to) by health care providers. In 1999, Cabana et al.[15] proposed a theoretical framework to understand why physicians do not adhere to guidelines, citing lack of awareness, disagreement with the guidelines recommendations, doubts about the effectiveness of the guidelines recommendations, lack of confidence in being able to carry out the best practice, inability to overcome the inertia of previous practice behaviors, and external barriers (e.g., time constraints during a visit, lack of user-friendly guidelines, patient preferences). There is a growing understanding that one of the shortcomings of asthma guidelines is the limited extent to which health care providers are provided with the tools and resources necessary to follow the recommended care.[16] There is a lack of interventions developed specifically to address the barriers outlined by Cabana et al. Awareness of asthma guidelines may have improved over time,[17,18] but certain barriers outlined by Cabana et al. would likely not be overcome as a result of increased exposure to asthma guidelines (e.g., the inability of health care providers to overcome practice inertia and external barriers).[19] Therefore, learning what strategies are available to overcome these barriers and improve adherence to asthma guidelines would be beneficial.

Most interventions targeting improvement of asthma care and outcomes have been patient-focused,[20-23] but there have also been provider-targeted interventions to improve adherence to guidelines (e.g., educational seminars, prompts, etc.).[24-29] However, there is no consensus on the most effective provider-targeted interventions that improve adherence to guidelines.

Scope and Key Questions

The objective of our systematic review was to assess whether interventions targeting health care providers improve adherence to asthma guideline recommendations for asthma care and if these interventions subsequently improve clinical outcomes for patients. We also sought to determine whether any observed changes in asthma care processes directly improve clinical outcomes. Successful interventions were those in which statistically significant improvements in a given outcome (e.g., prescriptions for controller medications) were observed. Ultimately results of this report will inform health care providers and policymakers regarding successful interventions or components of specific interventions that may be translated into clinical practice with the goal to improve health care provider adherence to asthma guidelines for their patients. It is important to note that the scope of this project does not include assessments of cost for implementation of the interventions reviewed. Therefore, users of this report will have to seek supplemental information to understand the complete implications of these interventions to patients, physicians, and organizations. This report has provided an organized systematic review of provider-focused interventions to improve asthma care and outcomes. Therefore, this report should provide a context in which to organize different types of interventions, their relative impact on a variety of outcomes, and considerations for what and how future studies should be planned. Our specific Key Questions (KQs) are listed below and are displayed graphically in Figure A.

KQ1: In the care of pediatric or adult patients with asthma, what is the evidence that interventions designed to improve health care provider adherence to guidelines impact health care process outcomes (e.g., receiving appropriate treatment)?

KQ2: In the care of pediatric or adult patients with asthma, what is the evidence that interventions designed to improve health care provider adherence to guidelines impact clinical outcomes (e.g., hospitalizations, patient-reported outcomes such as symptom control)?

KQ3: In the care of pediatric or adult patients with asthma, what is the evidence that interventions designed to improve health care provider adherence to guidelines impact health care process outcomes that then affect clinical outcomes?

Figure A. Analytic framework for guidelines on the care of adults and children with asthma

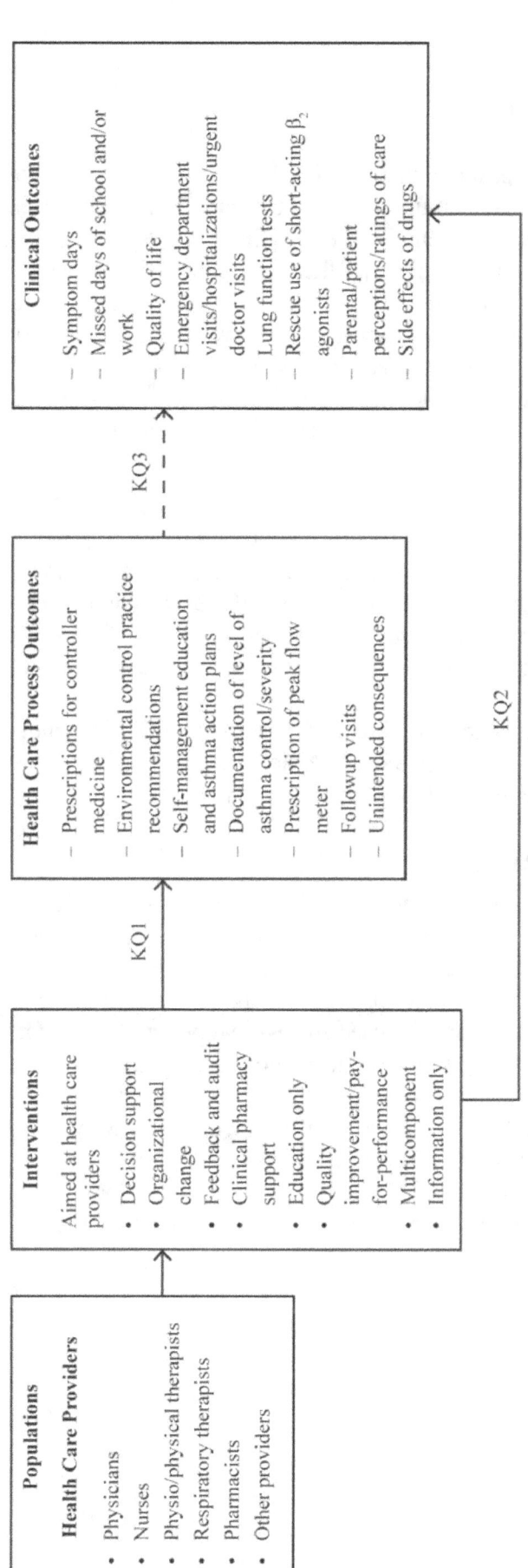

| Populations | | Interventions | | Health Care Process Outcomes | | Clinical Outcomes |

Populations

Health Care Providers

- Physicians
- Nurses
- Physio/physical therapists
- Respiratory therapists
- Pharmacists
- Other providers

Interventions

Aimed at health care providers

- Decision support
- Organizational change
- Feedback and audit
- Clinical pharmacy support
- Education only
- Quality improvement/pay-for-performance
- Multicomponent
- Information only

Health Care Process Outcomes

– Prescriptions for controller medicine
– Environmental control practice recommendations
– Self-management education and asthma action plans
– Documentation of level of asthma control/severity
– Prescription of peak flow meter
– Followup visits
– Unintended consequences

Clinical Outcomes

– Symptom days
– Missed days of school and/or work
– Quality of life
– Emergency department visits/hospitalizations/urgent doctor visits
– Lung function tests
– Rescue use of short-acting β_2 agonists
– Parental/patient perceptions/ratings of care
– Side effects of drugs

KQ1

KQ3

KQ2

KQ = Key Question

Methods

Literature Search Strategy

We searched the following databases for primary studies: MEDLINE®, Embase®, and the Cochrane Central Register of Controlled Trials, Cumulative Index to Nursing and Allied Health Literature (CINAHL®), Educational Resources Information Center (ERIC^SM), PsycINFO®, and Research and Development Resource Base in Continuing Medical Education (RDRB/CME) through July 2012. We developed a search strategy for MEDLINE, accessed via PubMed®, based on an analysis of the medical subject headings (MeSH), terms, and text words of eligible articles identified a priori (Appendix B). This strategy was translated for use in the other electronic sources. No limits were imposed based on language or date of publication. Searches were conducted in July 2012. We also completed backward citation searching using Scopus for each included article.

Study Selection

Title and abstracts were screened independently by two trained investigators, and were excluded if both investigators agreed that the article met one or more of the exclusion criteria (see inclusion and exclusion criteria listed in Table A and the Abstract Review Form in Appendix C). Differences between investigators regarding abstract eligibility were resolved through consensus.

Citations promoted on the basis of title and abstract screen underwent another independent paired-reviewer screen using the full-text article (Appendix C, Article Review Form). Differences regarding article inclusion were resolved through consensus.

Data Abstraction and Data Management

We used DistillerSR (Evidence Partners, 2010) to manage the screening process. DistillerSR is a Web-based database management program that manages all levels of the review process. We uploaded to the system all citations identified by our search.

We created standardized forms for data extraction (Appendix C) and pilot tested the forms prior to the beginning the process of data extraction. We used Access (Microsoft, Redmond, WA) for the data abstraction process. Reviewers extracted information on general study characteristics, study participants, eligibility criteria, interventions, and the outcomes. One reviewer completed data abstraction and the second reviewer confirmed the first reviewer's data abstraction for completeness and accuracy. Reviewers completed risk of bias assessment independently. Reviewer pairs included personnel with both clinical and methodological expertise. We resolved differences between reviewer pairs through consensus among the larger group of investigators.

Table A. Study inclusion and exclusion criteria

PICOTS Framework	Inclusion	Exclusion
Populations	Participants: human subjects. Health care providers: physicians, nurses, physiotherapists/physical therapists, respiratory therapists, pharmacists, and other health care providers treating children or adults <u>with asthma.</u>	• Animal models/simulations.
Intervention	Interventions to improve adherence to guidelines including decision support (health information technology and paper-based), organizational change, feedback and audit, clinical pharmacy support, education only, quality improvement/pay-for-performance, multicomponent, information only.	Studies that do not: • Assess an intervention. • Address adherence to asthma guidelines. • Target health care providers.
Comparisons of interest	Usual care, as defined in each eligible study, and comparisons between interventions.	Studies lacking a comparison.

Outcomes	**Health care process outcomes:**
	  ➤ Prescriptions for controller medicine
	  ➤ Environmental control practice recommendations
	  ➤ Self-management education and asthma action plans
	  ➤ Documentation of level of asthma control/severity
	  ➤ Prescription of peak flow meter
	  ➤ Followup visits
	  ➤ Unintended consequences
	Clinical outcomes:
	  ➤ Symptom days
	  ➤ Missed days of school and/or work
	  ➤ Quality of life
	  ➤ Emergency department visits/hospitalizations/urgent doctor visits
	  ➤ Lung function tests
	  ➤ Rescue use of short-acting B2 agonists
	  ➤ Parental/patient perceptions/ratings of care
	  ➤ Side effects of drugs
	The outcomes were nondirectional; that is, all outcomes were considered whether they were beneficial or caused potential harms or unintended consequences.
		Studies that do not report an outcome of interest (e.g., studies reporting acceptability of intervention only).

Type of Study	Randomized and quasi-randomized controlled trials and cross-over studies. Nonrandomized studies with comparison groups including nonrandomized controlled trial or crossover studies, controlled pre-post studies, historically controlled studies, cohort studies, case-control studies, and cross-sectional studies. Nonrandomized studies without a separate comparison group, including interrupted-time-series, noncontrolled and pre-post studies.	We excluded meeting abstracts, studies with no original data (e.g., reviews, editorials, comments, and letters) and noncomparative studies.
Timing and Setting	Studies of any duration followup that occurred in an outpatient setting employing healthcare providers were eligible for inclusion.	We excluded studies exclusively addressing inpatient or emergency department settings or guidelines.

Risk of Bias Assessment

We used the Cochrane Collaboration's tool for assessing the risk of bias of controlled studies. Two reviewers independently assessed the included studies according to the guidelines in Chapter 8 of the Cochrane Handbook for Systematic Reviews of Interventions[30] using the following criteria: sequence generation and allocation concealment (selection bias), blinding of health care providers, investigators, and outcome assessors (detection bias), incomplete outcome data (attrition bias), selective outcome reporting (reporting bias), and other sources of bias. We report judgments for each criterion as "Low risk of bias," "High risk of bias," or "Unclear risk of bias (information is insufficient to assess)."

For pre-post studies, we added the two relevant criteria from the Cochrane Effective Practice and Organization of Care (EPOC) data collections checklists.[31]

Data Synthesis

For each KQ, we created a detailed set of evidence tables containing all information abstracted from eligible studies. We grouped the information for each KQ by intervention(s) being assessed:

1. Decision support interventions are health information technology- and/or paper-based-interventions designed to support/facilitate health care provider treatment decisionmaking (e.g., classify asthma severity);
2. Organizational change interventions are designed to change the way in which an organization provides asthma care (e.g., having an asthma "champion");
3. Feedback and audit interventions are based upon providing performance data to health care providers about their quality of asthma care;
4. Clinical pharmacy service support: interventions targeting pharmacists' delivery of asthma care;
5. Education-only interventions are focused on educating health care providers about the content of asthma clinical practice guidelines;
6. Quality improvement/pay-for-performance interventions are focused on quality improvement initiatives or pay-for-performance as the primary intervention;
7. Multicomponent interventions use more than one type of intervention; and
8. Information-only interventions are designed only to provide information to health care providers about asthma guideline recommendations (e.g., provide a pocket guide to asthma guidelines).

Studies implementing combinations of interventions were categorized by the predominant intervention. Studies using multiple interventions in which no single intervention could be characterized as predominant were grouped into a separate category.

Based on input from key informants and public comment, the following outcomes were abstracted.

The health care process outcomes included:
- Prescriptions for controller medicine
- Environmental control practice recommendations
- Self-management education and asthma action plans
- Documentation of level of asthma control/severity
- Prescription of peak flow meter

- Followup visits
- Unintended consequences

The clinical outcomes, assessed in patients, included:

- Symptom days
- Missed days of school and/or work
- Quality of life
- Emergency department (ED) visits/hospitalizations/urgent doctor visits
- Lung function tests
- Rescue use of short-acting β_2 agonists
- Parental/patient perceptions/ratings of care
- Side effects of drugs

To answer Key Question 3, we sought to identify studies providing evidence on the link between changes in health care provider behavior (health care process outcomes) to changes in clinical outcomes. Ideally, relevant studies suitably answering Key Question 3 would measure both health care process and clinical outcomes, as well as measure the strength of association between the changes in health care process to the change in clinical outcomes observed in a given study.

To focus our synthesis, we selected outcomes we considered the most commonly used in practice; those relied upon by clinicians to guide decisionmaking; and those endorsed by the NIH Workshop on Asthma Outcomes.[32] These critical outcomes identified were prescription of asthma controller medicines, provision of asthma action plan/self-management education, ED visits/hospitalizations, and missed days of school or work.[33] Data abstracted for all outcomes can be found in Appendix E.

We conducted a qualitative synthesis of the evidence. The heterogeneity of the studies, related to measures of outcomes, population included, and specifics of the interventions, precluded quantitative synthesis.

In the absence of national qualitative standards to determine magnitude of effect in clinical asthma studies, we chose magnitudes of effect by group consensus among the investigators that were felt to be clinically meaningful changes. Magnitude of effect for studies addressing each outcome was described as small (less than 10 percent change or difference), moderate (10–30 percent change or difference), and large (over 30 percent change or difference). These judgments were made by one reviewer and checked by another, with disagreements discussed with the full team.

Strength of the Body of Evidence

Two reviewers graded the strength of evidence for each outcome for each of the Key Questions using the grading scheme recommended by the "Methods Guide for Effectiveness and Comparative Effectiveness Reviews."[34] In assigning evidence grades we considered four domains: risk of bias, directness, consistency, and precision. We classified evidence into four basic categories: (1) "high" grade (indicating high confidence that the evidence reflects the true effect, and further research is very unlikely to change our confidence in the estimate of the effect); (2) "moderate" grade (indicating moderate confidence that the evidence reflects the true effect, and further research may change our confidence in the estimate of the effect and may change the estimate); (3) "low" grade (indicating low confidence that the evidence reflects the true effect, and further research is likely to change our confidence in the estimate of the effect and is likely to change the estimate); and (4) "insufficient" grade (evidence is unavailable or does not permit a conclusion). Our judgments were first based on the ability to make a conclusion (if not able to make a conclusion, then "insufficient" was assigned) and then on the confidence in the conclusion (classified as low, moderate, or high with increasing certainty). The author of the section first graded the evidence and this was reviewed by the principal investigator. Any disagreements were discussed with the full team.

Applicability

An applicability statement was created in order to help different key stakeholders understand what key implications to take away from this document, to inform future relevant activities. Applicability was assessed separately for the different outcomes of benefit and harm for the entire body of evidence guided by the PICOTS framework as recommended in the "Methods Guide for Effectiveness and Comparative Effectiveness Reviews."[34] We considered factors that may limit applicability of the findings (e.g., a study conducted in a non-U.S. health care setting, providers not common to the U.S. health care system).

Results

Results of Literature Searches

We identified 4,217 unique citations. We excluded 3,892 citations during the abstract screening. During full-text article screening, we excluded an additional 249 articles that did not meet one or more of the inclusion criteria. Seventy-three articles were eligible for inclusion and 68 addressed 1 of the 4 critical outcomes (prescription of asthma controller medicines, provision of asthma action plan/self-management education, ED visits/hospitalizations, and missed days of school or work) and are thus included in the narrative of the report.

Organization of Results

The results are organized according to each KQ, the four critical outcomes, and each type of intervention. For each KQ, a description and summary of the key findings from each type of intervention are presented, along with a table summarizing the strength of evidence.

Results by Key Questions

KQ1: In the care of pediatric or adult patients with asthma, what is the evidence that interventions designed to improve health care provider adherence to guidelines impact health care process outcomes (prescription of controller medications; providing asthma education/asthma action plans)?

Outcome: Prescription of Controller Medicines

Decision Support

Fifteen studies of decision support interventions evaluated the effects on prescription of asthma controller medications: six RCTs[5,35-39] and nine pre-post studies.[40-48] The types of decision support interventions varied, including the provision of asthma guidelines in a more accessible format (e.g., "pocket" versions),[37,44,46] use of a specific algorithm, pathway or flow sheet,[37,45-47] a structured template for taking a history,[40,41] or a reminder system to raise awareness of the health care provider about the patient's asthma status.[5,36,42] The decision support interventions were often combined with other strategies, including education,[35,37-39,42,47,49,50] reminders,[36,39-41,44] feedback,[5,44] and/or organizational change.[43] Computer-based interventions served to guide the health care provider through a guideline-consistent assessment and/or treatment approach.[36,38,39,42,44,48,51]

Ten studies reported that a decision support intervention significantly increased prescribing of asthma controller medicines by health care providers,[5,35,39-42,44,45,47,48] while the remaining studies did not.[36-38,43,46] Eight of the studies in which increased prescribing was observed used a pre-post study design, while three of the five RCTs observed no benefit from decision support interventions.[36-38] The increase in prescribing of asthma controller medicines ranged from 2 percent to 34 percent in the pre-post design studies and ranged from 2 percent to 17 percent in RCTs. The absolute difference in effect observed between control and interventions arms of the RCT studies was generally less than 10 percent. In summary, moderate evidence supports the use of decision support interventions to increase prescribing of asthma controller medications.

Organizational Change

Two studies[52,53] examined the impact of organizational change on the prescribing of asthma controller medications by health care providers. One study was an RCT,[52] while the other used a pre-post study design.[53] Both studies focused the intervention on pediatric health care providers. Both studies utilized additional personnel to facilitate organizational change, as well as education for the participating health care providers. One study used an asthma nurse educator,[52] while the pre-post study used a community health worker.[53] The RCT found that neither the peer-led education arm nor the planned care intervention (utilizing an asthma nurse educator) arms resulted in a significantly higher proportion of prescriptions for inhaled steroids or asthma controller medications compared with the control arm of the study.[52] Notably, prescribing increased in all arms of the study, including the control arm. The improvement in prescribing any type of controller medication ranged from 8 to 16 percent among all patients with asthma and 4 to 11 percent among asthma patients with persistent asthma In the pre-post study, investigators observed a 12 percent increase (absolute change from 44 percent to 56 percent) in prescriptions for inhaled steroids among all asthma patients (no p-value reported).[53] Low strength of evidence supports the effectiveness of organizational change in increasing the prescribing of asthma controller medicines.

Feedback and Audit

We identified six RCTs,[54-59] four pre-post studies,[60-63] and one nonrandomized controlled study[64] evaluating the effect of feedback and audit interventions on the prescription of controller medications. Most feedback and audit interventions were part of a multifaceted intervention combined with provider education,[54,57,59-63] prioritized review criteria for audit,[56] benchmarking or comparison with peers or other practices[56,58] or pharmacy monitoring of fill data and feedback.[64]

Of the six RCTs,[54-59] four demonstrated positive effects from the intervention.[54,56,57,59] Increased prescribing of asthma controller medicines was reported for audit and feedback interventions using targeted key guideline messages about the inflammatory nature of asthma (such as, "use inhaled corticosteroids promptly") (5 percent to 12 percent increase from baseline, p=0.05),[54] prioritized guideline review criteria on single card,[56] medical record prompts for annual review of asthma management with guideline prompts,[57] and individualized feedback on prescribing and decision strategies.[59] The two RCTs reporting no effect on prescribing of asthma controller medications involved feedback of prescribing data[55] and a trial of performance feedback.[58] Of the studies using a pre-post or nonrandomized controlled design, two studies reported an increase in prescribing of controller medicines.[62,64] The increase reported in these studies ranged from 52 to 104 percent.[62,64] The magnitude of effect for feedback and audit support on the prescription of controller medications is moderate. The positive effect sizes, measured as an increase in patients on inhaled corticosteroids from baseline to outcome and between intervention and control groups, ranged from a low (0.12) to a moderate (0.66) effect size.[54] A significant increase in the change of percentage of patients treated with inhaled steroid from baseline to 12 months post intervention between three groups (guidelines alone, prioritized guideline review criteria and review criteria plus feedback on actual prescribing behavior) was noted as a positive increase of 15.9 percent in controller prescribing in the review criteria plus feedback group as compared with an increase of 11 percent in the review criteria only and no change (0 percent) in the guideline only group.[56] A positive but nonsignificant difference (2.7 percent difference in proportion of patients) was noted in the proportions of patients in practice with asthma "prophylaxis" after one year as compared with practices provided with diabetes guidelines (Difference in asthma prophylaxis: 2.7 [95% CI: -14.4 to19.7]).[57]

Two RCTs reported no effect on prescribing asthma controller medications, based on low hazard ratios of 0.77 (95% CI: 0.59, 1.01) and 1.08 (95% CI: 0.90, 1.3).One study used a mailed prescriber feedback intervention.[55] In the other study, there was no difference in percentage of patients prescribed medication consistent with guidelines (3.2 to 8 percent, p=0.19) between a "benchmark" group (their prescribing behavior was compared with a performance benchmark or with other prescribers) versus a traditional or individual feedback group (who did not receive comparison with other prescribers).[58] Of the five pre-post design studies, only three reported an increase in prescribing controller medications, ranging from 52 percent to 104 percent; change in prescribing over time (52 percent change over 6 months), increase of 104.4 percent in patients with intermittent asthma but a decrease of ICS by 10.0 percent in patients with persistent asthma. The strength of the evidence of feedback and audit support on the prescription of asthma controller medications is moderate with several caveats. Factors that lessen the confidence in the results include inconsistent definitions of controller medication prescribing behavior (controller only, controller + rescue medication, and prophylaxis asthma medication), wide variation in feedback and audit intervention protocols, use of varying clinical asthma and GP guidelines over a long period (1990–2007), inconsistent followup periods ranging from 3-12 months, and inconsistent control in the analysis for asthma severity. The strength of the evidence in support of feedback/audit interventions to increase prescribing of controller medicines by health care providers is moderate.

Clinical Pharmacy Support

Three studies—one RCT,[65] one nonrandomized study[66] and a controlled pre-post study[67]—evaluated the effect of clinical pharmacy support on the prescription of asthma controller medications. In the RCT, pharmacists trained in risk assessment, medication adherence, and spirometry reported increases in the dispensation of asthma controller medicines (odds ratio: 3.80 [95% CI: 1.40, 10.32]; p=0.01).[65] In the two non-RCTs, increases in controller medication prescribing of 20 percent[67] and 6 percent[66] were observed (p<0.05 for both studies). In the controlled pre-post study, the intervention was a specialized asthma service provided by community pharmacies; components included seeing patients by appointment, assessment and intervention in responses to patient medication needs, and goal-setting with the patient.[67] In the latter study, pharmacists were encouraged to hold meetings with local general practitioners to discuss guidelines for the care of children with asthma.[66] The strength of the evidence of clinical pharmacy support on the prescription of asthma controller medications is moderate because of consistent and precise results, though the risk of bias was high. The one RCT evaluating the effect of clinical pharmacy support on the prescription of asthma controller medications versus rescue medication for children, indicated a large shift from the use of rescue medication only to rescue medication plus controller medication (OR 3.80 [95% CI: 1.40, 10.32], p=0.01).[65] The evidence from this study is of high quality due to its large sample size (n=50 pharmacies and n=351/396 patients completing study), blinding of pharmacists and high rates of followup (intervention: 86 percent and control: 91 percent). Still, it is the only RCT evaluating a pharmacy intervention. The two non-RCTs reported moderate effect size defined as change in percentage of patients prescribed controller medication between pre and post intervention periods (6 percent to 21 percent);[66,67] however, the studies either lacked a large sample size and/or reported inconsistent description of controller medication use ("no inhaled corticosteroid use while on long-acting betamimetics"[74] or ideal profile was reliever + preventer + symptom controller medication).[66]

In summary, the strength of the evidence is moderate for an effect of clinical pharmacy support on the prescription of asthma controller medications with a moderate increase in prescribing of controller medications.

Education Only

Ten studies of education alone as an intervention examined prescribing asthma controller medication as an outcome. Six were RCTs[26,68-72] and four were pre-post designs.[73-76] Nearly all of the studies targeted primary care physicians (GPs, FPs, pediatricians) or nurses. One study recruited pharmacists.[71] The education interventions were varied and included small group asthma education programs,[69] structured training,[76] seminars (including interactive),[70] and grand rounds.[76] Besides delivering specific asthma content, certain interventions also emphasized more general skills, such as training in communication.[68,70] The findings from all studies were consistently in the positive direction, reporting increases in controller medicines prescribing from 3.5 percent to 50.3 percent, though statistically significant differences were reported in only three of the studies. Provider education does not appear to increase the prescription of asthma controller medications. However, our confidence in this conclusion is low (low strength of evidence).

Quality Improvement and Pay-for-Performance

No studies examined the effect of quality improvement strategies on prescription of asthma controller medications. Therefore, there is insufficient evidence for this outcome.

Multicomponent

Seven studies evaluated the impact of multicomponent interventions.[77-83] All interventions included *information, education,* and at least two of the following; *organizational change, decision support,* and *feedback and audit.* Four[78-80,83] were cluster-randomized controlled trials (randomizing primary care practices) and three[77,81,82] were pre-post studies with no comparison group. Only two of the pre-post studies[77,81] and one of the three RCTs[78] found an impact of their multicomponent intervention on rates of inhaled corticosteroid prescriptions. The two pre-post studies found large positive effects on ICS prescribing rates (25 percent to 49 percent increases). Among the four experimental studies, three found effects in a positive direction, but only one reached statistical significance, and the magnitude of effect was small (0.1 puff per day per patient between groups). In summary, there is low strength of evidence supporting the effectiveness of multicomponent interventions to increase prescribing of controller medications for asthma.

Information Only

Two RCTs[84,85] evaluated the provision of information to health care providers (without an accompanying educational intervention) on rates of controller medication prescribing. One study, which randomized patients to have asthma management information and treatment guidelines inserted into their medical records for provider use, reported no benefit.[85] The second study[84] included providers randomly selected to participate in developing local asthma guidelines, which were then mailed to providers in both intervention and comparison groups. This study reported a negative effect on controller medication prescribing, with providers in the intervention group writing 8 fewer prescriptions per 1,000 patients than those in the comparison group ($p<0.01$). This is the only unintended consequence that we identified. In summary, because of inconsistent results between only two studies, there is insufficient evidence to evaluate the effect of information alone on rates of controller medication prescribing in asthma.

Outcome: Self-Management Education and Asthma Action Plans

Decision Support

Ten studies evaluated the impact of decision support interventions on the provision of patient education/asthma action plans.[27,38,39,43,44,46,49,86-88] Four of the studies were RCTs,[38,39,87,88] while the remainder employed a pre-post study design.[49,27,43,44,46,86] The interventions included computerized support,[38,39,43,44,88] a flow sheet/algorithm,[27,86] and/or the provision of guidelines.[46] These studies all focused on primary care settings and involved general practitioners,[38] pediatricians,[49,87] or family practitioners.[27]

Seven of these studies reported a positive effect of decision support on the provision of patient education/asthma action plans.[27,43,44,46,49,86,87] The increase in self-management education/use of asthma action plans ranged from 14 percent to 84 percent (all reported as statistically significant). Of the four RCTs, only one showed a positive impact from decision support intervention.[87] In summary, moderate evidence supports the use of decision support interventions to increase the provision of asthma education/asthma action plans by health care providers.

Organizational Change

Two studies examined how organizational change influenced the provision of patient self-management education and/or asthma action plans; one used an RCT design[89] and the other a pre-post design.[90] In the pre-post study, the investigators[90] instituted a registry to track asthma patients and an asthma case manager, while in the RCT[89] the investigators restructured the clinical protocol for how asthma patients are cared for during ambulatory care encounters ("3+ visit plan"). In general, the effect of organizational changes to increase self-management education/asthma action plan use by health care providers was small. Investigators in the pre-post study observed a 10 percent increase in documentation of patient education ($p<0.001$) and a 14 percent increase in documentation of home asthma action plan dispensations ($p<0.001$), while in the RCT, there was a 10 percent increase in asthma education ($p=0.01$). In summary, low strength of evidence supports the use of organizational change as a method to increase the provision of self-management education/asthma action plan by health care providers.

Feedback and Audit

Five studies—three RCTs[56-58] and two pre-post studies[61,63]—evaluated the effect of feedback and audit interventions on the provision of self-management education and asthma action plans by health care providers. Statistically significant increases in provision of self-management education/asthma action plans ranging from 1 to 40 percent were reported in four of the five studies.[57,58,61,63] The magnitude of effect for feedback and audit support to increase the provision of self-management education/asthma action plans is low based on a range of negative to low differences in proportions for practices recording peak flow meter use after a feedback/audit intervention. A negative change for peak flow meter use was noted in the guideline review criteria plus feedback group (decrease 3.6 percent)[56] and a minimal increase of 0.7 difference in proportion (95% CI: -15.2, 16.7) after practices received asthma guidelines.[57] A moderate increase was noted for inhaler technique—12.9 (95% CI: 1.9, 23.9)[57]—and a small increase in change of asthma action plan use (7.6 percent) in a benchmarking feedback group.[58] In summary, the strength of evidence is low for support of the use of feedback and audit interventions to increase the provision of self-management education/asthma action plans by health care providers.

Clinical Pharmacy Support

We identified one RCT[65] evaluating the effect of clinical pharmacy support on self-management education/asthma action plan use by health care providers. Patients receiving care by pharmacists enrolled in the Pharmacy Asthma Care Program had increased asthma action plan possession (mean change from baseline: 40.4 percent [95% CI: 31.9, 48.9; $p=0.001$]), however there are no comparison data for the control group.[65] In summary, the strength of the evidence is moderate in support of the use of clinical pharmacy interventions to increase self-management education/asthma action plan use by health care providers.

Education Only

There were five RCTs of education-only interventions[26,68,70,91,92] that reported provision of a written asthma action plan as an outcome. Most targeted general practitioners and one focused on pediatricians. The educational strategies included small group asthma education programs, structured training, and interactive seminars. Two studies showed increased use of asthma action plans of 10 percent ($p=0.03$)[70] and 15 percent ($p=0.046$).[68] The other three studies[26,91,92] reported no benefit from their educational intervention on the provision of asthma action plans.

In summary, low strength of evidence suggests that educational interventions can increase use of asthma action plans by health care providers.

Quality Improvement and Pay-for-Performance

Three studies examined the effect of quality improvement strategies on receipt of asthma action plans.[93-95] The design of the studies included an RCT,[95] a pre-post study,[93] and a controlled, pre-post study.[94] All three studies involved pediatric health care providers, including nurses, nurse practitioners, and physicians. Two studies assessed participation in a Breakthrough Series collaborative,[94,95] and one study assessed a combination of continuous quality improvement and the addition of a community health worker.[93]

Overall, the results are inconsistent, with a -3 to 33 percent change in the proportion of patients provided an asthma action plan. Two of the three studies,[93,94] both pre-post studies, showed a 19 to 33 percent improvement in the proportion of patients who had received an asthma action plan. One of these studies,[94] the controlled pre-post study, showed a 19 percent increase by survey and a difference of difference of 33 percent by medical record review in the intervention arm. The second study[93] showed a 28.2 percent increase in the proportion of patients who had received an asthma action plan. These two nonrandomized studies that demonstrated a beneficial effect enrolled practices that had already joined a quality improvement initiative[94] or were part of a demonstration project.[93]

The third study[95]—an RCT—showed no effect, with a 1 percent increase in the intervention group and 4 percent increase in the control group for a -3 percent difference of difference.[95] However, there was some evidence of poor adherence to the quality improvement intervention in the RCT, with decreases in participation in the learning sessions and in outcome reporting over time.[95]

One controlled pre-post study examined the effect of a quality improvement initiative on asthma self-management education in addition to asthma action plans.[94] In this study, documented self-management education increased by 21 percent, although there was no definition of what constituted self-management education and how it was documented.

In summary, there is low strength of evidence that quality improvement leads to moderate increases in the provision of self-management education/asthma action plans in select populations of health care providers, based on two observational studies and one negative RCT with evidence of suboptimal engagement by participants.

Multicomponent

Six studies[77,79,81-83,96] examined the impact of multimodal interventions on rates at which providers created asthma action plans for their patients. Two studies[79,83] were cluster-randomized trials of primary care practices, while the remaining four studies[77,81,82,96] were pre-post studies. The interventions varied in their content, but most included an educational component. Other elements of these interventions included: (1) training in communication techniques, provision of a spirometer and training in use of the spirometer;[77] (2) laminated posters of asthma guidelines and medications, feedback on asthma action plan use, and monthly calls from an intervention team to troubleshoot communication problems;[96] (3) asthma kits (peak flow meters, spacers, educational materials) and systems-level changes (flow sheets and standing medication orders);[79] (4) systematic use of a patient questionnaire and an asthma management algorithm;[81] (5) an asthma coordinator and feedback on performance as part of continuous quality improvement efforts; and (6) an educational toolbox, seminars, teleconferences, mini fellowships, opinion leader visits, clinician-specific feedback, and pay for performance.[83] All four pre-post studies reported a large and statistically significant positive impact on asthma action plans over time (ranging from 27 percent to 46 percent of providers, median 42 percent). Both RCTs reported changes in the provision of patient education/asthma action plans in a positive direction, (one reporting an increase among 7 percent of providers, the other reporting RR=1.82) but neither result achieved statistical significance. Based on the use of weak study designs among studies observing an intervention effect, combined with the inconsistency of results among studies, there is low evidence to support the effectiveness of multicomponent interventions in increasing the provision of patient education/asthma action plans.

Information Only

No studies examined the impact of information provision alone on self-management education or asthma action plans. Therefore, there is insufficient information to assess the effect of information-only strategies on self-management education/asthma action plan use by health care providers.

KQ2: In the care of pediatric or adult patients with asthma, what is the evidence that interventions designed to improve health care provider adherence to guidelines impact clinical outcomes (ED visits/hospitalizations; missed days of school/work)?

Outcome: Emergency Department Visits/Hospitalizations

Decision Support

Ten studies examined the effect of decision support interventions on patient use of emergency department (ED) visits or hospitalizations for asthma.[5,37,43,44,46,50,51,86,88,97] The decision support interventions included computer systems,[43,44,51,88] checklists,[97] supplemental feedback protocols,[5] and structured pathways/algorithms.[37,50] These interventions were combined with educational interventions, organizational changes, and/or reminders. Of the 10 studies evaluating the effect of decision support on ED visits/hospitalizations, 4 were RCTs,[5,37,88,97] while the others were pre-post studies.[43,44,46,50,51,86] The populations in these studies were a mix of adult[43,44,46,86,88,97] and pediatric patients.[5,37,50,51,86]

Nine studies reported a reduction in ED visits or hospitalizations[5,37,43,44,46,50,51,86,97] ranging from 5 percent to 60 percent (all statistically significant) among the studies using a pre-post study design. Among the RCTs reporting a difference, the difference between intervention and control arms ranged from 1 percent to 7 percent.[5,37,97] The one study reporting no difference was an RCT.[88]

In summary, there is moderate evidence that decision support interventions targeting health care provider adherence to guidelines reduce ED visits/hospitalizations.

Organizational Change

Four studies evaluating organizational change measured the impact on patient ED visits and/or hospitalizations.[52,53,89,90] Two of these were RCTs,[52,89] while the other two were pre-post studies.[53,90] Three of the studies were focused on pediatric health care providers.[52,53,89] One of the studies restructured asthma care visits,[89] while the remaining three studies utilized supplemental trained personnel as part of the intervention.[52,53,90] Three of the studies also incorporated an educational component provided to health care providers.[52,53,90]

Two studies reported reductions in ED visits and/or hospitalizations. The first study reported 41 percent reduction in ED visits and 54 percent reduction in hospitalizations (p-value <0.001 for both outcomes).[90] The second study reported a 4 percent reduction in hospitalizations (no p-value reported).[53] The two RCTs did not report statistically significant reductions in ED visits/hospitalizations (1 percent, p>0.05[52] and 7 percent, p=0.06[89]) compared with the control arms in the study. In summary, organizational change does not reduce ED visits/hospitalizations. The strength of evidence for this conclusion is low.

Feedback and Audit

We identified one RCT[58] and one pre-post study[63] that evaluated the effect of health care provider feedback and audit on ED visits and hospitalizations of patients. The interventions were: (1) a traditional quality circle (TQC) intervention, in which providers were given feedback on their individual performance and the aggregate performance of group providers, compared with a benchmark quality circle (BQC) intervention, in which feedback on providers' individual performance was explicitly compared with a performance benchmark,[58] and (2) an intervention comparing individual primary care provider's guideline practice patterns with their peers plus providing asthma education to office staff.[63] Clinicians in both studies were primary care practitioners. Patients whose providers participated in a benchmark quality circle (BQC) and received prescribing feedback with comparison with other providers had a 6.7 point decrease in ED visits (from 17.6 percent at baseline to 10.9 percent 12 months post intervention), but this decrease was smaller than that seen among patients whose provider participated in a traditional quality circle (TQC) (19.7 percent at baseline to 6.1 percent or a 12.2 point decrease; p=0.064).[58]

No change in ED visits (baseline: 82 percent, 6 months: 81 percent) or hospitalizations (baseline: 96 percent, 6 months: 94 percent) was reported in the pre-post study.[63] No conclusions could be made because of conflicting results among a small number of studies. The strength of the evidence is insufficient to determine the effect of feedback and audit interventions on ED visits/hospitalizations.

Clinical Pharmacy Support

We identified one RCT[98] evaluating the effect of clinical pharmacy support on the number of ED visits and hospitalizations in patients with asthma. In this RCT, patients seen by pharmacists provided with patient specific clinical data, training about asthma management, patient educational materials, resource guides, and pragmatic strategies were more likely to have a reduction in ED visits/hospitalizations at 12 months compared with patients seen by pharmacists who received peak flow meter (PFM) instruction only (odds ratio 2.16 [95% CI: 1.76 to 2.63]). However, patients in the clinical pharmacy support intervention group did not experience a decline in ED visits/hospitalizations compared with patients of the usual care control group (odds ratio 1.08 [95% CI: 0.93 to 1.25]).[98] In summary, we are unable to make a conclusion regarding the benefit of clinical pharmacy support on ED visits and hospitalizations. The strength of evidence was insufficient.

Education Only

There were seven studies, five RCTs[25,26,70,71,92] and two pre-post studies,[74,76] that examined the impact of health care provider education on ED visits and/or hospitalizations. The educational interventions included interactive seminars, structured training, and medical grand rounds. The effects reported were inconsistent. One of the studies did not find a statistically significant effect for the intervention group overall, but did report statistically significant findings in a subgroup of low-income participants (-1.23 visits per year, p=0.001).[26] For hospitalization, one study reported statistically significant reduction in the annual rate,[26] while the other five studies reported no reduction on the rates of hospitalization. Overall, education only interventions do not reduce asthma ED visits and/or hospitalizations. The strength of evidence for this conclusion is low.

Quality Improvement and Pay-for-Performance

One RCT[95] examined the effect of quality improvement on ED visits and hospitalizations and one controlled pre-post study evaluated the effect on the combined number of ED visits and hospitalizations.[94] Both studies evaluated a Breakthrough Series collaborative quality improvement strategy. These studies focused on pediatric health care providers working in community health center settings. The patients were primarily African American or Hispanic.

Neither study showed a statistically significant reduction in any outcome, with a 5 percent reduction in ED visits,[95] a 2 percent reduction in hospitalizations,[95] and an increase of 0.3 combined ED visits and hospitalizations[94] reported in the quality improvement arms.

However, there was some evidence of poor adherence to the quality improvement intervention in the RCT, with decreases in participation in the learning sessions and in outcome reporting over time.[95] When analyses were limited to the nine practices that attended all three learning sessions, they report that there was a significant reduction in ED visits.

There is low strength of evidence to suggest that quality improvement does not significantly reduce ED visits/hospitalizations based on one controlled pre-post study and one RCT with evidence of suboptimal engagement by participants.

Multicomponent

One study[82] evaluated the impact of a multicomponent intervention in pediatric clinics on rates of ED visits and hospitalizations. This study implemented an intervention that included elements of quality improvement, decision support, organizational change, and feedback-and-audit. Among a longitudinal cohort of patients, this study found large and statistically significant reductions in rates of ED visits and hospitalizations (69 percent reductions for both outcomes). However, 44 percent of the patient sample was lost to followup, and significant heterogeneity in results was seen across participating clinical sites.

The strength of evidence is insufficient to determine the effect of multicomponent interventions on ED visits and/or hospitalizations.

Information Only

Only one RCT study[85] examined the impact of information provision on rates of ED visits and hospitalizations for asthma. This study randomized patients to have information about asthma guidelines inserted in their medical records for provider use; each provider thus managed patients in both intervention and control arms simultaneously. This study found no differences in rates of either ED visits or hospitalizations between study groups. In summary, based on a single study with a high risk of bias, there is insufficient evidence to determine the effect of information-only interventions on ED visits/hospitalizations.

Outcome: Missed Days of Work/School

Decision Support

There were two studies that examined the impact of decision support interventions on missed work or school. One study used an RCT design,[5] while the other used a pre-post design.[86] Both studies involved children, although one study[86] also included adult patients. The RCT study[5] reported no significant reduction in missed school (0.05 school days; p=0.4) in their study of mailing patient-specific asthma morbidity information to their health care provider. The pre-post design study[86] reported a 49 percent reduction (p<0.001) in school absenteeism and a 51 percent reduction in the odds of missed work (odds ratio: 0.49 [95% CI: 0.34, 0.71]) among the patient populations in a study that utilized a combination of an asthma care map, a treatment flow chart, program standards, management flow chart, and action plan.

In summary, there is insufficient evidence for the effect of decision support on the number of missed days due to inconsistent results from two studies.

Organizational Change

One RCT of organizational change based on restructuring the clinical protocol for asthma patient care during ambulatory care encounters ("3+ visit plan"), evaluated the impact on missed school days.[89] More specifically, at 12 months, the percentage of children who missed no school was 52 percent in the intervention group and 45 percent in the control group (odds ratio 0.8 [95% CI: 0.5 to 1.2]; p=0.3). In summary, organizational change does not reduce missed school days from asthma. The strength of evidence for this conclusion is low.

Feedback and Audit

We identified one pre-post study[63] that evaluated the impact of feedback and audit on days of missed work/school. This study provided asthma education to office staff and observed an 11 percent reduction in school days missed (percent reporting no school absences due to asthma in past 6 months: baseline: 49 percent; 6 months: 38 percent). The magnitude of the effect is low (11 percent reduction in school days missed). There was 0 percent reduction in parent work days missed due to child's asthma. In summary, there is insufficient evidence to evaluate the effect of feedback/audit interventions on the number of missed days of school or work.

Clinical Pharmacy Support

We identified no studies evaluating the effect of clinical pharmacy support on the outcome of missed days of work and school. Therefore, there is insufficient evidence to evaluate the effect of clinical pharmacy support interventions on the number of missed days of school or work.

Education Only

There were five studies that evaluated the effect of health care provider education on missed school or missed work as outcomes. There were three RCTs that included missed school days as an outcome.[26,68,71] The interventions targeted GPs, pediatricians, and pharmacists and included structured training, seminars, and workshops. In all three trials there was consistent evidence of small non-statistically-significant reductions in missed school (0.6 days to 4 days).

Two RCTs[68,91] and one pre-post study[74] examined missed work as an outcome. The interventions included workshops and training in how to perform spirometry and one study compared asthma program development with a nurse educator program or continuing education. There were no significant reductions in missed work in any studies (range: 10 percent reduction to a 5 percent increase in missed days of work; p>0.05).

In summary, the study results were inconsistent and had imprecise estimates of the effect of these education interventions. Therefore there is insufficient evidence to evaluate the effect of education-only strategies on the number of missed days of work from asthma.

Quality Improvement and Pay-for-Performance

One controlled pre-post study examined the effect of quality improvement on missed school and missed parental work.[94] This study evaluated health care provider participation in a Breakthrough Series collaborative quality improvement strategy. This study showed no significant reduction in the mean number of school days (0.2 school days; p=0.4) or parental work days (0 work days; p=0.7) missed due to a child's asthma. In summary, with only one study at high risk of bias, there is insufficient evidence to determine the effect of quality improvement interventions on school or work absenteeism.

Multicomponent

One study[82] evaluated the impact of a multicomponent intervention in pediatric clinics on rates of ED visits and hospitalizations. This study implemented an intervention that included elements of quality improvement, decision support, organizational change, and feedback-and-audit. Among a longitudinal cohort of patients, this study found large and statistically significant reductions in rates of missed days of school (53 percent reduction) and work (72 percent reduction). However, 44 percent of the patient sample was lost to followup, and significant heterogeneity in results was seen across participating clinical sites. Therefore, the strength of evidence is insufficient to determine the effect of multicomponent interventions on missed days of school or work

Information Only

No studies examined the impact of information provision alone on missed days of work or school (insufficient strength of evidence).

KQ3: In the care of pediatric or adult patients with asthma, what is the evidence that interventions designed to improve health care provider adherence to guidelines impact health care process outcomes that then affect clinical outcomes?

No studies evaluated how interventions designed to change health care provider adherence to asthma guidelines impacts clinical outcomes.

Discussion

We identified a number of different strategies designed to improve health care provider adherence to asthma guidelines. The studies we reviewed evaluated these strategies either in terms of their impact on health care processes and/or clinical outcomes. We found a large degree of variability in the frequency with which certain interventions were studied and in the frequency with which certain outcomes were evaluated. More specifically, decision support, feedback/audit and education only interventions were the most common and were tested for each of the critical outcomes we evaluated in this report. Conversely, organizational change, clinical pharmacy support, quality improvement/pay-for-performance, information-only, and multicomponent strategies were less consistently tested for each of the outcomes.

In terms of the outcomes we evaluated, there was much more evaluation of the health care process outcomes than the clinical outcomes. Most common was the evaluation of prescribing of asthma controller medications, which arguably has been a frequently reported problem in the management of asthma in primary care settings. Least common was evaluations of missed days of work/school (we noted three types of interventions in which no data were available to evaluate the impact on missed days of work/school), which has significant implications for patient quality of life.

We identified few RCTs testing these interventions. Most of the interventions were studied using a pre-post design, which more often reported a beneficial effect than the few RCTs we identified. We found that there was insufficient evidence to comment on the effectiveness of many of the interventions on health care process outcomes or clinical outcomes. The inability to draw conclusions due to inadequate evidence was particularly striking for the outcome of missed school or work days, where there was insufficient evidence to evaluate the effect of any of these interventions.

Table B summarizes the strength of evidence in support of eight interventions.

Table B. Summary of the strength of evidence in support of eight interventions designed to modify clinician adherence to asthma guidelines

Intervention	Outcome: Prescription of Controller Medications	Outcome: Patient Education/Asthma Action Plans	Outcome: ED Visits/ Hospitalizations	Outcome: Missed Days of Work/School
Decision support	Benefit with large magnitude of effect. SOE moderate.	Studies consistently favor intervention with large magnitude of effect. SOE moderate.	Benefit with moderate magnitude of effect (larger in pre-post studies). SOE moderate.	Unable to conclude due to inconsistent results. SOE insufficient.
Organizational change	Benefit with small magnitude of effect. SOE low.	Two studies show benefit with moderate magnitude of effect. SOE low.	No benefit with range of magnitudes of effect. SOE low.	No benefit (for missed school days). SOE low.
Feedback and audit	Benefit with moderate magnitude of effect. SOE moderate.	Benefit with low magnitude of effect. SOE low.	No conclusion could be made due to conflicting results in few studies. SOE insufficient.	No conclusion due to inconsistent results in one included study. SOE insufficient.
Clinical pharmacy support	Benefit within three studies with moderate magnitude of effect. SOE moderate.	Benefit in one study with moderate magnitude of effect. SOE moderate.	Unable to make a conclusion based on one study with imprecise results. SOE insufficient.	No studies. SOE insufficient.
Education only	No benefit. SOE low.	Small to moderate increases in a minority of studies. SOE low.	No benefit. Inconsistent results (reductions and increases). Low SOE.	No conclusion due to inconsistent and imprecise estimates of effect in five studies. SOE insufficient.
QI and pay-for-performance	No studies. SOE insufficient.	Observational studies showed benefit, while the RCT did not. Benefit with moderate magnitude of effect. SOE low.	No benefit. Low SOE.	Unable to draw conclusions. One study (with high risk of bias) reported a nonsignificant reduction in school days missed. SOE insufficient.
Multicomponent interventions	Benefit with moderate magnitude of effect. SOE low.	Benefit, with moderate magnitude of effect (larger in observational studies). SOE low.	Unable to make conclusion; while the one study reported a large reduction, the study quality was low. Insufficient SOE.	No conclusion; One study reported a large reduction, but study quality was low. SOE insufficient.
Information only	No studies. SOE insufficient.	No studies. SOE insufficient.	Unable to make conclusion; no difference seen, but study quality was low. SOE insufficient.	No studies. SOE insufficient.

ED = emergency department; QI = quality improvement; RCT = randomized controlled trial; SOE = strength of evidence

KQ1: In the care of pediatric or adult patients with asthma, what is the evidence that interventions designed to improve health care provider adherence to guidelines impact health care process outcomes (prescription of controller medications; providing asthma education/asthma action plans)?

The key findings are summarized in Table C.

Table C. Summary of strength of evidence for included studies for KQ1

Outcomes	Intervention	No. of Studies/No. of Health Care Providers	Strength of Evidence	Conclusions
Prescriptions for controller medications	Decision support	15/1,635 6 RCTs, 9 pre-post	Moderate	Most of the evidence supporting the use of decision support interventions comes from a number of nonrandomized studies consistently showing that decision support interventions can increase health care provider prescriptions for asthma controller medications. The magnitude of effect is large: 2%–34% in pre-post studies; 2%–17% in RCTs.
	Organizational change	2/228 1 RCT, 1 pre-post	Low	Although far fewer studies performed using organizational change (in comparison with decision support or feedback/audit), the findings consistently showed that organizational change can increase health care provider prescriptions for controller medicines. The effect on prescriptions by health care providers is smaller. The magnitude of effect is small. In the RCT: 8%–16% for all asthma patients; 4%–11% for patients with persistent asthma; 4%–9% for inhaled steroids (ICS) for all asthma patients; 13%–19% for ICS for patients with persistent asthma. In the pre-post study: 12% increase in ICS.
	Feedback and audit	11/1,831 6 RCTs, 4 pre-post and 1 nonrandomized controlled	Moderate	These studies consistently showed that feedback/audit interventions effectively increase prescriptions for controller medicines by health care providers. The magnitude of the effect is moderate. Effect size: 0.12–0.66. Increases in prescribing controller medications ranged from 15.9% to 52–104%. Hazard ratio range: 0.77–1.08.

Table C. Summary of strength of evidence for included studies for KQ1 (continued)

Outcomes	Intervention	No. of Studies/ no. of Health Care Providers	Strength of Evidence	Conclusions
Prescriptions for controller medications (continued)	Clinical pharmacy support	3/91 1 RCT, 1 pre-post, 1 nonrandomized	Moderate	The three studies were consistent in showing that clinical pharmacy support interventions increase asthma controller medication prescribing. The magnitude of the effect is moderate. OR: 3.80 (95% CI: 1.4, 10.32) and percent increase in patients prescribed controller meds pre and post: 6–21%.
	Education only	10/451 6RCTs, 4 pre-post	Low	The evidence suggests that interventions based only on education of clinicians do not improve prescription of asthma controller medications. The magnitude of effect is small to large in studies (3.5–50.3% increase in prescribing controller medicines).
	Quality improvement and pay-for-performance	0	Insufficient	No studies identified.
	Multicomponent interventions	7/>1,141 4 cluster randomized, 3 pre-post	Low	Two pre-post studies and one RCT reported a significant increase in prescribing (25–49% in pre-post studies), while all other effects were null. Overall, the magnitude of effect is small.
	Information only	2/107 1 RCT, 1 quasi-experimental	Insufficient	Due to inconsistency across studies, evidence is insufficient to determine the effect of information alone on prescribing of asthma controller medication.
Patient education/asthma action plans	Decision support	10/122-124 4RCTs, 6 pre-post	Moderate	A majority of nonrandomized studies consistently favor the use of decision support interventions to improve the provision of self-management education/asthma action plans by health care providers. The magnitude of effect is large: 14%–84%.
	Organizational change	2/24 1 RCT, 1 pre-post	Low	Both studies favor the use of organizational change to increase patient education/asthma action plan use by health care providers. The magnitude of effect is moderate: 10%–14%.

Table C. Summary of strength of evidence for included studies for KQ1 (continued)

Outcomes	Intervention	No. of Studies/ no. of Health Care Providers	Strength of Evidence	Conclusions
Patient education/asthma action plans (continued)	Feedback and audit	5/336 3 RCTs, 2 pre-post	Low	Despite a number of studies examining feedback/audit, inconsistent results lead to a low strength of evidence for the use of feedback/audit to improve self-management education/ asthma action plan use. The magnitude of the effect is low. Self-management education: difference in proportions range from low of 0.7 (95% CI: -15.2, 16.7) for peak flow meter use to 12.9 (95% CI: 1.9, 23.9) for inhaler technique education. Asthma Action Plans: Increase of 7.6% in feedback with benchmark as compared with traditional: 4.5%. Asthma Education: Range pre to post 46–133% increase.
	Clinical pharmacy support	1/82 1 RCT	Moderate	The one study demonstrated a positive effect in the use of clinical pharmacy support to improve self-management education/asthma action plan use by health care providers. The magnitude of the effect is moderate. Asthma Action Plans: 40–45% increase from baseline.
	Education only	5/470 5 RCTs	Low	Small increases in asthma self-management education were observed in a minority of studies, resulting in an overall low strength of evidence regarding this outcome. The magnitude of effect is small to moderate: 10%–15%. OR: 1.00; RR: 1.40.
	Quality improvement and pay-for-performance	3/63 practices (providers not reported) 1 RCT, 2 pre-post	Low	Inconsistent results with a -3 to 33% change in the provision of asthma action plans. Both observational studies reported increases of 19–33% while the negative RCT had evidence of suboptimal practice engagement.
	Multicomponent interventions	6/>937 2 RCT, 4 pre-post	Low	Magnitude of effect is moderate. Provision of asthma action plan increased 27%-46% in observational studies. Smaller effect sizes were seen in RCTs (7% of providers and RR: 1.82).
	Information only	0	Insufficient	No studies identified.

CI = confidence interval; OR = odds ratio; RCT = randomized controlled trial; RR = relative risk

Note: If the number of health care provider participants was not reported for a particular study, the "NR" value was treated as zero for that particular intervention and outcome category.

KQ2: In the care of pediatric or adult patients with asthma, what is the evidence that interventions designed to improve health care provider adherence to guidelines impact clinical outcomes (e.g., hospitalizations, patient-reported outcomes such as symptom control)?

The key findings are summarized in Table D.

Table D. Summary of strength of evidence for included studies for KQ2

Outcomes	Intervention	No. of Studies/ No. of Health Care Providers	Strength of Evidence	Conclusions
ED Visits/Hospitalizations	Decision support	10/820 4 RCTs, 6 pre-post	Moderate	Nine of 10 studies reported that decision support interventions reduce ED visits/hospitalizations. The magnitude of effect is large in pre-post studies (5%–60%) and small in RCTs (1%–7%).
	Organizational change	4/252 2 RCTs, 2 pre-post	Low	Inconsistent results account for the low strength of evidence for organizational change to reduce ED visits/hospitalizations. Magnitude of effect is large in pre-post studies (41%–54%) and small in RCTs (1%–7%).
	Feedback and audit	2/125 1 RCT, 1 pre-post	Insufficient	No conclusions could be made because of conflicting results and low magnitude of effect.
	Clinical pharmacy support	1/36 1 RCT	Insufficient	No conclusion could be made because of imprecise results from one study.
	Education only	7/343 5 RCTs, 2 pre-post	Low	Overall, due to conflicting results among a number of studies, the low strength of evidence suggests that education only interventions do not reduce asthma ED visits and/or hospitalizations. Magnitude of effect is low. Reductions and increases in ED visits were observed. One study demonstrated significant decreases; in hospitalizations; others showed no change or an increase in hospitalizations (+5 to 10.5%).
	Quality improvement and pay-for-performance	2/56 practices (providers not reported) 1 RCT, 1 pre-post	Low	Two studies found no significant change in ED visits and hospitalizations. The RCT had evidence of suboptimal practice engagement. Magnitude of effect is low. ED visits: 5% reduction. Hospitalizations: 2% reduction.
	Multicomponent	1/17 clinics (providers not reported) 1 cohort	Insufficient	There is insufficient evidence to determine the effect of multicomponent interventions on ED visits/ hospitalizations due to high rates of participant attrition (low study quality) in the single study included.
	Information only	1/13 1 RCT	Insufficient	Based on a single study with a high risk of bias, there is insufficient evidence to determine the effect of information-only interventions on ED visits/hospitalizations.

Table D. Summary of strength of evidence for included studies for KQ2 (continued)

Outcomes	Intervention	No. of Studies/ No. of Health Care Providers	Strength of Evidence	Conclusions
Missed days of work/school	Decision support	2/435 1 RCT, 1 pre-post	Insufficient	There is insufficient evidence to evaluate the effect of decision support interventions on the number of missed days of work/school due to inconsistent results across the two studies analyzed.
	Organizational change	1/24 1 RCT	Low	Organizational change does not reduce missed school days from asthma. The strength of evidence for this conclusion is low.
	Feedback and audit	1/29 1 pre-post	Insufficient	There is insufficient evidence to evaluate the effect of feedback and audit interventions on the number of missed days of work and school from asthma due to inconsistent results and study design.
	Clinical pharmacy support	0	Insufficient	No studies identified.
	Education only	5/1,767 4 RCTs, 1 pre-post	Insufficient	There is insufficient evidence to evaluate the effect of education only strategies on the number of missed days of work/school from asthma due to imprecise estimates and inconsistent results.
	Quality improvement and pay-for-performance	1/13 practices (providers not reported) 1 pre-post	Insufficient	There is insufficient evidence to evaluate the effect of quality improvement/pay-for-performance interventions on the number of missed days of work/school from asthma because of high risk of bias in the single study analyzed.
	Multicomponent	1/17 clinics (providers not reported) 1 cohort	Insufficient	There is insufficient evidence to determine the effect of multicomponent interventions on the number of missed days of work/school from asthma due to risk of bias (high rates of attrition) and inconsistent results across clinical sites.
	Information only	0	Insufficient	No studies identified.

ED = emergency department; RCT = randomized controlled trial
Note: If the number of health care provider participants was not reported for a particular study, the "NR" value was treated as zero for that particular intervention and outcome category.

Future Research

Future health care provider interventions aimed at improving adherence to national asthma guidelines should take a more *active* role in the asthma care process (e.g., provide asthma action plans, patient education, environmental control practices), particularly processes associated with a low risk of harm and those inhibited by specific barriers such as time constraints, poor self-efficiency, and lack of provider awareness. Interventions are needed that address all elements of the asthma care process including prescription for controller medication and peak flow meter, environmental control practice education, self-management education and asthma action plans, documentation of asthma severity, and control and automated scheduling of followup visit within 3 months. This also suggests that systems-level interventions that address barriers external to the health care provider would be an important approach to effecting positive changes in health care provider behavior. In addition to further evaluating interventions for which we found insufficient evidence, there are a variety of study design elements that may be considered to strengthen future research of health care provider-targeted interventions. Such design considerations include: standardization of presentation of data and outcome measures, particularly controller medication adherence; more comprehensive measurement of health care process and clinical outcomes within a given study; more information about the intensity (dose and frequency of the intervention); improved description of the comparator and the intervention populations; and more use of RCT study designs to isolate the effectiveness of each intervention. Cost implications of specific interventions may be associated with reduced use but this was not addressed in this report. Lastly, testing the efficacy of the more potent multifaceted interventions in targeted populations (i.e., adolescents, obese patients, high asthma severity, or high health care utilizers) may lead to identification of novel preventive and therapeutic strategies for high risk patients.

Conclusion

In summary, we found more information about the effectiveness of interventions on improving health care process outcomes than for clinical outcomes. There is a need for further evaluations of how these interventions may improve clinical outcomes for patients with asthma. There is low to moderate evidence to support the use of decision support tools, feedback and audit, and clinical pharmacy support to improve the adherence of health care providers to asthma guidelines, as measured through health care process outcomes, and to improve clinical outcomes. There is a need to further evaluate health care provider-targeted interventions with a focus on standardized measures of outcomes, more rigorous study designs and addition of cost measures.

References

1. Vital signs: asthma prevalence, disease characteristics, and self-management education: United States, 2001--2009. MMWR Morb Mortal Wkly Rep 2011; 60(17):547-52. Centers for Disease Control and Prevention (CDC).

2. Akinbami L. The state of childhood asthma, United States, 1980-2005. Adv Data 2006; (381):1-24. Centers for Disease Control and Prevention National Center for Health Statistics.

3. Expert Panel Report 3 (EPR-3): Guidelines for the Diagnosis and Management of Asthma-Summary Report 2007. J Allergy Clin Immunol. 2007;120(5 Suppl):S94-138. National Asthma Education and Prevention Program.

4. Evans R 3rd, Gergen PJ, Mitchell H et al. A randomized clinical trial to reduce asthma morbidity among inner-city children: results of the National Cooperative Inner-City Asthma Study. J Pediatr. 1999;135(3):332-8.

5. Kattan M, Crain EF, Steinbach S et al. A randomized clinical trial of clinician feedback to improve quality of care for inner-city children with asthma. Pediatrics. 2006;117:e1095-103.

6. Szefler SJ, Mitchell H, Sorkness CA et al. Management of asthma based on exhaled nitric oxide in addition to guideline-based treatment for inner-city adolescents and young adults: a randomised controlled trial. Lancet. 2008;372(9643):1065-72.

7. Wisnivesky JP, Lorenzo J, Lyn-Cook R et al. Barriers to adherence to asthma management guidelines among inner-city primary care providers. Ann Allergy Asthma Immunol. 2008;101(3):264-70.

8. Halterman JS, Aligne CA, Auinger P, et al. Inadequate therapy for asthma among children in the United States. Pediatrics. 2000;105(1 Pt 3):272-6.

9. Halterman JS, Yoos HL, Kaczorowski JM et al. Providers underestimate symptom severity among urban children with asthma. Arch Pediatr Adolesc Med. 2002;156(2):141-6.

10. Cabana MD, Slish KK, Nan B, et al. Asking the correct questions to assess asthma symptoms. Clin Pediatr. 2005;44(4):319-25.

11. Cabana MD, Bruckman D, Meister K, et al. Documentation of asthma severity in pediatric outpatient clinics. Clin Pediatr. 2003;42(2):121-5.

12. Ortega AN, Gergen PJ, Paltiel AD, et al. Impact of site of care, race, and Hispanic ethnicity on medication use for childhood asthma. Pediatrics. 2002;109(1):E1.

13. Akinbami LJ, Moorman JE, Garbe PL, et al. Status of childhood asthma in the United States, 1980-2007. Pediatrics. 2009;123 Suppl 3:S131-45.

14. Flores G, Snowden-Bridon C, Torres S et al. Urban minority children with asthma: substantial morbidity, compromised quality and access to specialists, and the importance of poverty and specialty care. J Asthma. 2009;46(4):392-8.

15. Cabana MD, Rand CS, Powe NR et al. Why don't physicians follow clinical practice guidelines? A framework for improvement. JAMA. 1999;282(15):1458-65.

16. Bracha Y, Brottman G, Carlson A. Physicians, guidelines, and cognitive tasks. Eval Health Prof. 2011;34(3):309-35.

17. Rastogi D, Shetty A, Neugebauer R, et al. National Heart, Lung, and Blood Institute guidelines and asthma management practices among inner-city pediatric primary care providers. Chest. 2006;129(3):619-23.

18. Bhogal SK, McGillivray D, Bourbeau J et al. Focusing the focus group: impact of the awareness of major factors contributing to non-adherence to acute paediatric asthma guidelines. J Eval Clin Pract. 2011;17(1):160-7.

19. Corrigan SP, Cecillon DL, Sin DD et al. The costs of implementing the 1999 Canadian Asthma Consensus Guidelines recommendation of asthma education and spirometry for the family physician. Can Respir J. 2004;11(5):349-53.

20. Butz AM, Eggleston P, Huss K, et al. Children with asthma and nebulizer use: parental asthma self-care practices and beliefs. J Asthma. 2001;38(7):565-73.

21. Coffman JM, Cabana MD, Yelin EH. Do school-based asthma education programs improve self-management and health outcomes? Pediatrics 2009;124(2):729-42.

22. Teach SJ, Crain EF, Quint DM, et al. Improved asthma outcomes in a high-morbidity pediatric population: results of an emergency department-based randomized clinical trial. Arch Pediatr Adolesc Med. 2006;160(5):535-41.

23. Wise RA, Bartlett SJ, Brown ED et al. Randomized trial of the effect of drug presentation on asthma outcomes: the American Lung Association Asthma Clinical Research Centers. J Allergy Clin Immunol. 2009;124(3):436-44, 444e1-8.

24. Bratton SL, Cabana MD, Brown RW et al. Asthma educational seminar targeting Medicaid providers. Respir Care. 2006;51(1):49-55.

25. Cabana MD, Slish KK, Evans D et al. Impact of physician asthma care education on patient outcomes. Pediatrics. 2006;117:2149-57.

26. Brown R, Bratton SL, Cabana MD, Kaciroti N, Clark NM. Physician asthma education program improves outcomes for children of low-income families. Chest. 2004;126:369-74.

27. Ruoff G. Effects of flow sheet implementation on physician performance in the management of asthmatic patients. Family Medicine. 2002;34:514-7.

28. Lozano P, Finkelstein JA, Carey VJ et al. A multisite randomized trial of the effects of physician education and organizational change in chronic-asthma care: health outcomes of the Pediatric Asthma Care Patient Outcomes Research Team II Study. Arch Pediatr Adolesc Med. 2004;158(9):875-83.

29. Halterman JS, McConnochie KM, Conn KM et al. A randomized trial of primary care provider prompting to enhance preventive asthma therapy. Arch Pediatr Adolesc Med. 2005;159(5):422-7.

30. Higgins JPT, Green S (editors).Cochrane Handbook for Systematic Reviews of Interventions Version 5.0.2 [updated September 2009]. The Cochrane Collaboration, 2009. Available from www.cochrane-handbook.org.

31. Cochrane Effective Practice and Organisation of Care Group. Data collection checklist. 2002. Available at http://epoc.cochrane.org/sites/epoc.cochrane .org/files/uploads/datacollectionchecklist. pdf. (Accessed 2012).

32. Akinbami LJ, Sullivan SD, Campbell JD et al. Asthma outcomes: healthcare utilization and costs. J Allergy Clin Immunol. 2012;129(3 suppl):s49-64.

33. Guyatt G, Oxman AD, Sultan S et al. GRADE guidelines 11. Making an overall rating of confidence in effect estimates for a single outcome and for all outcomes. J Clin Epidemiol. 2012.

34. Owens DK et al. AHRQ series paper 5: grading the strength of a body of evidence when comparing medical interventions--Agency for Healthcare Research and Quality and the effective health-care program. J Clin Epidemiol. 2010;63(5): p. 513-23.

35. Fairall L, Bachmann MO, Zwarenstein M et al. Cost-effectiveness of educational outreach to primary care nurses to increase tuberculosis case detection and improve respiratory care: economic evaluation alongside a randomised trial. Trop Med Int Health. 2010;15:277-86.

36. Martens JD, van der Weijden T, Severens JL et al. The effect of computer reminders on GPs' prescribing behaviour: a cluster-randomised trial. Int J Med Inform. 2007;76 Suppl 3:S403-16.

37. Mitchell EA, Didsbury PB, Kruithof N et al. A randomized controlled trial of an asthma clinical pathway for children in general practice. Acta Paediatr. 2005;94:226-33.

38. Eccles M, McColl E, Steen N et al. Effect of computerised evidence based guidelines on management of asthma and angina in adults in primary care: cluster randomised controlled trial. BMJ. 2002;325:941.

39. Bell LM, Grundmeier R, Localio R et al. Electronic health record-based decision support to improve asthma care: a cluster-randomized trial. Pediatrics. 2010;125:e770-7.

40. Rance K, O'Laughlen M, Ting S. Improving asthma care for African American children by increasing national asthma guideline adherence. J Pediatr Health Care. 2011;25:235-49.

41. Shapiro A, Gracy D, Quinones W et al. Putting guidelines into practice: improving documentation of pediatric asthma management using a decision-making tool. Arch Pediatr Adolesc Med. 2011;165:412-8.

42. Cho SH, Jeong JW, Park HW et al. Effectiveness of a computer-assisted asthma management program on physician adherence to guidelines. J Asthma. 2010;47:680-6.

43. Newton WP, Lefebvre A, Donahue KE et al. Infrastructure for large-scale quality-improvement projects: early lessons from North Carolina Improving Performance in Practice. J Contin Educ Health Prof. 2010;30:106-13.

44. Horswell R, Butler MK, Kaiser M et al. Disease management programs for the underserved. Dis Manag. 2008;11:145-52.

45. Cloutier MM, Hall CB, Wakefield DB et al. Use of asthma guidelines by primary care providers to reduce hospitalizations and emergency department visits in poor, minority, urban children. Pediatr. 2005;146:591-7.

46. Lesho EP, Myers CP, Ott M et al. Do clinical practice guidelines improve processes or outcomes in primary care? Mil Med. 2005;170:243-6

47. Cloutier MM, Wakefield DB, Carlisle PS et al. The effect of Easy Breathing on asthma management and knowledge. Arch Pediatr Adolesc Med. 2002;156:1045-51.

48. Davis AM, Cannon M, Ables AZ et al. Using the electronic medical record to improve asthma severity documentation and treatment among family medicine residents. Family Medicine. 2010;42:334-7.

49. Ragazzi H, Keller A, Ehrensberger R et al. Evaluation of a practice-based intervention to improve the management of pediatric asthma. J Urban Health. 2011;88 Suppl 1:38-48.

50. Cloutier MM, Grosse SD, Wakefield DB et al. The economic impact of an urban asthma management program. Am J Manag Care. 2009;15:345-51.

51. Shiffman RN, Freudigman M, Brandt CA et al. A guideline implementation system using handheld computers for office management of asthma: effects on adherence and patient outcomes. Pediatrics. 2000;105:767-73.

52. Finkelstein JA, Lozano P, Fuhlbrigge AL et al. Practice-level effects of interventions to improve asthma care in primary care settings: the Pediatric Asthma Care Patient Outcomes Research Team. Health Serv Res. 2005;40:1737-57.

53. Thyne SM, Marmor AK, Madden N et al. Comprehensive asthma management for underserved children. Paediatr Perinat Epidemiol. 2007;21:29-34.

54. Veninga CCM, Lagerlav P, Wahlström R et al. American Journal of Respiratory and Critical Care Medicine: Evaluating an educational intervention to improve the treatment of asthma in four European countries. 1999;160:1254-62.

55. Sondergaard J, Andersen M, Vach K. Detailed postal feedback about prescribing to asthma patients combined with a guideline statement showed no impact: a randomised controlled trial. Pharmacol. 2002;58:127-32.

56. Baker R, Fraser RC, Stone M et al. Randomised controlled trial of the impact of guidelines, prioritized review criteria and feedback on implementation of recommendations for angina and asthma. Br J Gen Pract. 2003;53:284-91.

57. Feder G, Griffiths C, Highton C et al. Do clinical guidelines introduced with practice based education improve care of asthmatic and diabetic patients? BMJ. A randomised controlled trial in general practices in east London. 1995;311:1473-8.

58. Schneider A, Wensing M, Biessecker K et al. Impact of quality circles for improvement of asthma care: results of a randomized controlled trial. J Eval Clin Pract. 2008;14:185-90.

59. Veninga CCM, Denig P, Zwaagstra R et al. Improving drug treatment in general practice. J Clin Epidemiol. 2000;53:762-72.

60. Hoskins G, Neville RG, Smith B et al. Does participation in distance learning and audit improve the care of patients with acute asthma attacks? The General Practitioners in Asthma Group. Health Bull (Edinb): 1997;55:150-5.

61. Coleman CI, Reddy P, Laster-Bradley NM et al. Effect of practitioner education on adherence to asthma treatment guidelines. Ann Pharmacother. 2003;37:956-61.

62. Suh DC, Shin SK, Okpara I et al. Impact of a targeted asthma intervention program on treatment costs in patients with asthma. Am J Manag Care. 2001;7:897-906.

63. Richman MJ, Poltawsky JS. Partnership for excellence in asthma care: evidence-based disease management. Stud Health Technol Inform. 2000;76:107-21.

64. Herborg H, Soendergaard B, Jorgensen T et al. Improving drug therapy for patients with asthma-part 2: Use of antiasthma medications. J Am Pharm Assoc (Wash). 2001;41:551-9.

65. Armour C, Bosnic-Anticevich S, Brillant M et al. Pharmacy Asthma Care Program (PACP) improves outcomes for patients in the community. Thorax. 2007;62:496-502.

66. de Vries TW, van den Berg PB, Duiverman EJ et al. Effect of a minimal pharmacy intervention on improvement of adherence to asthma guidelines. Arch Dis Child. 2010;95:302-4.

67. Saini B, Krass I, Armour C. Development, implementation, and evaluation of a community pharmacy-based asthma care model. Annals of Pharmacotherapy. 2004;38:1954-60.

68. Shah S, Sawyer SM, Toelle BG et al. Improving paediatric asthma outcomes in primary health care: a randomised controlled trial. Med J Aust. 2011;195:405-9.

69. Smeele IJ, Grol RP, van Schayck CP et al. Can small group education and peer review improve care for patients with asthma/chronic obstructive pulmonary disease? Qual Health Care. 1999;8:92-8.

70. Clark NM, Gong M, Schork MA et al. Impact of education for physicians on patient outcomes. Pediatrics. 1998;101(5):831-6.

71. Stergachis A, Gardner JS, Anderson MT et al. Improving pediatric asthma outcomes in the community setting: does pharmaceutical care make a difference? J Am Pharm Assoc. (Wash). 2002;42.743-52.

72. Premaratne UN, Sterne JA, Marks GB et al. Clustered randomised trial of an intervention to improve the management of asthma: Greenwich asthma study. BMJ. 1999;318:1251-5.

73. Mahi-Taright S, Belhocine M, Ait-Khaled N. Can we improve the management of chronic obstructive respiratory disease? The example of asthma in adults. Int J Tuberc Lung Dis. 2004;8:873-81.

74. Cowie RL, Underwood MF, Mack S. The impact of asthma management guideline dissemination on the control of asthma in the community. Can Respir J. 2001;8 Suppl A:41A-5A.

75. Davis RS, Bukstein DA, Luskin AT et al. Changing physician prescribing patterns through problem-based learning: an interactive, teleconference case-based education program and review of problem-based learning. Ann Allergy Asthma Immunol. 2004;93:237-42.

76. Blackstien-Hirsch P, Anderson G, Cicutto L et al. Implementing continuing education strategies for family physicians to enhance asthma patients' quality of life. J Asthma. 2000;37:247-57.

77. Bender BG, Dickinson P, Rankin A et al. The Colorado Asthma Toolkit Program: a practice coaching intervention from the High Plains Research Network. J Am Board Fam Med. 2011;24:240-8.

78. Hagmolen of ten Have W, van den Berg NJ, van der Palen J et al. Implementation of an asthma guideline for the management of childhood asthma in general practice: a randomised controlled trial. Prim Care Respir J. 2008;17:90-6

79. Daniels EC, Bacon J, Denisio S et al. Translation squared: improving asthma care for high-disparity populations through a safety net practice-based research network. J Asthma. 2005;42:499-505.

80. Lundborg CS, Wahlstrom R, Oke T et al. Influencing prescribing for urinary tract infection and asthma in primary care in Sweden: a randomized controlled trial of an interactive educational intervention. J Clin Epidemiol. 1999;52:801-12.

81. Yawn BP, Bertram S, Wollan P. Introduction of asthma APGAR tools improve asthma management in primary care practices. J Asthma Allergy. 2008;1-10.

82. Lob SH Boer JH, Porter PG et al. Promoting best-care practices in childhood asthma: quality improvement in community health centers. Pediatrics. 2011;128;20; Originally Published Online June 13, 2011; DOI: 10.1542/Peds.2010-1962.

83. Cloutier MM, Tennen H, Wakefield DB et al. Improving clinician self-efficacy does not increase asthma guideline use by primary care clinicians. Acad Pediatr. 2012;12(4):312-8.

84. Martens JD, Winkens RA, van der Weijden T et al. Does a joint development and dissemination of multidisciplinary guidelines improve prescribing behaviour: a pre/post study with concurrent control group and a randomised trial. BMC Health Serv Res. 2006;6:145.

85. Bryce FP, Neville RG, Crombie IK et al. Controlled trial of an audit facilitator in diagnosis and treatment of childhood asthma in general practice. BMJ.1995; 310:838-42.

86. To T, Cicutto L, Degani N et al. Can a community evidence-based asthma care program improve clinical outcomes?: a longitudinal study. J Med Care. 2008;46:1257-66.

87. Halterman JS , Fisher S, Conn KM et al. Improved preventive care for asthma: a randomized trial of clinician prompting in pediatric offices. Arch Pediatr Adolesc Med. 2006;160:1018-25.

88. McCowan C, Neville RG, Ricketts IW et al. Lessons from a randomized controlled trial designed to evaluate computer decision support software to improve the management of asthma. Med Inform Internet Med. 2001;26:191-201.

89. Glasgow NJ, Ponsonby AL, Yates R et al. Proactive asthma care in childhood: general practice based randomised controlled trial. BMJ. 2003;327:659.

90. Patel PH, Welsh C, Foggs MB. Improved asthma outcomes using a coordinated care approach in a large medical group. Dis Manag. 2004;7:102-11.

91. Holton C, Crockett A, Nelson M et al. Does spirometry training in general practice improve quality and outcomes of asthma care? Int J Qual Health Care. 2011;23:545-53.

92. Sulaiman ND, Barton CA, Liaw ST et al. Do small group workshops and locally adapted guidelines improve asthma patients' health outcomes? A cluster randomized controlled trial. Fam Pract. 2010;27:246-54.

93. Fox P, Porter PG, Lob SH et al. Improving asthma-related health outcomes among low-income, multiethnic, school-aged children: Results of a demonstration project that combined continuous quality improvement and community health worker strategies. Pediatrics. 2007;120:e902-e911.

94. Mangione-Smith R, Schonlau M, Chan KS et al. Measuring the effectiveness of a collaborative for quality improvement in pediatric asthma care: Does implementing the chronic care model improve processes and outcomes of care? Ambul Pediatr. 2005;5:75-82.

95. Homer CJ, Forbes P, Horvitz L et al. Impact of a quality improvement program on care and outcomes for children with asthma. Arch Pediatr Adolesc Med. 2005;159:464-9.

96.   Frankowski BL, Keating K, Rexroad A et al. Community collaboration: concurrent physician and school nurse education and cooperation increases the use of asthma action plans. J Sch Health. 2006;76:303-6.

97.   Renzi PM, Ghezzo H, Goulet S et al. Paper stamp checklist tool enhances asthma guidelines knowledge and implementation by primary care physicians. Can Respir J. 2006;13:193-7.

98.   Weinberger M , Murray MD, Marrero DG et al. Effectiveness of pharmacist care for patients with reactive airways disease: A randomized controlled trial. JAMA. 2002;288:1594-602.

Introduction

Background

Burden of Asthma

Asthma is a respiratory disease characterized by variable and recurring symptoms, airflow obstruction, bronchial hyper-responsiveness, and inflammation of the airways. In the U.S., an estimated 24.6 million people (8.2 percent) currently have asthma.[1] Students with asthma miss more than 14 million school days every year due to illness. Furthermore, certain U.S. population subgroups have higher prevalence rates of asthma in comparison with the national average: children (9.6 percent), poor children (13.5 percent), non-Hispanic black children (17.0 percent), women (9.7 percent), and poor adults (10.6 percent).[1]

Treatment of Asthma and Clinical Practice Guidelines

The current approach to asthma management includes monitoring symptoms and lung function, encouraging the use of medications that control and prevent symptoms, controlling the triggers of asthma, educating the patient, and maintaining a collaborative patient-provider relationship that includes the use of written action plans.[2] The main goals of therapy are to minimize current impairment and future risk.

A number of different organizations and countries have published clinical practice guidelines to guide health care providers in the diagnosis and management of asthma. For example, the National Asthma Education and Prevention Program (NAEPP) of the National Heart, Lung, and Blood Institute (NHLBI) has published comprehensive guidelines for diagnosing and managing asthma. The most recent guidance was published in 2007 (previous versions were published in 1991, 1997, and 2002): "Expert Panel Report 3: Guidelines for the Diagnosis and Management of Asthma" is also known as EPR-3.[2] This guideline provides treatment recommendations with the strength of the evidence base for children 0 to 4, 5 to11, and over 12 years of age and adults. EPR-3 is based on a systematic review and expert opinion.

Clinical trials have shown that treatment in alignment with asthma guideline recommendations improves clinical patient outcomes in a variety of populations, including among high-risk populations, such as inner-city, poor, and/or African American populations.[3-5] The available evidence suggests that most people with asthma can be symptom-free if they receive appropriate medical care, use inhaled corticosteroids when prescribed, and modify their environment to reduce or eliminate exposure to allergens and irritants. It is not known how best to prioritize the many recommendations of asthma guidelines, though it should be noted that the evidence supporting varies considerably. For example, medication recommendations tend to be supported by multiple randomized controlled trials, while some environmental control practices, such as avoidance of furry pets, are based only on expert opinion.

Current Asthma Management Practices

Despite the evidence of efficacy in improving outcomes, their long-standing presence (>20 years) and their wide availability, there is extensive evidence that guideline recommendations are not routinely followed by health care providers.[6,7] In one study, only 34.2 percent of patients reported being given a written asthma action plan, while only 68.1 percent had been taught the appropriate response to symptoms of an asthma attack.[7] In the same study, only about one-third of children or adults were using long-term control medicine such as inhaled corticosteroids. Health care providers do not appropriately assess asthma control in most children,[8-11] resulting in substandard care. Minority children are up to half as likely as Caucasian children to receive inhaled steroids.[12] The significance of these studies is that suboptimal outcomes persist, such as 2-fold higher rates of emergency room visits for African American children compared with their Caucasian counterparts.[13]In 2005, there were approximately 679,000 emergency room visits in the U.S. due to asthma in children under 15 years of age.[14] Currently, asthma is the third leading cause of hospitalization among children in this age group.[14]

With the growing evidence that health care providers are poorly adherent to the asthma management recommendations in published clinical practice guidelines (CPGs), there has been more focused attention on the lack of adherence to best practices. In 1999, Cabana et al[15] proposed a theoretical framework to understand why health care providers do not adhere to CPGs: lack of awareness of CPGs, disagreement with the CPG recommendations (e.g., use of inhaled corticosteroids), doubts about the effectiveness of the CPG recommendations (e.g., efficacy of inhaled steroids to reduce the likelihood of asthma attacks), lack of confidence in being able to carry out the best practice (e.g., confidence in ability to provide smoking cessation counseling(e.g., inability to overcome the inertia of previous practice behaviors (e.g., changing from prescribing orally administered Albuterol to prescribing inhaled Albuterol), and external barriers (e.g., time constraints during a visit, the CPGs are not user-friendly, patient preferences, organizational constraints). There is a growing understanding that the shortcomings in health care providers' adherence to asthma CPGs may also relate to the content of asthma CPGs, which do not provide health care providers with the tools and strategies necessary to follow the recommended care.[16] It is possible that with the publication of additional asthma CPGs over the past 20 years, more physicians have been exposed to the asthma CPGs, resulting in greater awareness of the CPGs, fewer disagreements with CPG recommendations, and greater confidence in carrying out recommended asthma care.[17,18] However, there are some barriers outlined by Cabana et al. that would not be solved by increased exposure to asthma CPGs, including the inability of health care providers to overcome practice inertia and external barriers (e.g., time constraints during a visit, CPGs that are not user-friendly, patient preferences).[19] These types of unaddressed barriers to the adherence by health care providers to asthma CPGs highlight the need to evaluate strategies that may improve adherence to asthma CPGs, including those aimed directly at health care providers as well as organizational changes that would indirectly change behavior.

Knowledge Gaps

Although most interventions targeted at improving asthma care and outcomes have been patient-focused,[20-23] there have been provider-targeted interventions to improve adherence to guidelines (e.g., educational seminars, prompts).[24,70,88,100,119,122] However, there is no consensus on the most effective health care provider-targeted interventions to improve adherence to guidelines.

Potential Impact of a Comparative Effectiveness Review

Good-quality guidelines are currently available for the care of children or adults with asthma. Systematic reviews have been published on patient-targeted interventions,[25,26] but little attention has been directed toward the effectiveness of clinician-focused strategies designed to

2

enhance the implementation of guidelines in clinical practice. In 2007, the Stanford University–University of California San Francisco Evidence-based Practice Center published a report on asthma care, titled "Closing the Quality Gap: A Critical Analysis of Quality Improvement Strategies: Volume 5—Asthma Care."[27] This report showed that, despite the availability of evidence-based guidelines for the management of pediatric and adult asthma, a significant gap remains between accepted best practices for asthma care and the actual care delivered to patients with asthma in the U.S. The report authors examined the published literature through May 2006 on quality improvement strategies to improve the processes and outcomes of outpatient care for children and adults with asthma. The interventions included from their search had been tested between 1976 and 2004, so studies published after 2004 would not have been included. Furthermore, the interventions used in those studies were directed at patient adherence to provider-prescribed care, rather than at provider adherence to asthma guidelines.

The purpose of this systematic review is to evaluate the effectiveness of interventions designed to improve health care provider adherence to asthma guidelines.

Key Questions

Our Key Questions (KQs) are listed below, with the PICOTS (Population, Intervention, Comparator, Outcomes, Timing, Setting) elements listed in Table 1 and the questions displayed in Figure 1.

KQ1: In the care of pediatric or adult patients with asthma, what is the evidence that interventions designed to improve health care provider adherence to guidelines impact health care process outcomes (e.g., receiving appropriate treatment)?

KQ2: In the care of pediatric or adult patients with asthma, what is the evidence that interventions designed to improve health care provider adherence to guidelines impact clinical outcomes (e.g., hospitalizations, patient reported outcomes such as symptom control)?

KQ3: In the care of pediatric or adult patients with asthma, what is the evidence that interventions designed to improve health care provider adherence to guidelines impact health care process outcomes that then affect clinical outcomes?

Table 1. Characteristics of the target studies according to the PICOTS framework

Population(s)	Physicians, nurses, physiotherapists/physical therapists, respiratory therapists, pharmacists and other health care providers treating children (0 to 18 years of age) or adults (over 18 years of age) with asthma.
Interventions	Interventions to improve adherence to guidelines. Includes: decision support (health information technology and paper-based), organizational change, feedback and audit, clinical pharmacy support, education only, quality improvement/pay-for-performance, multicomponent, information only.
Comparators	Usual care, as defined by eligible study, and comparisons between interventions.
Outcomes	Health care process outcomes (including: prescriptions for controller medicine, environmental control practice recommendations, self-management education, asthma action plans, documentation of level of asthma severity, prescription of peak flow meter, and follow-up visits) Clinical outcomes (including: symptom days, missed days of school and/or work, quality of life, emergency department visits/hospitalizations/urgent doctor visits, lung function tests, rescue use of short-acting β_2 agonists, parental/patient perceptions/ratings of care, and side effects of drugs). The outcomes are nondirectional. That is, outcomes deemed good, as well as those deemed to be potential harms or unintended consequences, were considered.
Timing	Studies with all duration of followup were considered for the review.
Setting	Outpatient settings in which health care providers work, but not emergency room or in-patient settings.

The relationship between each Key Question and the PICOTS format is depicted in Figure 1, below.

Figure 1. Analytic framework for guidelines on the care of adults and children with asthma

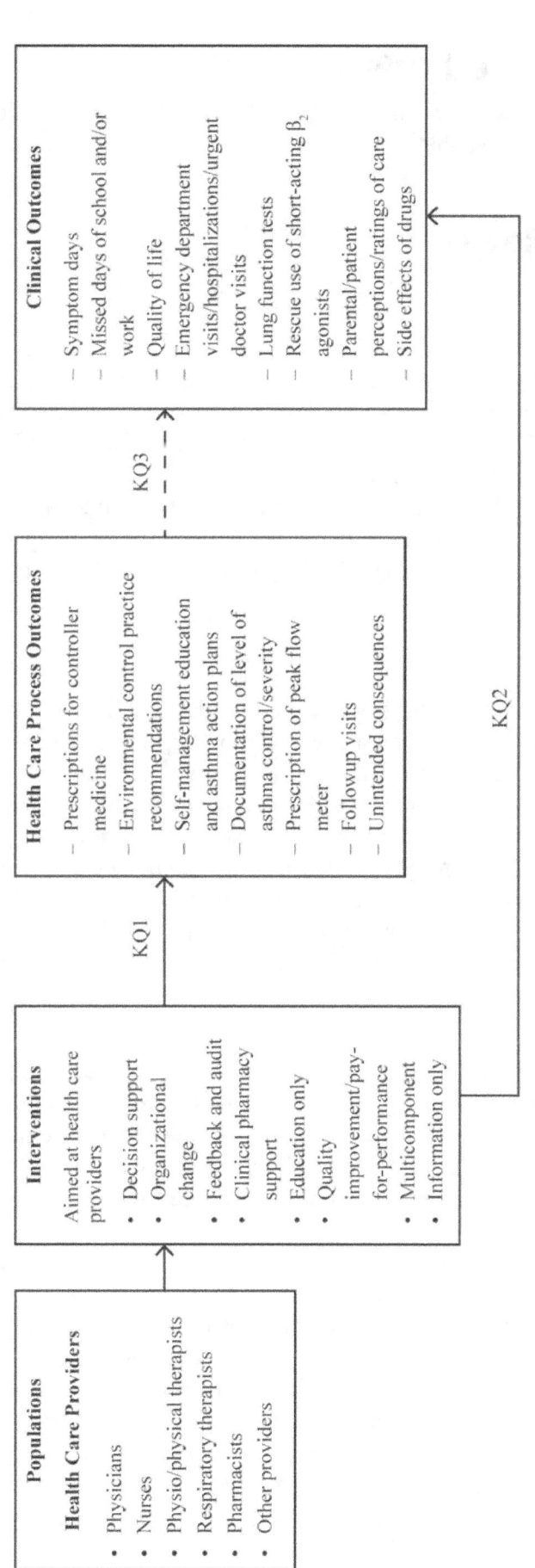

KQ = Key Question

Methods

The methods for this systematic review follow the AHRQ Methods Guide for Effectiveness and Comparative Effectiveness Reviews (available at: www.effectivehealth care.ahrq.gov/methods guide.cfm).

Topic Development and Review Protocol

The topic for this report was nominated in a public process by a staff member of the Ohio Department of Health. We recruited six key informants to provide input on the selection and refinement of the questions for the systematic review. To develop the Key Questions, we reviewed existing systematic reviews, developed an analytic framework and solicited input from our key informants through email and conference calls. Our draft Key Questions were posted on Effective Health Care Program Web site for public comment on October 14th, 2011. The Key Questions were revised, as necessary, based on comments.

We drafted a protocol and recruited a panel of technical experts, including guidelines and methods experts, pediatricians and asthma specialists. We finalized the protocol with input from the technical expert panel and representatives from AHRQ. The protocol was posted on the Effective Health Care Program Web site on March 2, 2012.

Search Strategy

We searched the following databases for primary studies: MEDLINE®, EMBASE®, and the Cochrane Central Register of Controlled Trials®, Cumulative Index to Nursing and Allied Health Literature (CINAHL®), Educational Resources Information Center (ERIC^sm), PsycINFO®, and Research and Development Resource Base in Continuing Medical Education (RDRB/CME) through July 2012. We developed a search strategy for MEDLINE, accessed via PubMed®, based on an analysis of the medical subject headings (MeSH), terms, and text words of eligible articles identified a priori (Appendix B). This strategy was translated for use in the other electronic sources. No limits were imposed based on language or date of publication. Searches were conducted in July 2012. We also completed backward citation searching using Scopus for each included article.

Study Selection

Title and abstracts were screened independently by two trained investigators, and were excluded if both investigators agreed that the article met one or more of the exclusion criteria (see inclusion and exclusion criteria listed in Table 2 and the Abstract Review Form in Appendix C). Differences between investigators regarding abstract eligibility were resolved through consensus.

Citations promoted on the basis of title and abstract screen underwent another independent paired-reviewer screen using the full-text article (Appendix C, Article Review Form). Differences regarding article inclusion were resolved through consensus. During full-text screen, we identified articles not in English for which we could not determine eligibility.

We included randomized and nonrandomized studies that included a comparison and that addressed interventions such as education, reminders, decision support, clinical pharmacy support, organization changes, etc. to improve adherence to guidelines in health care providers. We excluded studies that were conducted in inpatient or emergency department settings only.

Table 2. Study inclusion and exclusion criteria

PICOTS Framework	Inclusion	Exclusion
Populations	Participants: human subjects. Health care providers: physicians, nurses, nurse practitioners, physiotherapists/physical therapists, respiratory therapists, pharmacists, and other health care providers treating children or adults <u>with asthma.</u>	• Animal models/simulations.
Intervention	Interventions to improve adherence to guidelines including decision support (health information technology and paper-based), organizational change, feedback and audit, clinical pharmacy support, education only, quality improvement/pay-for-performance, multicomponent, information only.	• Intervention does not address adherence to asthma guidelines. • Intervention does not target health care providers.
Comparisons of interest	Usual care, as defined in each eligible study, and comparisons between interventions.	Studies lacking a comparison

Outcomes	**Health care process outcomes:**
	  ➢ Prescriptions for controller medicine
	  ➢ Environmental control practice recommendations
	  ➢ Self-management education and asthma action plans
	  ➢ Documentation of level of asthma control/severity
	  ➢ Prescription of peak flow meter
	  ➢ Follow-up visits
	  ➢ Unintended consequences
	
	Clinical outcomes:
	  ➢ Symptom days
	  ➢ Missed days of school and/or work
	  ➢ Quality of life
	  ➢ Emergency department visits/hospitalizations/urgent doctor visits
	  ➢ Lung function tests
	  ➢ Rescue use of short-acting B2 agonists
	  ➢ Parental/patient perceptions/ratings of care
	  ➢ Side effects of drugs
	The outcomes were nondirectional; that is, all outcomes were considered whether they were beneficial or caused potential harms or unintended consequences.
		Studies that do not report an outcome of interest (e.g., studies reporting acceptability of intervention only).

Type of Study	Randomized and quasi-randomized controlled trials and crossover studies. Nonrandomized studies with comparison groups including nonrandomized controlled trial or cross-over studies, controlled pre-post studies, historically controlled studies, cohort studies, case-control studies, and cross-sectional studies. Nonrandomized studies without a separate comparison group, including interrupted-time-series, noncontrolled and pre-post studies.	We excluded meeting abstracts, studies with no original data (e.g., reviews, editorials, comments, and letters) and noncomparative studies.
Timing and Setting	Studies of any duration followup that occurred in an outpatient setting employing healthcare providers were eligible for inclusion.	We excluded studies exclusively addressing inpatient or emergency department settings or guidelines.

Data Abstraction and Data Management

We used DistillerSR (Evidence Partners, 2010) to manage the screening process. DistillerSR is a Web-based database management program that manages all levels of the review process. We uploaded to the system all citations identified by the search strategies.

We created standardized forms for data extraction. (Appendix C) We pilot tested the forms prior to the beginning the process of data extraction. We used Access (Microsoft, Redmond, WA) for the data abstraction process. Reviewers extracted information on general study characteristics, study participants, eligibility criteria, interventions, and the outcomes. One reviewer completed data abstraction and the second reviewer confirmed the first reviewer's data abstraction for completeness and accuracy. Reviewers completed risk of bias assessment independently. Reviewer pairs included personnel with both clinical and methodological expertise. We resolved differences between reviewer pairs regarding data through discussion and, as needed through consensus among the larger group of investigators.

Risk of Bias Assessment

We used the Cochrane Collaboration's tool for assessing the risk of bias of controlled studies. Two trained reviewers independently assessed the included studies according to the guidelines in Chapter 8 of the Cochrane Handbook for Systematic Reviews of Interventions[28] using the following criteria: sequence generation and allocation concealment (selection bias), blinding of health care providers, investigators, and outcome assessors (detection bias), incomplete outcome data (attrition bias), selective outcome reporting (reporting bias), and other sources of bias. We reported judgments for each criterion as "Low risk of bias," "High risk of bias" or "Unclear risk of bias (information is insufficient to assess)" per criteria provided by tool. Disagreements were resolved through team discussion.

For pre-post studies, we added the two relevant criteria from the Cochrane Effective Practice and Organization of Care (EPOC) data collections checklists.[29] Specifically, the questions ask if the intervention was likely to affect data collection, and if the intervention was independent of other changes.

Data Synthesis

For each KQ, we created a detailed set of evidence tables containing all information abstracted from eligible studies. We categorized the interventions being assessed in the studies, and synthesized information by KQ based on these categories:

1. Decision support interventions are health information technology- and/or paper-based-interventions designed to support/facilitate health care provider treatment decisionmaking (e.g., classify asthma severity);
2. Organizational change interventions are designed to change the way in which an organization provides asthma care (e.g., having an asthma "champion");
3. Feedback and audit interventions are based upon providing performance data to health care providers about their quality of asthma care;
4. Clinical pharmacy support: interventions targeting pharmacists' delivery of asthma care;
5. Education only interventions are focused on educating health care providers about the content of asthma clinical practice guidelines;
6. Quality improvement/pay-for-performance interventions are focused on quality improvement initiatives or pay-for-performance as the primary intervention;

7. Multicomponent interventions use more than one type of intervention, with no intervention clearly identifiable as the predominant intervention.
8. Information only interventions provide only information to health care providers about asthma guideline recommendations (e.g., provide a pocket guide to asthma guidelines)

Several studies utilized more than one of the above interventions. For these studies, intervention descriptions were carefully reviewed to identify the predominant interventions. Studies in which the predominant intervention was unclear were reviewed and discussed among team members until consensus on the predominant intervention was reached. Some studies used multicomponent interventions in which no intervention could be clearly identified as predominant. All of these multicomponent studies included provision of information and provider education plus two or more of the following: decision support, organizational change, feedback-and-audit, or quality improvement interventions.

Based on feedback from key informants and public comment, a variety of health care process and clinical outcomes were selected to evaluate the effectiveness of interventions.

The health care process outcomes included:
- Prescriptions for controller medicine
- Environmental control practice recommendations
- Self-management education and asthma action plans
- Documentation of level of asthma control/severity
- Prescription of peak flow meter
- Follow-up visits
- Unintended consequences

The clinical outcomes, assessed in patients, included:
- Symptom days
- Missed days of school and/or work
- Quality of life
- Emergency department visits/hospitalizations/urgent doctor visits
- Lung function tests
- Rescue use of short-acting β_2 agonists
- Parental/patient perceptions/ratings of care
- Side effects of drugs

To answer Key Question 3, we sought to identify studies providing evidence on the link between changes in health care provider behavior (health care process outcomes) to changes in clinical outcomes. Ideally, relevant studies suitably answering Key Question 3 would measure health care process and clinical outcomes, as well as a measure of strength of association between the changes in health care process to the change in clinical outcomes observed in a given study.

We selected outcomes we considered as the most commonly used in practice; those relied upon by clinicians to guide decisionmaking; and those endorsed by the NIH Workshop on Asthma Outcomes on which to focus our synthesis.[30] These critical outcomes identified were prescription of asthma controller medicines, provision of asthma action plan/self-management education, ED visits/hospitalizations, and missed days of school or work.[31] Data abstracted for all outcomes can be found in Appendix E.

We conducted qualitative synthesis of the evidence. Our team felt that the heterogeneity in the studies, including the measures of outcomes, population included, and specifics of the interventions, precluded quantitative synthesis.

In the absence of national qualitative standards to determine magnitude of effect in clinical asthma studies, we chose magnitudes of effect by group consensus among the investigators that were felt to be clinically meaningful changes. Magnitude of effect for studies addressing each outcome was considered as: small (less than 10 percent change or difference), moderate (10-30 percent change or difference) and large (over 30 percent change or difference). These judgments were made by one reviewer, checked by another, with disagreements discussed with the full team.

Strength of the Body of Evidence

We graded the strength of evidence for each outcome for each of the Key Questions using the grading scheme recommended by the Methods Guide for Conducting Comparative Effectiveness Reviews.[32] In assigning evidence grades, we considered the four required domains including risk of bias, directness, consistency and precision. We classified the strength of evidence into four basic categories: (1) "high" grade (indicating high confidence that the evidence reflects the true effect, and further research is very unlikely to change our confidence in the estimate of the effect); (2) "moderate" grade (indicating moderate confidence that the evidence reflects the true effect, and further research may change our confidence in the estimate of the effect and may change the estimate); (3) "low" grade (indicating low confidence that the evidence reflects the true effect, and further research is likely to change our confidence in the estimate of the effect and is likely to change the estimate); and (4) "insufficient" grade (evidence is unavailable or does not permit a conclusion). Our judgments were first based on the ability to make a conclusion (if not able to make a conclusion, then "insufficient" was assigned) and then on the confidence in the conclusion (classified as low, moderate or high with increasing certainty). The author of the section first graded the evidence and this was reviewed by the principal investigator. Any disagreements were discussed with the full team.

Applicability

An applicability statement was created in order to help different key stakeholders understand what key implications to take away from this document, to inform future activities (e.g., research studies; implementing policies). Applicability was assessed separately for the different outcomes for the entire body of evidence guided by the PICOTS framework as recommended in the Methods Guide for Comparative Effectiveness Reviews of Interventions.[32] We considered factors that may limit applicability of the findings (e.g., a study conducted in a non-U.S. health care setting, providers not common to the U.S. health care system).

Peer Review and Public Comment

A full draft report was reviewed by experts and posted for public commentary from August 8, 2012, through September 5, 2012. Comments received from either invited reviewers or through the public comment website were compiled and addressed. A disposition of comments will be posted on the Effective Healthcare Program Web site 3 months after the release of the evidence report.

Results

Results of the Search

Figure 2 summarizes the results of our search. We identified 4,217 unique citations. We excluded 3,892 citations during the abstract screening. During full-text article screening, we excluded an additional 249 articles that did not meet one or more of the inclusion criteria. (Listing of excluded studies is included in Appendix D.) Seventy-three articles were eligible for inclusion and sixty eight addressed one of the critical outcomes and are thus included in the narrative of the report. We selected four outcomes as critical to making a decision on which to focus our synthesis: prescription of asthma controller medicines, provision of asthma action plan/self-management education, ED visits/hospitalizations, and missed days of school or work. Data abstracted for all outcomes can be found in Appendix E.

Figure 2. Summary of search (number of articles)

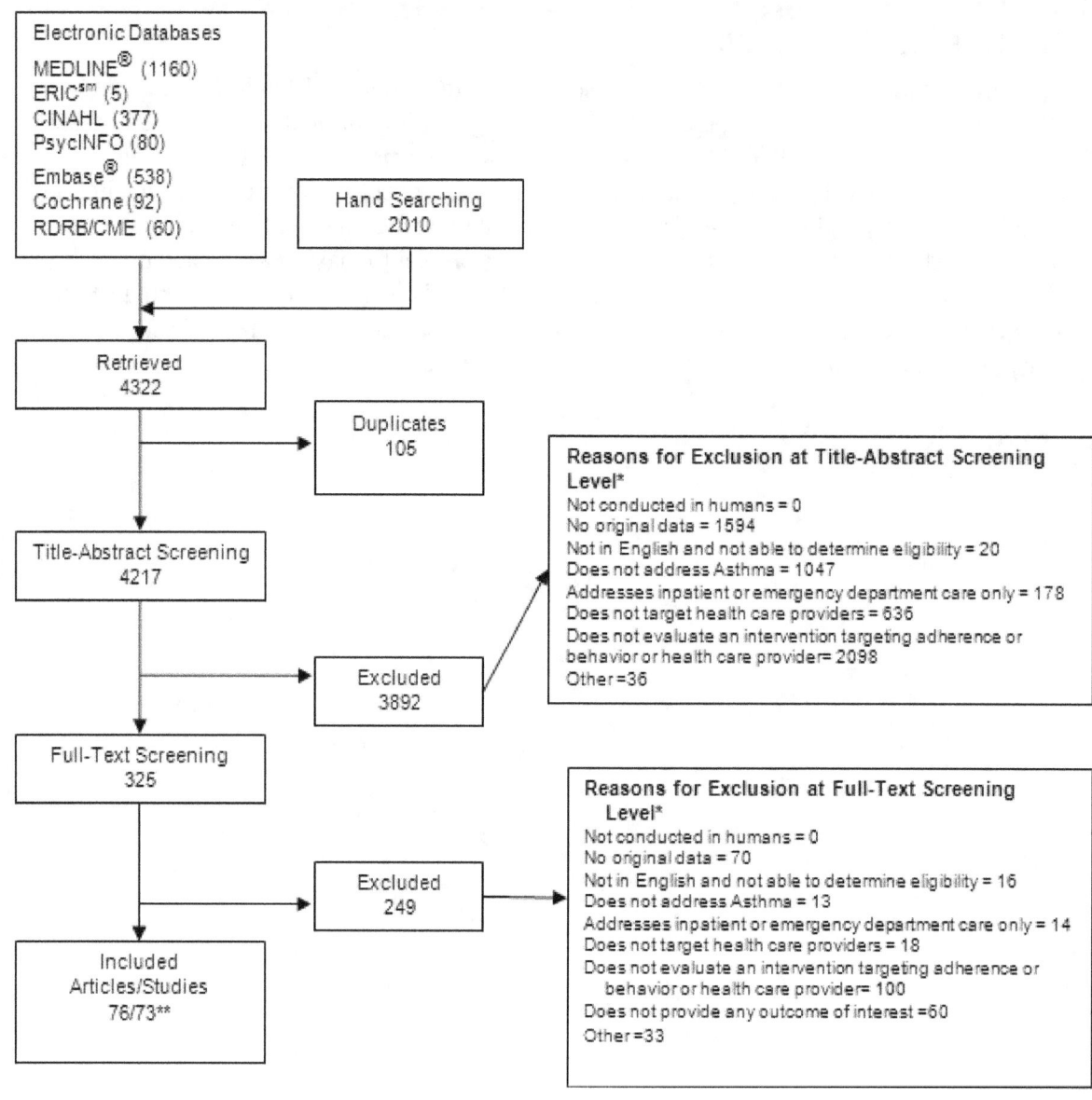

*Total exceeds the # in the exclusion box, as reviewers did not need to agree on reason for exclusion.
**Three distinct pairs of articles described a single intervention or cohort. For the purposes of this review, each pair was counted as a single study, yielding 73 studies reported in 76 articles.

Description of Types of Studies

Of the 73 studies identified, 38 (52.1 percent) were based in the U.S. and 35 (47.9 percent) were international (Table 7). Studies were classified by predominant intervention using the process described in the Methods, into the following groups: Decision Support (n=24), Organizational Change (n=4), Feedback and Audit (n=12), Clinical pharmacy support (n=4), Education only (n=16), Quality Improvement (n=3), Multicomponent (n=8), Information Only (n=2) (Table 3). Roughly half of the studies were randomized trials (n=34), 29 were pre-post, and the remainder were cluster-randomized (n=4), controlled pre-post (n=3), cohort (n=1). (Table 4) Most interventions targeted general practitioners (n=24) or primary healthcare providers. To a lesser extent, studies involved midlevel practitioners (nurse practitioners, physician assistants), pharmacists and different combinations of providers. The most frequently reported health care process outcome was prescription of controller medication (n=44), followed by provision of an asthma action plan (n=18), prescription of a peak flow meter (n=17), and self-management education (n=12) (Table 5). Common clinical outcomes included emergency department visits (n=30) and hospitalizations (n=27), followed by use of short-acting $\beta 2$ agonists (n=9), missed school days (n=8), lung function tests (n=6), symptom days (n=6), quality of life (n=6) and urgent doctor visits (n=5) (Table 6).

Table 3. Studies stratified by intervention

Intervention Type	Number of Studies
Decision support	24
Organizational change	4
Feedback and audit	12
Clinical pharmacy support	4
Education only	16
Quality improvement	3
Multicomponent	8
Information only	2

Table 4. Studies stratified by study design

Study Design	Number of Studies
Cluster-randomized	4
Controlled pre-post	3
Nonrandomized controlled	2
Pre-post	29
Randomized	34
Cohort	1

Table 5. Studies stratified by health care process outcome

Health Care Process Outcome	Number of Studies (n)
Asthma action plan	18
Documentation of asthma control/severity	9
Environmental control practice recommendations	6
Followup visits	8
Prescription of peak flow meter	17
Prescriptions for controller medicine	44
Proportion of patients on inhaled corticosteroids	1
Self-management education	12
Nonurgent care asthma visit	1

Table 6. Studies stratified by clinical outcome

Health Care Clinical Outcome	Number of Studies (n)
Emergency department visits	30
Hospitalizations	27
Lung function tests	6
Missed days of school	8
Missed days of work	4
Parental/patient perceptions	2
Quality of life	6
Use of short-acting β_2 agonists	9
Symptom days	6
Symptom score	3
Urgent doctor visits	5

Table 7. Studies stratified by setting

International vs. Domestic	Number of Studies, n (%)
U.S.	00 (52.1)
International	35 (47.9)

Organization of Results

The results are organized according to each KQ, the four critical outcomes (prescription of asthma controller medicines, provision of asthma action plan/self-management education, ED visits/hospitalizations, and missed days of school or work) and each type of intervention. For each KQ, a description and summary of the key findings from each type of intervention are presented, along with a table summarizing the strength of evidence.

KQ1: In the care of pediatric or adult patients with asthma, what is the evidence that interventions designed to improve health care provider adherence to guidelines impact health care process outcomes (e.g., receiving appropriate treatment)?

Outcome: Prescription of Controller Medicines

Key Points and Evidence Grades

- There is moderate evidence for the effectiveness of decision support interventions to increase prescribing of asthma controller medicines by health care providers. Most of the evidence supporting the use of decision support interventions comes from nonrandomized studies.
- Low strength of evidence supports the effectiveness of organizational change to increase the prescribing of asthma controller medicines by health care providers.
- There is moderate evidence to support feedback/audit interventions as an effective means to increase prescribing of asthma controller medications. Most feedback and audit interventions were multifaceted, limiting our ability to discern whether the feedback and audit component was effective in increasing controller medication prescribing by practitioners.
- There is moderate evidence that clinical pharmacy support interventions increase prescribing of asthma controller medications.
- Low evidence suggests that education interventions do not increase prescription of asthma controller medications by clinicians.
- No studies examined the effect of quality improvement strategies on prescription of asthma controller medications.
- Low strength of evidence supports the effectiveness of multicomponent interventions to increase the prescribing of asthma controller medicines by health care providers.
- There is insufficient evidence to determine if information alone is effective in improving rates of asthma controller medication prescribing in asthma.

Decision Support

Fifteen studies of decision support interventions evaluated prescription of asthma controller medications as an outcome. These studies included six RCTs[33-38] and nine pre-post studies.[39-47] The control condition for the RCTs was usual care[33,35,36,38] or the provision of decision support for nonasthma conditions.[34,37] The health care provider participants all worked in primary care settings (i.e., no allergists, pulmonologists or other sub-specialists). Most studies did not focus the intervention on one type of health care provider, but involved a combination of physicians, nurse practitioners/physician assistants and other nonphysician employees.[40,42,44,46] A minority of studies involved pediatric health care providers.[35,39,44] With few exceptions, there was little description of the patient populations by race/ethnicity,[35,38,44] gender,[35,40,44,47] or disease severity/control.[39,47] The reported racial/ethnic make-up in those studies providing such data reported that a majority of patients cared for as African American, Latino and/or requiring public health insurance.[35,38,39,44,46-48]

The types of decision support interventions varied, and included the provision of asthma guidelines in a more accessible format (e.g., "pocket" versions),[36,43,45] use of a specific algorithm, pathway or flow sheet,[36,44-46] a structured template for taking a history,[39,40] or a reminder system to raise awareness of the health care provider about the patient's asthma status.[34,35,41] The decision support interventions were often combined with other strategies, including education,[33,36-38,41,46,48,49] reminders,[34,38-40,43] feedback,[35,43] and/or organizational change.[42] A minority of interventions were computer-based.[34,37,38,41,43,47,50]

Ten studies found that a decision support intervention significantly increased prescribing asthma controller medicines by health care providers,[33,35,38-41,43,44,46,47] while the remaining studies did not.[34,36,37,42,45] Eight of the studies in which increased prescribing was observed used a pre-post study design, while 3 of the 5 RCTs observed no benefit from decision support interventions.[34,36,37] The increase in prescribing of controller medicines ranged from 2 percent to 34 percent in the studies using the pre-post design, while the difference between intervention and control conditions in the RCT studies ranged from 2 percent to 17 percent. The absolute difference in increased prescribing observed in the RCT studies was generally less than 10 percent. The impact of these decision support interventions to increase the prescribing of controller medicines by health care providers was modest and was observed primarily in pre-post study designs and not as consistently in RCT studies (Table 10).

In summary, moderate evidence supports the use of decision support interventions to increase prescribing of asthma controller medications (Table 8).

Organizational Change

Two studies[51,52] examined the impact of organizational change on the prescribing of asthma controller medications by health care providers. One study was an RCT,[51] while the other was a pre-post study.[52] Both studies included pediatric health care providers. Both studies utilized the addition of personnel to facilitate organizational change. The former study used an asthma nurse educator,[51] while the latter study used a community health worker.[52] Both studies also incorporated provider education as part of the organizational change intervention. The two studies reported beneficial effects on the prescribing practices of health care providers. The former study[51] found that neither the peer-led education arm nor the planned care intervention (utilizing an asthma nurse educator) arms resulted in a statistically significantly higher proportion of prescriptions for inhaled steroids or asthma controller medications compared with the control arm of the study. Notably, prescribing improved in all arms of the study, including the control arm. The improvement in prescribing any type of controller medications ranged from 8 to 16 percent among all patients with asthma and 4 to 11 percent among asthma patients with persistent asthma. For inhaled steroids, the ranges of improved prescribing were 4 to 9 percent and 13 to 19 percent, respectively. In the pre-post study, the investigators[52] observed a 12 percent increase (an absolute change from 44 percent to 56 percent) in prescriptions for inhaled steroids among all asthma patients. The effect of organizational change on increasing prescribing asthma controller medications ranges from small to moderate in the two eligible studies reviewed (Table 10).

In summary, a low strength of evidence supports the effectiveness of organizational change in increasing the prescribing of asthma controller medicines (Table 8).

Feedback and Audit

We identified six RCTs[53-58] and four pre-post studies[59-62] and one nonrandomized controlled study[63] evaluating the effect of feedback and audit on prescribing controller medications. Most feedback and audit studies were conducted in Europe[53-59,63] or the U.S.[60-62,64] Clinicians included primarily general practitioners[53-59] along with primary care physicians[57,62] unidentified prescribers,[60] pharmacists,[63] and pharmacist and physicians[61]. No studies addressed specialty care such as allergy, pediatrics or pulmonary medicine. There was little description of the clinician populations by race/ethnicity, gender, or years of experience.

Most feedback and audit interventions were combined with another intervention; 7 included provider education,[53,56,58-62] one included prioritized review criteria for audit,[55] two included benchmarking or comparison with peers or other practices[55,57] and one included pharmacy monitoring of fill data and feedback to providers as part of a therapeutic outcomes monitoring (TOM) intervention, in which pharmacists also provided counseling and medication monitoring to patients.[63] For each of these studies, however the feedback and audit component was the predominant provider intervention. Comparison groups included feedback unrelated to asthma, control groups located in another community/country, or pre-post comparisons. Implementation many of the interventions appeared complex and may potentially influence the effectiveness of the interventions.

Of the six RCTs[53-58] four demonstrated positive effects of the intervention[53,55,56,58]. Increased prescribing of asthma controller medicines was reported for audit and feedback interventions using targeted key guideline messages about the inflammatory nature of asthma (such as, "use inhaled corticosteroids promptly, treat severe exacerbations with oral corticosteroids") (5 percent to 12 percent increase from baseline, p=0.05),[53] prioritized guideline review criteria on single card,[55] medical record prompts for annual review of asthma management with guideline prompts,[56] and individualized feedback on prescribing and decision strategies.[58] The two RCTs reporting no increase in prescribing of asthma controller medications involved feedback of prescribing data[54] and a trial of performance feedback.[57] Of the studies using a pre-post design and a nonrandomized controlled design, two studies reported an increase in prescribing of controller medicines ranging from 52 to 104 percent.[61,63] No significant increase was observed in an RCT of unsolicited mailed prescriber feedback of individual patient pharmacy count data (Incidence Rate 0.013 [95% CI: 0.01, 0.017]) versus group practice aggregate prescribing data (Incidence Rate 0.014 [95% CI: 0.01, 0.018]) as compared with controls who received feedback regarding another disease (Incidence Rate 0.018 [95% CI: 0.015,0.021]).[54] No significant increase in prescribing of controller medications was also noted in an RCT comparing a traditional quality circle (TQC) intervention, in which providers were given feedback on their individual performance and the aggregate performance of group providers, with a benchmark quality circle (BQC) intervention, in which feedback on providers' individual performance was explicitly compared with a performance benchmark (the highest-performing 10 percent of providers in the benchmark arm).[57]

In a pre-post study of a physician education and mailed asthma management fact sheet + patient pharmacy profile for patients with short-acting bronchodilator over use or no anti-inflammatory medication use demonstrated a strong positive effect (Mean difference in number of long-acting controllers over 9 months: Intermittent asthma: 0.37 (95% CI: 0.25,0.47, p<0.001; Persistent asthma: -0.29 (95% CI: -0.47, -0.12, p=0.009).[61] Yet, a mailed educational and feedback of specific patient pharmacy profile with copy of guidelines showed no effect on inhaled corticoid steroid fills post intervention, despite targeting patients with poorly controlled asthma, i.e. high short acting beta agonist users.[60]

The magnitude of effect for feedback and audit support on prescribing controller medications is moderate based on evidence presented in 4 of the 6 RCTs with positive effect sizes and a significant increase in the percent of patients prescribed or record of use noted for a controller medication before and after interventions. The positive effect sizes, measured as an increase in patients on inhaled corticosteroids from baseline to outcome and between intervention and control groups, ranged from a low effect size of 0.12 (relative effect size defined as [Int $_{outcome}$ – Int $_{baseline}$]/ Int $_{baseline}$] – [(Control $_{outcome}$ –Control $_{baseline}$)/Control $_{baseline}$][58] to a moderate effect size of 0.66 (standard effect size defined as [(Int $_{outcome}$ – Int $_{baseline}$) – (Control $_{outcome}$ – Control $_{baseline}$)]/pooled standard deviation). A significant increase in the change of percentage of patients treated with inhaled steroid from baseline to 12 months post intervention between three groups (guidelines alone, prioritized guideline review criteria and review criteria plus feedback on actual prescribing behavior) was noted as a positive increase of 15.9 percent in controller prescribing in the review criteria plus feedback group as compared with an increase of 11percent in the review criteria only and no change (0 percent) in the guideline only group.[55] A positive but nonsignificant difference (2.7 difference in proportion of patients) was noted in the proportions of patients in practice with asthma "prophylaxis" after one year as compared with practices provided with diabetes guidelines (Difference in asthma prophylaxis: 2.7 (95% CI -14.4 to 19.7).[56]

Two RCTs reported no effect based on low hazard ratios of 0.77 (95% CI: 0.59, 1.01) to 1.08 (95% CI: 0.90, 1.3) on prescribing asthma controller medications, in a study using a mailed prescriber feedback intervention[54] and no before and after differences in percentage of patients with full adherence to guideline defined as prescribed medication consistent with guidelines was low (3.2 to 8 percent, p=0.19) between a "benchmark" group who had their prescribing behavior compared with a performance benchmark or comparison with other prescribers versus a traditional or individual feedback group who did not receive comparison with other prescribers.[57] Of the five pre-post and nonrandomized controlled design studies, only two reported an increase in prescribing controller medications[61,63] ranging from 52 percent to 104 percent; change in prescribing over time (52 percent change over 6 months) in a therapeutic outcomes monitoring program,[63] increase of 104.4 percent in patients with intermittent asthma but a decrease of ICS by 10.8 percent in patients with persistent asthma.[61] The strength of the evidence of feedback and audit support on prescribing asthma controller medications is moderate with several caveats. Factors that lessen the confidence in the results include inconsistent definitions of controller medication prescribing behavior (controller only, controller + rescue medication, and prophylaxis asthma medication), wide variation in feedback and audit intervention protocols, use of varying clinical asthma and GP guidelines over a long period (1990-2007), inconsistent follow-up periods ranging from 3-12 months, and inconsistent control in the analysis for asthma severity (Table 10).

In summary, a number of feedback/audit studies show a small to moderate increase in prescribing of controller medicines by health care providers. Most feedback/audit interventions were multifaceted, thereby limiting our ability to discern if the specific feedback/audit component was effective in increasing controller medication prescribing by health care providers. In summary, moderate evidence supports the use of feedback/audit to increase the prescribing of controller medicines (Table 8).

Clinical Pharmacy Support

We identified one RCT[65], a nonrandomized study[66] and a controlled pre-post study[67] evaluating the effect of clinical pharmacy support on prescribing asthma controller medications. All interventions included a pharmacist education component. All were conducted at international sites including Australia[65,67] and Netherlands.[66]

Clinicians in all studies were pharmacists.[65-67] Only one study included clinician characteristics such as gender (control: female 56 percent, intervention: female 44 percent) and most pharmacists 35 years of age or older.[65]

The one RCT implemented a pharmacy care program training pharmacists in risk assessment, medication adherence and spirometry use and compared with a control group of usual care.[65] Among the non-RCTs, only one intervention of a specialized asthma service by community pharmacies including seeing patients by appointment, assessing and intervening on patient medication needs and goal setting was compared with two groups of control patients was strong.[67] The nonrandomized study tested a minimal intervention that encouraged pharmacists to hold meetings with local general practitioners to discuss guideline care for children with asthma.[66]

The one RCT reported a statistically significant increase in dispensing asthma controller and reliever medication versus reliever only medications in the intervention group when compared with controls (odds ratio 3.80 (95% CI: 1.40, 10.32, p=0.01).[65] Of the two other studies, increased asthma controller medication use at 6 months follow-up was also reported in an intervention of a specialized asthma service by community pharmacies including seeing patients by appointment, assessing and intervening on patient medication needs and goal setting with the patient as compared with control patients in two control groups (Preventive medication use: control 1: 90.9 percent, control 2: 78.6 percent, intervention: 97.4 percent; p=0.04), however an analysis was not reported for comparison of control 1 with intervention group.[67] The second study was of a minimal intervention, encouraged pharmacists to hold meetings with local general practitioners to discuss guideline care for children with asthma. This study reported an increase in controller medications (2.7 percent children with no use of an inhaled corticosteroid medication at 12 months, p<0.05).[66]

The strength of evidence that clinical pharmacy support increases prescription of asthma controller medications is moderate due to consistent and precise results, despite medium risk of bias. There was a notable lack of RCTs addressing this intervention and outcome. The one RCT evaluating the effect of clinical pharmacy support on prescribing asthma controller medications versus rescue medication for children indicated a large shift from the use of rescue medication only to rescue medication plus controller medication (OR 3.80 (95% CI: 1.40, 10.32, p=0.01).[65] The evidence from this study is strong based on a large sample size (n=50 pharmacies and n=351/396 patients completing study), blinding of pharmacists and high follow-up rates (Intervention: 86 percent and Control 91 percent), yet this is the only RCT evaluating a pharmacy intervention. Two studies reported moderate effect size defined as change in percentage of patients prescribed controller medication between pre and post intervention periods (6 percent to 21 percent),[66,67] However the studies either lacked a large sample size and/or reported inconsistent description of controller medication use ("no inhaled corticosteroid use while on long-acting betamimetics" or "ideal asthma medication profile was reliever + preventer + symptom controller medication") (Table 10).

In summary, moderate evidence suggests that the use of clinical pharmacy support increases prescribing of controller medications (Table 8).

Education Only

Ten studies of education alone as an intervention examined prescribing asthma controller medication as an outcome, including six RCTs[68-73] and four with pre-post designs.[74-77] Nearly all of the studies targeted primary care physicians (GPs, FPs, pediatricians) or nurses and one recruited pharmacists.[72] The education interventions were varied and included small group asthma education programs,[69] structured training[77] seminars (including interactive),[71] and grand rounds.[77] Besides delivering specific asthma content, certain interventions also emphasized more general skills, such as training in communication.[68,71] The studies examined prescription of asthma controller medications, including "anti-inflammatory" medications generally, as well as specific classes such as inhaled corticosteroid, leukotriene modifiers and cromolyn. The findings from all studies were consistently in the positive direction, reporting increases in controller medicines prescribing by 3.5 percent to 50.3 percent, though statistically significant increases were reported only in 3 of the studies. Most studies were at high risk of bias and the strength of the evidence was low overall. Thus, the evidence is not sufficient to conclude that the education of health care providers would increase prescribing of controller medications. A majority of provider education intervention studies showed no significant increase in prescribing of asthma controller medicines (Table 10).

In summary, provider education does not increase the prescription of asthma controller medications. However, our confidence in this conclusion is low (low strength of evidence) (Table 8).

Quality Improvement and Pay-for-Performance

No studies examined the effect of quality improvement strategies on prescription of asthma controller medications. Therefore, there is insufficient evidence for this outcome (Table 8).

Multicomponent

Seven studies evaluated the impact of multicomponent interventions.[64,78-83] All interventions included a copy of the guidelines (*information*) and an educational component (*education*); additional interventions included onsite staff to aid in reorganization of practice flow (*organizational change*); feedback to individual providers based on chart reviews (*feedback and audit*), and toolkits with materials for provider use and/or distribution by providers for patient use. Four[79-81,83] were cluster-randomized controlled trials (randomizing primary care practices) and three[64,78,82] were pre-post studies with no comparison group. Only two of the pre-post studies[64,78] and one of the three RCTs[79] found an impact of their multicomponent intervention on rates of inhaled corticosteroid prescriptions. The magnitudes of effect reported by the two pre-post studies were large (reporting a 25 percent increase and a 49 percent increase, respectively, in prescribing rates); however, these studies utilized the weakest available study design. Furthermore, one of these two studies measured this outcome via provider self-report, thus introducing a substantial risk of bias. In the single RCT reporting a statistically significant impact, the magnitude of effect was small, with investigators reporting a difference of only 0.1 puffs per day per patient between groups. Two other RCTs[80,81] observed an effect in the positive direction, but the observed effect did not reach statistical significance. In both these studies, the lack of statistical significance could be attributed to a comparable increase in ICS prescribing rates in the comparison group, thus raising questions about the true impact of the intervention as reported by the two uncontrolled studies (Table 10).

In summary, there is low strength of evidence supporting the effectiveness of multicomponent interventions to increase prescribing of controller medications for asthma (Table 8).

Information Only

Two RCTs[84,85] evaluated the provision of information to providers as the only intervention. One study was a trial in which patients were randomized to have information about asthma management and treatment guidelines inserted in their medical records for provider use.[85] Individual providers thus cared for patients in both arms simultaneously. This study found no difference in rates of inhaled corticosteroid prescribing between study groups. The other study[84] randomized providers to be involved in guideline development or not, prior to the distribution of the guidelines to all study providers. This study reported a decrease, rather than an increase, in inhaled corticosteroid prescribing rates that was statistically significantly larger in the intervention group than the comparison group (9 fewer prescriptions per 1000 patients in the intervention group versus 1 fewer prescription per 1000 patients in the control group, p<0.01). This was the only unintended consequence we identified from the included studies in our review (Table 10).

In summary, because of inconsistent results between only two studies, there is insufficient evidence to determine if information alone is effective in improving rates of controller medication prescribing in asthma (Table 8).

Table 8. Prescriptions for controller medications—strength of evidence for KQ1

Intervention	No. of Studies/No. Of Health Care Providers	Risk of Bias	Consistency	Directness	Precision	Strength of Evidence (SOE) & Magnitude of Effect (MOE)
Decision support	15/1,635 6 RCTs,9 pre-post	Medium	Consistent	Direct	Precise	SOE: Moderate MOE: Large: 2%–34% in pre-post studies; 2%–17% in RCTs
Organizational change	2/228 1RCT, 1 pre-post	Medium	Consistent	Direct	Precise	SOE: Low MOE: Small: In the RCT: 8%–16% for all asthma patients; 4%–11% among patients with persistent asthma; 4%–9% for inhaled steroids (ICS) for all asthma patients; 13%–19% for ICS for patients with persistent asthma. In the pre-post study: 12% increase in ICS
Feedback and audit	11/ 1,831 6 RCTs, 4 pre-post and 1 nonrandomized controlled	Medium	Consistent	Direct	Imprecise	SOE: Moderate MOE: Moderate Effect size: 0.12-0.66. Percent increase in patients treated with ICS: 15.9% feedback vs. 11% review guideline and 0% guideline only. Pre-post studies of therapeutic outcomes monitoring or a mailed fact sheet + pharmacy profile feedback study increased ICS prescribing: 52-104%, Hazard ratio range: 0.77-1.08
Clinical Pharmacy Support	3/ 91 1 RCT, 1pre-post, 1 non randomized	Medium	Consistent	Direct	Precise	SOE: Moderate MOE: Moderate OR: 3.80 (95% CI: 1.4, 10.32) Percent increase in patients prescribed controller meds pre and post: 6-21%.
Education only	10/ 451 6RCTs, 4 pre-post	Medium	Consistent	Direct	Imprecise	SOE: Low MOE: Small to large in studies: 3.5-50.3% increase in prescribing controller medicines [no benefit].
Quality improvement and Pay-for-performance	0					SOE: Insufficient MOE: N/A
Multicomponent interventions	7/ >1141 4 Cluster randomized, 3 pre-post	High	Consistent	Direct	Imprecise	SOE: Low MOE: Moderate. Of 7 studies, only two pre-post studies and one RCT reported significant increases in prescribing of controller medicines (25%-49% in pre-post study; small positive MOE in RCT). Other effects were null.
Information Only	2/107, 1 RCT, 1 quasi-experimental	High	Inconsistent	Direct	Imprecise	SOE: Insufficient

MOE = magnitude of evidence; RCT = randomized controlled trial; SOE = strength of evidence

Outcome: Self-Management Education and Asthma Action Plans

Key Points and Evidence Grades

- Moderate evidence supports the effectiveness of decision support interventions to increase the provision of self-management education/asthma action plans by health care providers. Most of the evidence supporting the use of decision support interventions comes from nonrandomized studies.
- The strength of evidence is low to support organizational change to increase provision of self-management education/asthma action plans by health care providers.
- The strength of evidence is low to support audit interventions to increase the use of self-management education/asthma action plans by health care providers.
- The strength of evidence is moderate to support the use of clinical pharmacy support interventions to increase the provision of self-management education and asthma action plans.
- The strength of evidence is low to support education-only interventions to increase the use of asthma action plans.
- The strength of evidence is low to support quality improvement interventions to increase prescribing of asthma action plans/self-management education by healthcare providers.
- The strength of evidence is low to support multicomponent interventions to increase the provision of self-management education/asthma action plans by health care providers.
- There is insufficient evidence to determine if information alone is effective in improving rates of provision of self-management education and asthma action plans by health care providers.

Decision Support

Ten studies evaluated the impact of decision support interventions on the provision of patient education/asthma action plans.[37,38,42,43,45,49,86-89] Four of the studies were RCTs,[37,38,87,89] while the remainder used a pre-post study design.[42,43,45,49,86,88] The interventions included computerized support,[37,38,42,43,89] a flow sheet/algorithm,[86,88] and/or the provision of guidelines.[45] These studies all focused on primary care settings and all studies involved a mix of primary care providers, such as general practitioners,[37] pediatricians,[49,87] or family practitioners.[88] Of the two studies that reported patient sociodemographic data,[38,87] the majority of patients were African American.

Seven of these studies reported a positive effect of decision support on the provision of patient education/asthma action plans.[42,43,45,49,86-88] The increase in self-management education/use of asthma action plans across these studies ranged from 14 percent to 84 percent. Of the four RCTs, only one showed a positive impact.[87] An increase in the provision of asthma education/asthma action plans by health care providers was observed primarily in pre-post studies (Table 10).

In summary, moderate evidence supports the use of decision support interventions to increase the provision of asthma education/asthma action plans by health care providers(Table 9).

Organizational Change

Two studies examined how organizational change influenced the provision of patient self-management education and/or asthma action plans, one using an RCT design[90] while the other used a pre-post design.[91] Investigators in the pre-post study[91] instituted a registry to track asthma patients and an asthma case manager, while investigators in the RCT[90] restructured the clinical protocol for how asthma patients are cared for during ambulatory care encounters ("3+ visit plan"). In general, the effect of organizational changes to increase self-management education/asthma action plan use by health care providers was small. In the pre-post study, there was a 10 percent increase in documentation of patient education (p<0.001) and a 14 percent increase in documentation of home asthma action plan (p<0.001), while in the RCT, the investigators observed a 10 percent increase in asthma education (p=0.01). (Table 10)

In summary, low strength of evidence supports the use of organizational change as a method to increase the provision of self-management education/asthma action plan by health care providers (Table 9).

Feedback and Audit

We identified three RCTs[55-57] and two pre-post studies [60,62] evaluating the effect of feedback and audit interventions on the self-management education and use of asthma action plans. Results of feedback and audit interventions for increasing use of self-management education and asthma action plans are positive. Statistically significant positive effects for recording inhaler technique were noted with an RCT of a medical record annual asthma and guideline audit with prompt intervention when compared with diabetes control group.[56] A significantly higher proportion of health care providers recording inhaler technique was reported in the audit and prompting intervention group (proportion difference between intervention and diabetes control group: 12.9 percent (95% CI: 1.9 percent, 23.9 percent).[56] A negative change for peak flow meter use was noted in the guideline review criteria plus feedback group (decrease 3.6 percent) . In this same study, no effect in self-management was observed[55] and a minimal increase of 0.7 difference in proportion (95% CI: -15.2, 16.7) after practices received asthma guidelines.[56]

Asthma action plan use was significantly increased in patients exposed to a benchmarking feedback intervention or benchmarking quality circle (BCQ), i.e. comparing own prescribing performance with performance of GP who performed best in the quality circles (benchmarking), as compared with Traditional Quality circles (TQC) intervention without benchmarking and compared over time between baseline (T1) and 12 months after implementing the intervention (T2) (T1-T2: Benchmark Quality Circle: increase percent use from 6.7 to14.3 percent (7.6 point increase), Traditional Quality Circle: 6.1 to 10.6 percent (4.5 point increase), p=0.008).[57]

There was no reported increase in providing self-management education in a benchmarking feedback intervention.[57]

Among the pre-post studies, spacer use was increased in patients enrolled an intervention that involved a letter based prescriber and pharmacist educational plus prescribing feedback intervention pre and post intervention (Feedback and pharmacy education intervention: increased 6-7 percent, vs. an 8-2 percent decrease in a comparator control group that received no feedback or pharmacy education with a decrease of 8-2 percent in spacer use in a comparison group with no intervention p=0.007) and no change in peak flow meter use between groups.[60] A 133 percent increase in the provision of patient asthma education was reported in a feedback intervention comparing individual primary care providers with peers and asthma education for their office staff (asthma education: baseline: 30 percent, 6 months:70 percent).[62]

Feedback/audit interventions increase asthma self-management education/asthma action plan use, although the amount of increase ranges is variable. The magnitude of effect for feedback and audit support to increase the provision of self-management education/asthma action plans is low based on a negative to low differences in proportions for practices recording peak flow meter use. A moderate increase was noted for inhaler technique: 12.9 (95% CI: 1.9, 23.9),[56] and a small increase in change of asthma action plan use (7.6 percent) in a benchmarking feedback group (Table 10).[57]

In summary, a low strength of evidence support of the use of feedback and audit interventions to increase the provision of self-management education/asthma action plans by health care providers (Table 9).

Clinical Pharmacy Support

We identified one RCT[65] evaluating the effect of clinical pharmacy support on the self-management education and asthma action plans. Patients receiving care by pharmacists enrolled in Pharmacy Asthma Care Program had increased asthma action plan noted as percent change from baseline to 6 months (asthma action plan provision mean change from baseline: 40.4 percent (95% CI: 31.9, 48.9), p=0.001, however there are no comparison data for the control group (Table 10).[65]

In summary, based on the one study, there is moderate evidence to support the use of clinical pharmacy interventions to increase self-management education/asthma action plan use by health care providers (Table 9).

Education Only

There were five RCTs of education only interventions[68,70,71,92,93] that examined provision of a written asthma action plan as an outcome. Most targeted general practitioners and one focused on pediatricians, with a variety of education only strategies. The education interventions were varied and included small group asthma education programs, structured training, and interactive seminars. Two studies reported statistically significant increases in receipt of an asthma action plan, with increases of 10 percent (p=0.03)[71] and 15 percent (p=0.046)[68] while the other three studies[70,92,93] reported no significant increase (relative risk: 1.40, +1.1 percent and OR 1.00).One study examined not only whether patients were more likely to receive an asthma action plan[93] but also whether the physicians in the intervention arm were more likely to report using a asthma action plan. However, in this study, no significant increase in physician report of asthma action plan was reported. These studies evaluating the use of health care provider education had mixed results in improving patient education/asthma action plan use by health care providers (Table 10).

In summary, low strength of evidence suggests that educational interventions can increase use of asthma action plans by health care providers (Table 9).

Quality Improvement and Pay-for-Performance

Three studies examined the effect of quality improvement strategies on receipt of asthma action plans.[94-96] The design of the studies included an RCT,[96] a pre-post study,[94] and a controlled, pre-post study.[95] All three studies involved pediatric health care providers, including nurses, nurse practitioners and physicians. Two studies assessed participation in a Breakthrough Series collaborative,[95,96] and one study assessed a combination of continuous quality improvement and the addition of a community health worker.[94]

Overall, the results are inconsistent, with a -3 percent to 33 percent change in the proportion of patients provided an asthma action plan. Two of the three studies[94,95], both pre post studies, showed a 19 percent to 33 percent improvement in the proportion of patients who had received an asthma action plan. One of these studies,[95] the controlled pre-post study, showed a 19 percent increase by survey and a difference of 33 percent by medical record review in the intervention arm. The second study showed a 28.2 percent increase in the proportion of patients who had received an asthma action plan. In one of the two pre-post studies, documented self-management education increased by 21 percent, although there was no definition of what constituted self-management education and how it was documented.[95]

The third study,[96] an RCT, showed no significant improvement in the use of asthma action plans by providers, with a 1 percent increase in the intervention group and 4 percent increase in the control group for a -3 percent difference of difference.[96] However, there was some evidence of poor adherence to the quality improvement intervention in the RCT, with decreases in participation in the learning sessions and in outcome reporting over time (Table 10).[96]

In summary, there is low strength of evidence that quality improvement leads to moderate increases the provision of self-management education/asthma action plans in select populations of health care providers, based on two positive observational studies and one negative RCT with evidence of suboptimal engagement by participants (Table 9).

Multicomponent

Six studies[64,78,80,82,83,97] examined the impact of multicomponent interventions on rates at which providers created asthma action plans for their patients. Two studies[80,83] were cluster-randomized trials of primary care practices, while the remaining four studies[64,78,82,97] were pre-post studies. The interventions varied in their content, but most included an educational component. Other elements of these interventions included: (1) training in communication techniques, provision of a spirometer and training in use of spirometer[78]; (2) laminated posters of asthma guidelines and medications, feedback on asthma action plan use, and monthly calls from an intervention team to troubleshoot communication problems[97]; (3) asthma kits (peak flow meters, spacers, educational materials) and systems-level changes (flow sheets and standing medication orders)[80]; (4) systematic use of a patient questionnaire and an asthma management algorithm; (5) an asthma coordinator and feedback on performance as part of continuous quality improvement efforts; (6) an educational toolbox, seminars, teleconferences, mini fellowships, opinion leader visits, clinician-specific feedback, and pay for performance.[83] All four pre-post studies reported a large and statistically significant positive impact on asthma action plans over time (ranging from 27 percent–46 percent of included providers, median 42 percent), but, in the absence of comparison groups, could not account for secular trends. Both RCTs reported changes in the provision of patient education/asthma action plans in a positive direction, (one reporting an increase among seven percent of providers, the other reporting a relative rate of 1.82) but neither result achieved statistical significance (Table 10).

Based on the use of weak study designs among studies observing an intervention effect, combined with the inconsistency of results among studies, there is low evidence to support the effectiveness of multicomponent interventions in increasing the provision of patient education/asthma action plans (Table 9).

Information Only

No studies examined the impact of information provision alone on self-management education or asthma action plans. Therefore, there is insufficient information to assess the effect of information-only strategies on self-management education/asthma action plan use by health care providers (Table 9).

Table 9. Self-management education and asthma action plans—strength of evidence for KQ1

Intervention	No. of Studies/No. Of Health Care Providers	Risk of Bias	Consistency	Directness	Precision	Strength of Evidence (SOE) & Magnitude of Effect (MOE)
Decision support	10/122-124 4 RCTs, 6 pre-post	Medium	Consistent	Direct	Precise	SOE : Moderate MOE: Large: 14% - 84%
Organizational change	2/24 1 RCT, 1 pre-post	Medium	Consistent	Direct	Precise	SOE: Low MOE: Moderate: 10% - 14%
Feedback and audit	5/336 3 RCTs, 2 pre-post	Medium	Inconsistent	Direct	Imprecise	SOE: Low MOE: Low _Self-management education:_ Peak Flow: difference in proportions between practice groups at follow-up range from low of 0.7 (95% CI: -15.2, 16.7) Inhaler technique education: 12.9% (95% CI: 1.9, 23.9) _Asthma Action Plans:_ Increase of 7.6 % in Feedback with Benchmark (Traditional: 4.5%) _Asthma Education:_ Pre to post: 133% increase.
Clinical pharmacy support	1/ 82 1 RCT,	Low	Consistent	Direct	Imprecise	SOE: Moderate MOE: Moderate _Asthma Action Plans:_ change from baseline to follow-up: 40%
Education only	5/470 5 RCTs	High	Inconsistent	Direct	Imprecise	SOE: Low MOE: Small – moderate _Asthma Action Plans:_ 10%-15% , OR/RR 1.40/1
Quality improvement and pay-for-performance	3/63 practices (providers not reported) 1 RCT, 2 pre-post	High	Inconsistent	Direct	Precise	SOE: Low MOE: Moderate: -3-33% increase
Multicomponent interventions	6/>937 2 RCT, 4 pre-post	High	Consistent	Direct	Imprecise	SOE: Low MOE: Moderate Pre-post studies: Positive impact on provision of Asthma action plans: 27-46% increase. RCTs: smaller effect sizes (7% of providers; RR²=1.82)
Information only	0	N/A	N/A	N/A	N/A	SOE: Insufficient MOE: N/A

SOE = strength of evidence; MOE = magnitude of effect; N/A = not applicable; OR = odds ratio; RCT = randomized controlled trial; RR = relative risk; RR² = relative rate

27

Table 10. Study characteristics for health care process outcomes

Intervention	Author, Year	Study Design	Type of Provider	No. of Providers	No. of Patients	Health Care Process Outcomes	
						Prescription for Controller Medicines	Self-Management Education/ Asthma Action Plan
	Mahi-Taright S., 2004[74]	Pre-post	General Practitioner	50	49	∅	N/A
	Cowie R. L., 2001[75]	Pre-post	NR	NR	Arm A (Basic Education): NR Arm (Intermediate Education): NR Arm C (Intensive Education): NR	∅	N/A
	Davis R. S., 2004[76]	Pre-post	Primary Healthcare	20	NR	↑	N/A
	Blackstien-Hirsch P., 2000[77]	Pre-post	Physician	59	195	∅	N/A
	Shah S., 2011[68]	RCT	General Practitioner	150	Arm A (control):107 Arm B: (PACE):110	↑	↑
Education Only	Smeele I. J., 1999[69]	RCT	General Practitioner	Arm A (Control):17 Arm B (Education):17	Arm A (Control):223 Arm B (Education):210	∅	N/A
	Brown R, 2004[70]	RCT	Pediatrician	Arm A(Control):11 Arm B(Education):12	Arm A(Control):122 Arm B(Education):157	∅	∅
	Clark NM, 1998[71]	RCT	Pediatrician, Physician	Arm A:37 Arm B(Education):37	637	↑	↑
	Stergachis A, 2002[72]	RCT	Pharmacist	Arm A(Control):NR Arm B(Education):35	Arm A(Control):177 Arm B(Education):153	∅	N/A
	Premaratne U. N., 1999[73]	RCT	Nurse practice nurses	NR	Arm A(control):14410 Arm B(Education):9900	∅	N/A
	Holton C., 2011[92]	RCT	General Practitioner	Arm A(Control):45 Arm B(Spirometry training):127	Arm A(Control):157 Arm B(Spirometry training):240	N/A	∅
	Sulaiman N. D., 2010[93]	RCT	General Practitioner	Arm A(Control):18 Arm B(Education and guidelines):18 Arm C(Guidelines): 15	Arm A(Control):121 Arm B(Education and guidelines):156 Arm C(Guidelines):134	N/A	∅

Table 10. Study characteristics for health care process outcomes (continued)

Intervention	Author, Year	Study Design	Type of Provider	No. of Providers	No. of Patients	Health Care Process Outcomes	
						Prescription for Controller Medicines	Self-Management Education/ Asthma Action Plan
	Bell, 2010[38]	RCT	Pediatrician	NR	Arm A (UP control): 5192 Arm B (UP intervention): 5040 Arm C (SP control): 3843 Arm D (up control): 5375	↑	∅
	Cho, S.H., 2010[41]	Pre-post	Allergist, general practitioner, physician	377	2042	↑	N/A
Decision Support	Cloutier M.M., 2002[46]	Pre-post	Nurse, nurse practitioner, other, pediatrician, physician, physician assistant advanced practice nurses, family practice	172	860	↑	N/A
	Cloutier M.M., 2005[44]	Pre-post	Nurse, nurse practitioner, pediatrician, physician assistant, primary health care pediatric residents, medical students	151	3748	↑	N/A
	Davis A.M., 2010[47]	Pre-post	Physician family medicine residents	NR	180	↑	N/A

Table 10. Study characteristics for health care process outcomes (continued)

Intervention	Author, Year	Study Design	Type of Provider	No. of Providers	No. of Patients	Health Care Process Outcomes	
						Prescription for Controller Medicines	Self-Management Education/ Asthma Action Plan
	Eccles M, 2002[37]	RCT	General practitioner	NR	Arm A (angina): 4851 Arm B (asthma): 4960	Ø	Ø
	Fairall L., 2010[33]	RCT	Nurse	148	Arm B (intervention): 1000	↑	N/A
	Halterman J.S., 2006[87]	RCT	Nurse practitioner, pediatrician, physician	NR	Arm A (control): 124 Arm B (intervention): 122	N/A	↑
	Horswell R.,2008[43]	Pre-post	Physician	NR	NR	↑	N/A
	Kattan M., 2006[35]	RCT	Nurse practitioner, physician assistant, primary healthcare	Arm A (standard practice): NR Arm B (decision support): 435	Arm A (standard practice): 466 Arm B (decision support): 471	↑	N/A
Decision Support (continued)	Lesho EP, 2005[45]	Pre-post	Primary healthcare	NR	330	Ø	↑
	Martens J.D.,2007[34]	RCT	General practitioner	Arm A (Control): 54 Arm B (Guidelines and involved in development): 53	Arm A: 24,160 Arm B: 35,748	Ø	N/A
	McCowan C., 2001[89]	RCT	General practitioner	NR	Arm A (control): 330 Arm B (decision support): 147	N/A	Ø
	Mitchell E.A.,2005[36]	RCT	General practitioner	270	NR	Ø	N/A
	Newton W.P., 2010[42]	Pre-post	Nurse, physician practice managers, other staff	NR	NR	Ø	↑
	Ragazzi H., 2011[49]	Pre-post	Nurse, pediatrician	Practices 1 and 2: 26-28 Practice 3: NR	Practice 1: 17 Practice 2: 26	N/A	↑

Table 10. Study characteristics for health care process outcomes (continued)

Intervention	Author, Year	Study Design	Type of Provider	No. of Providers	No. of Patients	Health Care Process Outcomes	
						Prescription for Controller Medicines	Self-Management Education/ Asthma Action Plan
Decision Support (continued)	Rance K., 2011[39]	Pre-post	Nurse practitioner, pediatrician	4	41	↑	
	Ruoff G., 2002[88]	Pre-post	Family physicians	17	122	N/A	↑
	Shapiro A., 2011[40]	Pre-post	Nurse, physician	25	Arm B (SBHC): 200 Arm C (NYCHP): 197	↑	N/A
	Shiffman R.N., 2000[50]	Pre-post	Pediatrician	11	Arm A (Sole physician arm; patient arm, pre): 91 Arm B (patient arm): 74	∅	N/A
	To T., 2008[86]	Pre-post	Primary healthcare	NR	1408	N/A	↑
	Veninga CCM, 1999[53]	RCT	General Practitioner	Arm A (Netherlands):181 Arm B (Sweden):204 Arm C (Norway):199 Arm D (Slovakia):81	NR	↑	N/A
Feedback and Audit	Sondergaard J., 2002[54]	RCT	General Practitioner	Arm A (control): 141 Arm B (Individual patient count data feedback):77 Arm C (Aggregate data feedback):74	6437	∅	N/A
	Baker R., 2003[55]	RCT	General Practitioner	Arm A (Guidelines only):27 Arm B (Guidelines with audit criteria):27 Arm C (Guidelines with audit criteria and feedback):27	Arm A (Guidelines only):483 Arm B (Guidelines with audit criteria):510 Arm C (Guidelines with audit criteria and feedback):489	↑	∅

31

Table 10. Study characteristics for health care process outcomes (continued)

Intervention	Author, Year	Study Design	Type of Provider	No. of Providers	No. of Patients	Health Care Process Outcomes	
						Prescription for Controller Medicines	Self-Management Education/ Asthma Action Plan
	Feder G, 1995[56]	RCT	General Practitioner	NR	Arm A (Diabetes Education):NR Arm B (Education, Reminders and Audit):NR	↑	↑
	Schneider A., 2008[57]	RCT	General Practitioner	96	Arm A (traditional quality circle):NR Arm B (benchmark quality circle):NR Arm C (combined arms):256	∅	↑
	Veninga CCM, 2000[58]	RCT	General Practitioner	Arm A (UTI):91 Arm B (Education and Feedback):90	Arm A (UTI):NR Arm B(Education and Feedback):NR	↑	N/A
Feedback and Audit (continued)	Coleman C. I., 2003[60]	Pre-post	Pharmacist Prescriber	NR	Arm A (Patient specific information: Prescribers with patients on 'high dose'):510 Arm B (Patient specific information: Prescribers with patients on 'low dose'):135	∅	↑
	Suh D. C., 2001[61]	Pre-post	NR	NR	Arm A: (566) Arm B(Feedback):1050	↑	N/A
	Richman M. J., 2000[62]	Pre-post	Pediatrician	29	228	N/A	↑
	Herborg H., 2001[63]	Non-RCT	General Practitioner, Other, Pharmacist Pharmacy assistant	Arm A (Control):64 Arm B (TOM):75	NR	↑	N/A
	Hoskins G., 1997[59]	Pre-post	General practitioner	91	Before intervention: 782 Education and feedback intervention: 669	N/A	N/A

Table 10. Study characteristics for health care process outcomes (continued)

Intervention	Author, Year	Study Design	Type of Provider	No. of Providers	No. of Patients	Health Care Process Outcomes	
						Prescription for Controller Medicines	Self-Management Education/ Asthma Action Plan
Clinical Pharmacy Support	Armour C., 2007[65]	RCT	Pharmacist	Arm A (control): 25 Arm B (PACP): 32	Arm A (Control): 186 Arm B (PACP): 165	↑	↑
	De Vries, 2010[66]	Nonrandomized pre-post	Arm A: General practitioner Arm B: General practitioner, pharmacists Arm C: General practitioner, pharmacists, pediatrictian	9	Arm A (control): 3527 Arm B (feedback): 1447	↑	N/A
	Saini B, 2004[67]	Pre-post	Arm A: General practitioner, pharmacist Arm B: pharmacist Arm C: pharmacist	Arm A (Control 1): 13 Arm B (Control 2):12 Arm C (Education): NR	Arm A (Control 1): 22 Arm B (Control 2):28 Arm C (Education): 52	↑	N/A
Information Only	Martens J. D., 2006[84]	RCT	General Practitioner	Arm A (Control):54 Arm B (Guidelines and involved in development):53 Arm C (Guidelines only):26	NR	→	N/A
	Bryce FP, 1995[85]	RCT	General Practitioner, Nurse	NR	Arm A (Control):1563 Arm B (Reminders and Tools):1585	∅	N/A

Table 10. Study characteristics for health care process outcomes (continued)

Intervention	Author, Year	Study Design	Type of Provider	No. of Providers	No. of Patients	Health Care Process Outcomes		
						Prescription for Controller Medicines	Self-Management Education/ Asthma Action Plan	
	Finkelstein J. A., 2005[51]	RCT	Pediatric medical provider	228	Arm A (Control):1531 Arm B (PLE Intervention):2003 Arm C (Planned Care Intervention):1635	∅	N/A	
Organizational Change	Thyne S.M., 2007[52]	Pre-post	Pediatric medical providers, "urgent care clinicians"	NR	Arm A (Time 1, 2002-2003):NR Arm B (Time 2, 2003-2004):NR Arm C (Time 3, 2004-2005):NR	↑	N/A	
	Glasgow N. J., 2003[90]	RCT	General Practitoner	Arm A (Control):12 Arm B (Intervention):12	Arm A (Control):73 Arm B (Intervention):101	N/A	↑	
	Patel P . H., 2004[91]	Pre-post	Physicians, Nurses	NR	451	N/A	↑	
	Fox P., 2007[94]	Pre-post	Nurse, Nurse Practitioner, Physician caregivers, administrative staff	NR	Chart review sample :280 Interview sample :405	N/A	↑	
Quality Improvement	Mangione-Smith R., 2005[95]	Pre-post	"Health care providers"	NR	Arm A (Control):126 Arm B (Learning collaborative):385	N/A	↑	
	Homer CJ, 2005[96]	RCT	Nurse, Physician Front office staff	NR	Arm A (Control):337 Arm B(Learning collaborative):294	N/A	∅	

34

Table 10. Study characteristics for health care process outcomes (continued)

Intervention	Author, Year	Study Design	Type of Provider	No. of Providers	No. of Patients	Health Care Process Outcomes	
						Prescription for Controller Medicines	Self-Management Education/ Asthma Action Plan
	Bender B. G., 2011[78]	Pre-post	Nurse, Physician, Physician Assistant Medical assistants, practice managers, office staff	372	15508	←	←
Multicomponent	Hagmolen, W., 2008[79]	RCT	General Practitioner	Arm A (Guidelines only):34 Arm B (Education and Guidelines):34 Arm C (Education and Guidelines and individualized treatment advice):38	Arm A (Guidelines only):98 Arm B (Education and Guidelines):133 Arm C (Education and Guidelines and individualized treatment advice):131	←	N/A
	Daniels E. C., 2005[80]	RCT	General Practitioner, Internist, Nurse Practitioner, Pediatrician, Physician, Physician Assistant staff	163	Arm A(Control): 136079 Arm B(Education): 90555	∅	∅

Table 10. Study characteristics for health care process outcomes (continued)

Intervention	Author, Year	Study Design	Type of Provider	No. of Providers	No. of Patients	Health Care Process Outcomes	
						Prescription for Controller Medicines	Self-Management Education/ Asthma Action Plan
Multicomponent (continued)	Lundborg C. S., 1999[81]	RCT	General Practitioner	Arm A (Control):104 Arm B (Education and Feedback):100	Arm A (Control):1333 Arm B (Education and Feedback):1121	Ø	N/A
	Yawn BP, 2008[64]	Pre-post	Nurse Practitioner, Physician, Physician Assistant	Education and Feedback: 211	Education and Feedback: 840	↑	↑
	Frankowski B. L., 2006[97]	Pre-post	Nurse, Pediatrician, Primary Healthcare	NR	Education and Feedback: 150	N/A	↑

N/A = not applicable; NR = not reported; PACE = Physician Asthma Care Education; RCT = randomized controlled trial
↑ — Statistically significant increase in outcome of interest.
↓ — Statistically significant decrease in outcome of interest.
Ø — Difference between intervention and control groups or between pre- and post-intervention *not* statistically significant.

36

KQ2: In the care of pediatric or adult patients with asthma, what is the evidence that interventions designed to improve health care provider adherence to guidelines impact clinical outcomes (e.g., hospitalizations, patient-reported outcomes such as symptom control)?

Outcome: Emergency Department Visits/Hospitalization

Key Points and Evidence Grades
- There is moderate strength of evidence supporting the effectiveness of decision support interventions to reduce ED visits/hospitalizations. Most of the evidence supporting the use of decision support interventions comes from nonrandomized studies.
- There is low strength of evidence that organizational change does not reduce ED visits and hospitalizations for asthma.
- The strength of evidence is insufficient to support the effectiveness of feedback and audit interventions reduce ED visits and hospitalizations.
- There is insufficient evidence to evaluate the effectiveness of clinical pharmacy support interventions to reduce ED visits and hospitalizations for asthma.
- There is low strength of evidence for no benefit of clinician education to reduce hospitalization/ED visits for asthma.
- There is low strength of evidence to suggest that quality improvement does not decrease ED visits and hospitalizations.
- There is insufficient evidence to evaluate the effect of multicomponent interventions on ED visits or hospitalizations for asthma.
- There is insufficient evidence to evaluate the effect of information-only strategies on ED visits or hospitalizations for asthma.

Decision Support
Of the ten studies evaluating the effect of decision support on ED visits/hospitalizations, four were RCTs,[35,36,89,98] while the others were pre-post studies.[42,43,45,48,50,86] The decision support interventions included computer systems,[42,43,50,89] checklists,[98] supplemental feedback protocols,[35] and structured pathways/algorithms.[36,48] These interventions were combined with educational interventions, organizational changes and/or reminders. The populations in these studies were a mix of adult[42,43,45,86,89,98] and pediatric patients.[35,36,48,50,86]

Nine studies reported a reduction in ED visits or hospitalizations,[35,36,42,43,45,48,50,86,98] ranging in impact from 5 percent to 60 percent (all statistically significant) among the studies using a pre-post study design. Among the RCTs, the difference between intervention and control arms ranged from 1 percent to 7 percent. One RCT reported no reduction in ED visits/hospitalizations (Table 13).[89]

In summary, there is moderate evidence that decision support interventions targeting health care provider adherence to guidelines reduce ED visits/hospitalizations (Table 11).

Organizational Change

Four studies evaluating organizational change measured the impact on patient ED visits and/or hospitalizations.[51,52,90,91] Two of these were RCTs,[51,90] while the other two were pre-post studies.[52,91] Three of the studies were focused on pediatric health care providers.[51,52,90] Little specific sociodemographic information is provided about the patient populations. One of the studies restructured asthma care visits[90], while the remaining three studies utilized supplemental trained personnel as part of the intervention.[51,52,91] Three of the studies also incorporated an educational component provided to health care providers.[51,52,91]

Reductions in ED visits and/or hospitalizations were reported by both of the pre-post studies (41 percent and 54 percent, respectively, p-value <0.001 for both outcomes[91] and 4 percent reduction in hospitalizations—no p-value reported[52]), while neither RCT (1 percent, p>0.05[51] and 7 percent, p=0.06[90]) reported statistically significant reductions in ED/hospitalization rates compared with the control arms in the study (Table 13).

In summary, organizational change does not reduce ED visits/hospitalizations. The strength of evidence for this conclusion is low (Table 11).

Feedback and Audit

We identified one RCT[57] and one pre-post study[62] that evaluated the effect of feedback and audit on ED visits and hospitalizations. Clinicians in both studies were primary care practitioners with one study providing asthma education to unspecified office staff.[62] No studies addressed specialty care such as allergy, pediatrics or pulmonary medicine. There was little description of the clinicians by race/ethnicity, gender or number of years of experience.

In the RCT[57], a traditional quality circle (TQC) intervention, in which providers were given feedback on their individual performance and the aggregate performance of group providers, was compared with a benchmark quality circle (BQC) intervention in which feedback on providers' individual performance was explicitly compared with a performance benchmark (the highest-performing ten percent of providers in the benchmark arm). The pre-post study[62] evaluated an intervention comparing individual primary care provider's guideline practice patterns with their peers plus providing asthma education to office staff.[62] The studies were conducted in Europe[57] and the U.S.[62]

There was a decrease in ED visits in the RCT.[57] Patients whose providers participated in a benchmark quality circle (BQC) had a 6.7 point decrease in ED visits (from 17.6 percent at baseline to 10.9 percent twelve months post intervention), but this decrease was smaller than the 13.6 percent decrease seen among patients whose provider participated in a traditional quality circle (TQC) (19.7 percent at baseline to 6.1 percent [p=0.064]).[57] The RCT did not report a change in hospitalizations.[57] A minimal reduction in ED visits (Baseline: 82 percent, 6 months: 81 percent) or hospitalizations (Baseline: 96 percent, 6 months: 94 percent) was reported in the pre-post study (Table 13).[62]

In summary, no conclusions could be made because of conflicting results among a small number of studies. The strength of the evidence is insufficient to determine the effect of feedback and audit interventions on ED visits/hospitalizations (Table 11).

Clinical Pharmacy Support

We identified one RCT[99] evaluating the effect of clinical pharmacy support on having an ED visit or hospitalizations over 12 months in adult patients with asthma. The RCT evaluated the effectiveness of a pharmaceutical care program for patients with asthma conducted at community drugstores. The three arms of the RCT included (1) a pharmaceutical care program intervention consisting of pharmacist computer alert of patient specific prescription fills + patient education materials and resources + pharmacy care support, (2) control group patients receiving peak flow meter instruction from pharmacist (PFM) and (3) a usual-care group. Patients assigned to the Pharmaceutical Care group were more likely to have an ED visit or hospitalization over 12 months as compared with PFM group: odds ratio 2.16 (95% CI: 1.76, 2.63), but no difference in ED or hospitalizations was noted when compared with the usual care control group (odds ratio 1.08; (95% CI: 0.93, 1.25) p > 0.05) (Table 13).[99]

In summary, there is insufficient evidence to determine the effect of clinical pharmacy support interventions on ED visits/hospitalizations due to imprecise results from a single study (Table 11).

Education Only

There were seven studies, 5 RCTs[70-72,93,100] and 2 pre-post studies,[75,77] that examined the impact of education only on ED visits and hospitalizations. One only considered ED visits.[93] A variety of educational approaches were used to influence general practitioners, pediatricians and pharmacists, including interactive seminars, structured training and medical grand rounds. The findings for both ED visits and hospitalizations were mixed. For ED visits, the findings included both reduction and increase in visits. One of the studies did not find a statistically significant effect for the intervention group overall, but did report statistically significant findings in a subgroup of low income participants (-1.23 visits per year, p=.001).[70] For hospitalization, one study showed significant reduction in the annual rate[70] (-.02 to-.03 visits per year)while the other 5 studies showed no reduction (0 change in visit rate) or increases of rates of hospitalization (+5 to 10.5 percent) (Table 13).

In summary, education-only interventions do not reduce asthma ED visit or hospitalizations. The strength of evidence for this conclusion is low (Table 11).

Quality Improvement and Pay-for-Performance

One RCT[96] examined the effect of quality improvement on ED visits and hospitalizations and one controlled pre-post study evaluated the effect of quality improvement on the combined number of ED visits and hospitalizations.[95] Both studies evaluated a Breakthrough Series collaborative quality improvement strategy. These studies focused on pediatric health care providers working in community health center settings. The patients were primarily African American or Hispanic.

Neither study showed a statistically significant reduction in ED visits/hospitalizations, with a 5 percent reduction in ED visits,[96] a 2 percent reduction in hospitalizations[96], and an increase of 0.3 combined ED visits and hospitalizations[95] reported in the quality improvement arms. However, there was some evidence of poor adherence to the quality improvement intervention in the RCT, with decreases in participation in the learning sessions and in outcome reporting over time.[96] When analyses were limited to the 9 practices that attended all three learning sessions, they report that there was a significant reduction in ED visits (Table 13).

In summary, there is low strength of evidence to suggest that quality improvement does not significantly reduce ED visits/hospitalizations based on one controlled pre-post study and one RCT with evidence of suboptimal engagement by participants (Table 11).

Multicomponent

One study[82] evaluated the impact of a multicomponent intervention in pediatric clinics on rates of ED visits and hospitalizations. This study implemented an intervention that included elements of quality improvement, decision support, organizational change, and feedback-and-audit. It recruited a cohort of patients across 17 participating sites, and collected ED and hospitalization rates using parent recall at multiple time points. This study reported large and statistically significant reductions in rates of ED visits and hospitalizations across the overall cohort of enrolled patients (69 percent reductions for both outcomes). However, 44 percent of the patient sample was lost to follow up, and significant heterogeneity in results was seen across participating clinical sites (Table 13).

In summary the strength of evidence is insufficient to determine the effect of multicomponent interventions on ED visits and/or hospitalizations (Table 11).

Information Only

Only one RCT study examined the impact of information provision alone.[85] The study was done in Australia and measured outcomes only in children ages 1-15.[85] Information was inserted into the charts of patients randomized to the intervention group. However, each provider managed patients in both intervention and control arms simultaneously. This study found no differences in rates of either ED visits or hospitalizations between study groups (Table 13).

In summary, based on a single study with a high risk of bias, there is insufficient evidence to evaluate the effect of information only interventions ED visits/hospitalizations (Table 11).

Table 11. Emergency department visits/hospitalization—strength of evidence for KQ2

Intervention	No. of Studies/No. of Health Care Providers	Risk of Bias	Consistency	Directness	Precision	Strength of Evidence (SOE) & Magnitude of Effect (MOE)
Decision support	10/820 4 RCTs 6 Pre-post	Medium	Consistent	Direct	Imprecise	SOE : Moderate MOE: Moderate: 5% - 60% in pre-post studies; 1% - 7% in RCTs
Organizational change	4/252 2 RCTs, 2 pre-post	Medium	Inconsistent	Direct	Imprecise	SOE: Low MOE: Large: 41% - 54% in pre-post studies; 1% - 7% in RCTs [no benefit]
Feedback and audit	2/125 1 RCT, 1 pre-post	Medium	Inconsistent	Direct	Precise	SOE: Insufficient MOE: N/A
Clinical pharmacy support	1/36 1 RCT	Low	Unknown	Direct	Imprecise	SOE: Insufficient MOE: N/A
Education only	7/343 5 RCTs, 2 pre-post	High	Inconsistent	Direct	Imprecise	SOE: Low MOE: Low [no benefit] ED visits: Findings included reductions and increases in ED visits. Hospitalizations: One study demonstrated significant decrease in hospitalizations; others showed no change or an increase (5 to 10.5%).
Quality improvement and pay-for-performance	2/56 practices (providers not reported) 1 RCT, 1 pre-post	Medium	Consistent	Direct	Imprecise	SOE: Low MOE: Low [no benefit] ED visits: 5% reduction Hospitalizations: 2% reduction ED visits/hospitalizations: 0.3 increase. Neither study demonstrated significant decreases in ED visits/hospitalization.
Multicomponent	1/17 clinics (providers not reported) 1 cohort	High	Unknown	Direct	Imprecise	SOE: Insufficient MOE: N/A
Information only	1/13 1 RCT	High	Unknown	Direct	Imprecise	SOE: Insufficient MOE: N/A

ED = emergency department; N/A = not applicable; SOE = strength of evidence; MOE = magnitude of effect; RCT = randomized controlled trial

Outcome: Missed Days of Work/School

Key Points and Evidence Grades

- There is insufficient evidence for the effect of decision support on the number of missed days of work/school from asthma, due to inconsistent results from two studies.
- Organizational change does not reduce missed school days from asthma. The strength of evidence for this conclusion is low.
- There is insufficient evidence for the effect of feedback and audit interventions on the number of missed work or school days due to inconsistent results in the one included study.
- There is insufficient evidence for the effect of clinical pharmacy support on the number of missed work or school days due to lack of any study addressing missed days of work and school.
- There is insufficient evidence to evaluate the effect of education only strategies on missed days of work/school from asthma due to inconsistent and imprecise results.
- There is insufficient evidence to evaluate the effect of quality improvement interventions on missed days of work/school from asthma.
- There is insufficient evidence to evaluate the effect of multicomponent interventions on missed days of work/school from asthma.
- There is insufficient evidence to evaluate the effect of provision of information to health care providers on the number of missed days of work/school from asthma.

Decision Support

The two studies examining the impact of decision support interventions on missed work or school had differing results. One study used an RCT design[35] while the other used a pre-post design.[86] Both involved children, although the pre-post study[86] also included adult patients. The RCT[35] reported no reduction in missed school in their study of providing supplemental morbidity information to health care providers. The pre-post study[86] reported a 49 percent reduction ($p<0.001$) in school absenteeism and a 51 percent reduction in the odds of missed work (odds ratio 0.49 [95% CI: 0.34, 0.71]) among the patient populations in a study that utilized a combination of an asthma care map, a treatment flow chart, program standards, management flow chart and action plan (Table 13).

In summary, there is insufficient evidence for the effect of decision support on the number of missed days due to inconsistent results from two studies (Table 12).

Organizational Change

One RCT of organizational change, based on restructuring the clinical protocol for how asthma patients are cared for during ambulatory care encounters ("3+ visit plan"), evaluated the impact on missed school days and observed no significant reduction.[90] More specifically, at 12 months, the percentage of children who missed no school was 52 percent in the intervention group and 45 percent in the control group (odds ratio 0.8 (95% CO: 0.5 – 1.2); p=0.3) (Table 13).

In summary, organizational change does not reduce missed school days from asthma. The strength of evidence for this conclusion is low (Table 12).

Feedback and Audit

We identified one pre-post study[62] that evaluated the effect of feedback and audit on work and school days missed. The study compared individual primary care provider's guideline practice patterns with their peers plus providing asthma education to office staff.[62] In the one study, the percent reporting no school absences due to asthma in past 6 months: baseline: 49 percent; 6 months: 38percent--no p-value was reported. There was zero percent reduction in parent work days missed due to child's asthma (Table 13).

In summary, the one study that evaluated feedback/audit did not report reduction in the number of missed days of work/school. The magnitude of the effect is low. In summary, there is insufficient evidence to evaluate the effect of feedback/audit interventions on the number of missed days of school or work (Table 12).

Clinical Pharmacy Support

We identified no studies evaluating the effect of clinical pharmacy support on the outcome of missed days of work and school. Therefore, there is insufficient evidence to evaluate the effect of clinical pharmacy support interventions on the number of missed days of school or work (Table 12).

Education Only

There were five studies that evaluated the effect of health care provider education on missed school or missed work as outcomes. There were 3 RCTs[68,70,72] that included children missing school as an outcome. The interventions targeted general practitioners, pediatricians and pharmacists and included structured training, seminars and workshops. In all 3 trials there was consistent evidence of small positive effects that were not of statistical significance (reductions of 4 percent and 0.6 to 3.96 days). Two RCTs[68,92] and one pre-post study[75] examined missed work as an outcome, including one study that had a compound outcome of missing either work or school. The interventions included workshops, training in how to perform spirometry and one study had compared asthma program development with a nurse educator program or continuing education. There were no significant reductions in missed work in any studies (ranging from -10 percent to + 5.6 percent) (Table 13).

In summary, the study results were inconsistent and had imprecise estimates of the effect of these education interventions. Therefore there is insufficient evidence to evaluate the effect of education only strategies on the number of missed days of work/school from asthma (Table 12).

Quality Improvement and Pay-for-Performance

One controlled pre-post study examined the effect of quality improvement on missed school and missed parental work.[95] This study evaluated health care provider participation in a Breakthrough Series collaborative quality improvement strategy. This study reported a nonsignificant reduction of 0.2 school days (p=0.4) and zero parental work days missed due to a child's asthma (p=0.7) (Table 13).

In summary, with only one study at high risk of bias, there is insufficient evidence to determine the effect of quality improvement interventions on school or work absenteeism (Table 12).

Multicomponent

One study[82] evaluated the impact of a multicomponent intervention in pediatric clinics on missed days of school in children and missed days of work in their parents. This study implemented an intervention that included elements of quality improvement, decision support, organizational change, and feedback-and-audit. It recruited a cohort of patients across 17 participating sites, and collected data on missed days of school and work using parent recall at multiple time points. This study reported large and statistically significant reductions in rates of missed days of school (53 percent reduction in patients with any missed days of school) and work (72 percent reduction in parents with any missed days of work) across the overall cohort of enrolled patients. However, 44 percent of the patient sample was lost to follow up, and significant heterogeneity in results was seen across participating clinical sites (Table 13).

In summary the strength of evidence is insufficient to determine the effect of multicomponent interventions on missed days of school or work (Table 12).

Information Only

No studies examined the impact of information provision alone on missed days of work or school (Table 12).

Table 12. Missed days of work/school—strength of evidence for KQ2

Intervention	No. of Studies/No. of Health Care Providers	Risk of Bias	Consistency	Directness	Precision	Strength of Evidence (SOE) & Magnitude of Effect (MOE)
Decision support	2/435 1 RCT, 1 pre-post	Medium	Inconsistent	Direct	Precise	SOE: Insufficient MOE: N/A
Organizational change	1/24 1 RCT	Low	Unknown	Direct	Imprecise	SOE: Low MOE: N/A
Feedback and audit	1/29 1 pre-post	High	Unknown	Indirect	Imprecise	SOE: Insufficient MOE: N/A
Clinical pharmacy support	0					SOE: Insufficient MOE: N/A
Education only	5/1767 4 RCTs, 1 pre-post	High	Inconsistent	Direct	Imprecise	SOE :Insufficient MOE: N/A
Quality improvement and pay-for-performance Information only	1/13 practices (providers not reported) 1 pre-post	High	Unknown	Direct	Imprecise	SOE: Insufficient MOE: N/A
Multicomponent	1/17 clinics (providers not reported) 1 cohort	High	Unknown	Direct	Imprecise	SOE: Insufficient MOE: N/A
Information only	0					SOE: Insufficient MOE: N/A

N/A = not applicable; SOE = strength of evidence; MOE = magnitude of effect; RCT = randomized controlled trial

45

Table 13. Study characteristics for clinical outcomes

Intervention	Author, Year	Study Design	Type of Provider	No. of Providers	No. of Patients	Clinical Outcomes	
						ED Visits/ Hospitalization	Missed Days of School/Work
	Cowie R. L., 2001[75]	Pre-post	NR	NR	Arm A (Basic Education):NR Arm (Intermediate Education):NR Arm C (Intensive Education):NR	Ø	Ø
	Blackstien-Hirsch P., 2000[77]	Pre-post	Physician	59	195	Ø	N/A
	Shah S., 2011[68]	RCT	General Practitioner	150	Arm A (control):107 Arm B (PACE):110	N/A	Ø
	Brown R., 2004[70]	RCT	Pediatrician	Arm A (Control):11 Arm B (Education): 12	Arm A (Control):122 Arm B (Education):157	↓*	Ø
Education Only	Clark NM, 1998[71]	RCT	Pediatrician, Physician	Arm A:37 Arm B (Education):37	637	Ø	N/A
	Stergachis A., 2002[72]	RCT	Pharmacist	Arm A (Control):NR Arm B (Education):35	Arm A (Control):177 Arm B (Education):153	Ø	Ø
	Holton C., 2011[92]	RCT	General Practitioner	Arm A (Control):45 Arm B (Spirometry training):127	Arm A (Control):157 Arm B (Spirometry training):240	N/A	Ø
	Sulaiman N. D., 2010[93]	RCT	General Practitioner	Arm A (Control):18 Arm B (Education and guidelines):18 Arm C (Guidelines):15	Arm A (Control):121 Arm B (Education and guidelines):156 Arm C (Guidelines):134	Ø	N/A
	Cabana M. D., 2006[100]	RCT	Primary Healthcare	Arm A (Control):43 Arm B (PACE):51	Arm A (Control):452 Arm B (PACE):418	Ø	N/A

Table 13. Study characteristics for clinical outcomes (continued)

Intervention	Author, Year	Study Design	Type of Provider	No. of Providers	No. of Patients	Clinical Outcomes	
						ED Visits/ Hospitalization	Missed Days of School/Work
	Cloutier M. M., 2009[48]	Pre-post	Pediatrician	NR	3298	↓	N/A
	Horswell R.,2008[43]	Pre-post	Physician	NR	NR	↓	N/A
	Kattan M, 2006[35]	RCT	Nurse practitioner, physician assistant, primary healthcare	Arm A (standard practice): NR Arm B (decision support): 435	Arm A (standard practice): 466 Arm B (decision support): 471	↓	∅
Decision Support	Lesho EP, 2005[45]	Pre-post	Primary healthcare	NR	330	↓	N/A
	McCowan C., 2001[89]	RCT	General practitioner	NR	Arm A (control): 330 Arm B (decision support): 147	∅	N/A
	Mitchell E.A., 2005[36]	RCT	General practitioner	270	NR	↓	N/A
	Newton W.P., 2010[42]	Pre-post	Nurse, physician practice managers, other staff	NR	NR	↓	N/A
	Renzi P.M., 2006[98]	RCT	Primary healthcare	NR	NR	↓	N/A
	Shiffman R.N., 2000[50]	Pre-post	Pediatrician	11	Arm A (Sole physician arm; patient arm, pre): 91 Arm B (patient arm): 74	↓	N/A
	To T., 2008[86]	Pre-post	Primary health care	NR	1408	↓	→
Feedback and Audit	Schneider A., 2008[57]	RCT	General Practitioner	96	Arm A (traditional quality circle):NR Arm B (benchmark quality circle):NR Arm C (combined arms):256	∅	N/A
	Richman M. J, 2000[62]	Pre-post	Pediatrician	29	228	∅	∅

47

Table 13. Study characteristics for clinical outcomes (continued)

Intervention	Author, Year	Study Design	Type of Provider	No. of Providers	No. of Patients	Clinical Outcomes ED Visits/ Hospitalization	Clinical Outcomes Missed Days of School/Work
Clinical Pharmacy Support	Weinberger M, 2002[99]	RCT	Pharmacist	NR	Arm A (control): 165 Arm B (Peak flow meter monitoring control group): 233	∅	N/A
Multicomponent	Lob, 2011[82]	Quasi-experimental (longitudinal at clinic level and cross-sectional at patient level)	Physician, nurse practitioner	NR	Longitudinal Evaluation Group – Patient-level Interview : 761 Cross-sectional Random Sample - Clinic-level Chart Review, T1: 680 Cross-sectional Random Sample - Clinic-level Chart Review, T2: 680 Cross-sectional Random Sample - Clinic-level Chart Review, T3: 680	→	N/A
Information only	Bryce FP, 1995[85]	RCT	General Practitioner, Nurse	NR	Arm A (Control):1563 Arm B (Reminders and Tools):1585	∅	N/A
	Finkelstein J. A., 2005[51]	RCT	Pediatric medical provider	228	Arm A (Control):1531 Arm B (PLE Intervention):2003 Arm C (Planned Care Intervention):1635	∅	N/A
Organizational Change	Thyne S.M., 2007[52]	Pre-post	Pediatric medical providers, "urgent care clinicians"	NR	Arm A (Time 1, 2002-2003):NR Arm B (Time 2, 2003-2004):NR Arm C (Time 3, 2004-2005):NR	↓**	N/A
	Glasgow N. J., 2003[90]	RCT	General Practitioner	Arm A(Control):12 Arm B(Intervention):12	Arm A (Control):73 Arm B (Intervention):101	∅	∅
	Patel P . H., 2004[91]	Pre-post	Physicians, Nurses	NR	451	→	N/A

Table 13. Study characteristics for clinical outcomes (continued)

Intervention	Author, Year	Study Design	Type of Provider	No. of Providers	No. of Patients	Clinical Outcomes	
						ED Visits/ Hospitalization	Missed Days of School/Work
Quality Improvement	Mangione-Smith R., 2005[95]	Pre-post	"Health care providers"	NR	Arm A (Control):126 Arm B (Learning collaborative):385	∅	∅
	Homer CJ, 2005[96]	RCT	Nurse, Physician Front office staff	NR	Arm A (Control):337 Arm B (Learning collaborative):294	∅	N/A

N/A = not applicable; NR = not reported; PACE = Physician Asthma Care Education; RCT = randomized controlled trial

↑ — Statistically significant increase in outcome of interest.

↓ — Statistically significant decrease in outcome of interest.

∅ — Difference between intervention and control groups, or between pre- and post-intervention *not* statistically significant.

*Reduction in ED visit for subgroup of low income participants only but reduction in annual rate of hospitalization for entire group.

**Reduction in ED visit but p value not reported in study.

49

KQ3: In the care of pediatric or adult patients with asthma, what is the evidence that interventions designed to improve health care provider adherence to guidelines impact health care process outcomes that then affect clinical outcomes?

We identified no studies providing evidence on the link between changes in health care provider behavior (health care process outcomes) to changes in clinical outcomes.

Discussion

The Discussion section is divided into the following topics: Applicability; Limitations of Review; Limitations of Evidence Base; Findings in Relationship to What Is Already Known; Future Research; Implications for Clinical and Policy Decisionmaking; and Conclusions. In these sections we discuss how our findings may be relevant to various asthma stakeholders, the limitations of our systematic review and future considerations for asthma stakeholders seeking to improve health care provider adherence to asthma guidelines.

Key Findings

The key findings from this report are outlined below, organized by general class of intervention. Subsequent tables summarize conclusions according to Key Question and by type of intervention (Tables 14–16).

Table 14. Summary of the strength of evidence in support of eight interventions designed to modify clinician adherence to asthma guidelines

Intervention	Outcome: Prescription of Controller Medications	Outcome: Patient Education/Asthma Action Plans	Outcome: ED Visits/ Hospitalizations	Outcome: Missed Days of Work/School
Decision support	Benefit with large magnitude of effect. SOE moderate.	Studies consistently favor intervention with large magnitude of effect. SOE moderate.	Benefit with moderate magnitude of effect (larger in pre-post studies). SOE moderate.	Unable to conclude due to inconsistent results. SOE inconsistent.
Organizational change	Benefit with small magnitude of effect. SOE low.	Two studies show benefit with moderate magnitude of effect. SOE low.	Inconsistent results. Benefit with large magnitude of effect in pre-post studies; smaller in RCTs. SOE low.	No benefit (for missed school days). SOE low.
Feedback and audit	Benefit with moderate magnitude of effect. SOE moderate.	Benefit with low magnitude of effect. SOE low.	Benefit with low magnitude of effect. SOE low.	No conclusion due to inconsistent results in one included study. SOE insufficient.
Clinical pharmacy support	Benefit within three studies with moderate magnitude of effect. SOE moderate.	Benefit in one study with moderate magnitude of effect. SOE moderate.	Unable to make a conclusion based on one study with imprecise results. SOE insufficient.	No studies. SOE insufficient.
Education only	No benefit. SOE low.	Small to moderate increases in a minority of studies. SOE low.	No benefit. Inconsistent results (reductions and increases). Low SOE.	No conclusion due to inconsistent and imprecise results in five studies. Insufficient SOE.
QI and pay-for-performance	No studies. SOE Insufficient.	Observational studies showed benefit, while the RCT did not. Benefit with moderate magnitude of effect. SOE low.	No benefit. Low SOE.	Unable to draw conclusions. One study (with high risk of bias) reported a nonsignificant reduction in school days missed. SOE insufficient.

51

Table 14. Summary of the strength of evidence in support of eight interventions designed to modify clinician adherence to asthma guidelines (continued)

Intervention	Outcome: Prescription of Controller Medications	Outcome: Patient Education/Asthma Action Plans	Outcome: ED Visits/ Hospitalizations	Outcome: Missed Days of Work/School
Multicomponent interventions	Benefit with moderate magnitude of effect. SOE low.	Benefit, with moderate magnitude of effect (larger in observational studies). SOE low.	Unable to make conclusion; while the one study reported a large reduction, the study quality was low. Insufficient SOE.	No conclusion; One study reported a large reduction, but study quality was low. SOE insufficient.
Information only	No studies. SOE Insufficient.	No studies. SOE Insufficient.	Unable to make conclusion; no difference seen, but study quality was low. SOE insufficient.	No studies. SOE insufficient.

ED = emergency department; QI = quality improvement; RCT = randomized controlled trial; SOE = strength of evidence

KQ1: In the care of pediatric or adult patients with asthma, what is the evidence that Interventions designed to improve health care provider adherence to guidelines impact health care process outcomes (e.g., receiving appropriate treatment)?

The key findings are summarized in Table 15.

Table 15. Summary of strength of evidence for included studies for KQ1

Outcomes	Intervention	No. of Studies/No. of Health Care Providers	Strength of Evidence	Conclusions
Prescriptions for controller medications	Decision support	15/1,635 6 RCTs, 9 pre-post	Moderate	Most of the evidence supporting the use of decision support Interventions comes from a number of nonrandomized studies consistently showing that decision support interventions can increase health care provider prescriptions for asthma controller medications. The magnitude of effect is large: 2%-34% in pre-post studies; 2%-17% in RCTs.
	Organizational change	2/228 1 RCT, 1 pre-post	Low	Although far fewer studies performed using organizational change (in comparison with Decision Support or Feedback/Audit), the findings consistently showed that organizational change can increase health care provider prescriptions for controller medicines, but the effect on prescriptions by health care providers is smaller. The magnitude of effect is small. In the RCT: 8%-16% for all asthma patients; 4%-11% for patients with persistent asthma; 4%-9% for inhaled steroids (ICS) for all asthma patients; 13%-19% for ICS for patients with persistent asthma. In the pre-post study: 12% increase in ICS.
	Feedback and audit	11/1,831 6 RCTs, 4 pre-post and 1 nonrandomized controlled	Moderate	These studies consistently showed that feedback/audit interventions effectively increase prescriptions for controller medicines by health care providers. The magnitude of the effect is moderate. Effect size: 0.12-0.66. Increase in prescribing controller medications ranging from 15.9% to 52-104% Hazard ratio range: 0.77-1.08.

Table 15. Summary of strength of evidence for included studies for KQ1 (continued)

Outcomes	Intervention	No. of Studies/No. of Health Care Providers	Strength of Evidence	Conclusions
Prescriptions for controller medications (continued)	Clinical pharmacy support	3/ 91 1 RCT, 1 pre-post, 1 nonrandomized	Moderate	The three studies were consistent in showing that clinical pharmacy support interventions increase asthma controller medication prescribing The magnitude of the effect is moderate. OR: 3.80 (95% CI: 1.4, 10.32) and percent increase in patients prescribed controller meds pre and post: 6-21%.
	Education only	10/451 6 RCTs, 4 pre-post	Low	The evidence suggests that interventions based only on education of clinicians do not improve prescription of asthma controller medications. The magnitude of effect is small to large in studies (3.5-50.3% increase in prescribing controller medicines.
	Quality improvement and pay-for-performance	0 studies	Insufficient	No studies identified.
	Multicomponent interventions	7/>1,141 4 Cluster randomized, 3 pre-post	Low	Two pre-post studies and one RCT reported a significant increase in prescribing (25-49% in pre-post studies), while all other effects were null. Overall, the magnitude of effect is small.
	Information only	2/107 1 RCT, 1 quasi-experimental	Insufficient	Due to inconsistency across studies, evidence is insufficient to determine the effect of information alone on prescribing of asthma controller medication.
Patient education/asthma action plans	Decision support	10/122-124 4 RCTs, 6 pre-post	Moderate	A majority of nonrandomized studies consistently favor the use of decision support interventions to improve the provision of self-management education/asthma action plans by health care providers. The magnitude of effect is large: 14%-84%.

Table 15. Summary of strength of evidence for included studies for KQ1 (continued)

Outcomes	Intervention	No. of Studies/No. of Health Care Providers	Strength of Evidence	Conclusions
Patient education/asthma action plans (continued)	Organizational change	2/24 1 RCT, 1 pre-post	Low	Both studies favor the use of organizational change to increase patient education/asthma action plan use by health care providers. However, more studies are needed to increase the strength of evidence. The magnitude of effect is moderate: 10%-14%.
	Feedback and audit	5/336 3 RCTs, 2 pre-post	Low	Despite a number of studies examining feedback/audit, inconsistent results lead to a low strength of evidence for the use of feedback/audit to improve self-management education/ asthma action plan use. The magnitude of the effect is low. Self-management education: difference in proportions range from low of 0.7 (95% CI: -15.2, 16.7) for peak flow meter use to 12.9 (95% CI: 1.9, 23.9) for inhaler technique education. Asthma Action Plans: Increase of 7.6 % in Feedback with Benchmark as compared with Traditional: 4.5%. Asthma Education: Range Pre to post 46-133% increase.
	Clinical pharmacy support	1/82 1 RCT	Moderate	The one study demonstrated a positive effect in the use of Clinical Pharmacy Support to improve self-management education/asthma action plan use by health care providers. The magnitude of the effect is moderate. Asthma Action Plans: 40-45% increase from baseline.
	Education only	5/470 5 RCTs	Low	Small increases in asthma self-management education were observed in a minority of studies, resulting in an overall low strength of evidence regarding this outcome. The magnitude of effect is small to moderate: 10%-15%. OR: 1.00; RR: 1.40.

Table 15. Summary of strength of evidence for included studies for KQ1 (continued)

Outcomes	Intervention	No. of Studies/No. of Health Care Providers	Strength of Evidence	Conclusions
Patient education/asthma action plans (continued)	Quality improvement and pay-for-performance	3/63 practices (providers not reported) 1 RCT, 2 pre-post	Low	Inconsistent results with a -3 to 33% change in the provision of asthma action plans. Both observational studies reported increases of 19-33% while the negative RCT had evidence of suboptimal practice engagement.
	Multicomponent interventions	6/>937 2 RCT, 4 pre-post	Low	Magnitude of effect is moderate. Provision of asthma action plan increased 27%-46% in observational studies. Smaller effect sizes were seen in RCTs (7% of providers and RR': 1.82).
	Information only	0	Insufficient	No studies identified.

OR = odds ration; RCT = randomized controlled trial, RR = relative risk; RR' = relative rate
Note: If the number of health care provider participants was not reported for a particular study, the "NR" value was treated as zero for that particular intervention and outcome category.

KQ2: In the care of pediatric or adult patients with asthma, what is the evidence that Interventions designed to improve health care provider adherence to guidelines impact clinical outcomes (e.g., hospitalizations, patient-reported outcomes such as symptom control)?

The key findings are summarized by outcome in Table 16.

Table 16. Summary of strength of evidence for included studies for KQ2

Outcomes	Intervention	No. of Studies/No. of Health Care Providers	Strength of Evidence	Conclusions
ED Visits/ Hospitalizations	Decision support	10/820 5 RCTs, 5 Pre-post	Moderate	9 of 10 studies reported that decision support interventions reduce ED visits/hospitalizations.
	Organizational change	4/252 2 RCTs, 2 pre-post	Low	Low strength of evidence organizational change does not reduce ED visits/hospitalizations.
	Feedback and audit	2/125 1 RCT, 1 pre-post	Insufficient	Inconsistent results from a limited number of studies have resulted in an insufficient grade of evidence to evaluate the impact of feedback and audit interventions on ED visits and hospitalizations. The magnitude of the evidence is low.
	Clinical pharmacy support	1/36 1 RCT	Insufficient	There is insufficient evidence available to determine the effect of clinical pharmacy support interventions on ED visits/hospitalizations.
	Education only	7/343 5 RCTs, 2 pre-post	Low	Overall, due to conflicting results among a number of studies, the low strength of evidence suggests that education-alone interventions do not reduce asthma ED visits and/or hospitalizations.

Table 16. Summary of strength of evidence for included studies for KQ2 (continued)

Outcomes	Intervention	No. of Studies/No. of Health Care Providers	Strength of Evidence	Conclusions
ED Visits/Hospitalizations (continued)	Quality improvement and pay-for-performance	2/56 practices (providers not reported) 1 RCT, 1 pre-post	Low	Two studies show that quality improvement does not reduce ED visits and hospitalizations. More studies are needed.
	Multicomponent	1/17 clinics (providers not reported) 1 cohort	Insufficient	There is insufficient evidence to determine the effect of multicomponent interventions on ED visits/ hospitalizations due to high rates of participant attrition (low study quality) in the single study included.
	Information only	1/13 1 RCT	Insufficient	Based on a single study with a high risk of bias, there is insufficient evidence to determine the effect of information-only interventions on ED visits/hospitalizations.
Missed days of work/school	Decision support	2/435 1 RCT, 1 pre-post	Insufficient	There is insufficient evidence to evaluate the effect of decision support interventions on the number of missed days of work/school.
	Organizational change	1/24 1 RCT	Low	Organizational change does not reduce missed school days from asthma. The strength of evidence for this conclusion is low.
	Feedback and audit	1/29 1 pre-post	Insufficient	There is insufficient evidence to evaluate the effect of feedback and audit interventions on the number of missed days of work and school from asthma due to inconsistent results and study design.
	Clinical pharmacy support	0	Insufficient	No studies identified.
	Education only	5/1,767 4 RCTs, 1 pre-post	Insufficient	There is insufficient evidence to evaluate the effect of education-only strategies on the number of missed days of work/school from asthma due to imprecise estimates and inconsistent results.
	Quality improvement and pay-for-performance	1/13 practices (providers not reported) 1 pre-post	Insufficient	There is insufficient evidence to evaluate the effect of quality improvement/pay-for-performance interventions on the number of missed days of work/school from asthma because of high risk of bias in the single study analyzed.
	Multicomponent	1/17 clinics (providers not reported) 1 cohort	Insufficient	There is insufficient evidence to determine the effect of multicomponent interventions on the number of missed days of work/school from asthma due to risk of bias (high rate of attrition) and inconsistent results across clinical sites.
	Information only	0	Insufficient	No studies identified.

ED = emergency department; RCT = randomized controlled trial

Note: If the number of healthcare provider participants was not reported for a particular study, the "NR" value was treated as zero for that particular intervention and outcome category.

Applicability

We assessed applicability of these studies to the potential users of this review using the PICOTS framework. The purpose of this section is to highlight the applicability of this report to various key stakeholders to whom this document may be of interest and used to direct future activities (e.g., implement policy or direct future research endeavors). We have detailed our assessment more specifically below (Table 17), according to each PICOTS element:

Table 17. Applicability

Domain	Description of Applicability of Evidence
Population - Provider	From a health care provider perspective, primary care providers were essentially the only targeted population of the studies we reviewed. The types of primary care providers were varied, but primarily focused on physicians, although some studies did include nurses, nurse practitioners and pharmacists. No studies targeted respiratory therapists and only one study included an asthma specialist (pulmonologist or allergist).
Population - Patients	A minority of studies described the patient population in detail—these often were U.S.-based studies that were conducted in settings with a high proportion of African American, Latino and/or poor patients. Therefore, we believe that at least some of the interventions reviewed could be implemented in settings that care for such patient populations.
Intervention	In terms of the interventions themselves, general descriptions of the content and administration were provided, but often without an explanation of dose or intensity needed—this would be important for: (1) those deciding what intervention to replicate for their own setting; (2) estimating the likelihood of successful implementation and long-term sustainability of a given intervention; (3) determining how likely health care providers are to buy-in and adhere to using these interventions in their routine clinical practice. In addition, three intervention types were most frequently studied: decision support, feedback/audit, and education accounted for 80% of the interventions we reviewed. There were relatively few studies of organizational change, quality improvement, information-only strategies or even using a combination of interventions.
Comparators	We often were not able to discern with any specificity what the comparative condition was in these studies, since the comparator was often described as "usual care". This limitation was true even among the RCTs we reviewed.
Outcomes	There were a number of different health care process and clinical outcomes evaluated in these studies, although these were heavily skewed to 2–3 outcomes: prescribing of asthma controller medicines; self-management education; asthma action plans; and emergency department visits/hospitalizations accounted for the vast majority of outcomes studied. Therefore, those seeking to impact these outcomes have data available to base an intervention choice upon, while those seeking to reduce missed days of school or other infrequently studied outcomes will not have sufficient evidence upon which to base this decision.
Setting	We observed a nearly equal distribution of studies conducted in the U.S. vs. outside of the U.S. The non-U.S. study locations were quite varied and included Africa, Asia, Australia, Canada and Europe. There was relatively little detail about the specific settings in which the studies were conducted, so applicability to a specific clinical type is limited.

Limitations of Review

There are a number of limitations of our review that should be acknowledged. First, we did not consider or search for reports of potentially relevant studies in the grey literature. This means that our evidence base could be open to publication bias. This may be particularly applicable to this topic, as many interventions aimed at changing health care provider behavior, particularly quality improvement efforts, may have been published in venues other than peer-reviewed literature. We did not complete formal assessment of publication bias as this is challenging, at best. It has been suggested that funnel plots be used to check for publication bias; however, these are difficult to interpret and considered unhelpful for comparisons and outcomes with less than 10 studies.[101]

We identified potentially eligible studies that were published in a language other than English (i.e., no restrictions by language in search) but were unable, due to resource limitations, to consider these articles for inclusion in the review. While this raises the possibility of introducing publication bias, we do not feel that the exclusion of the non-English reports of studies influenced our conclusions or ability to draw conclusions. In addition, there were only 20 of 3,846 abstracts and 16 of 244 articles excluded because they were not in English and we could not determine eligibility, thus representing a minority of the studies excluded. Furthermore, it is unclear if these studies would be relevant to the U.S. health care setting or U.S. health care provider.

Many studies implemented more than one intervention. We made a concerted effort to categorize studies by the predominant intervention, based on review and discussion by team members; however, our classifications may not always be identical to those intended by the original investigators. Furthermore, the frequent use of multiple interventions within a single study means that intervention-specific categories may appear to be missing some studies, as they may have been categorized with another intervention or with multicomponent interventions.

We determined that the heterogeneity in the studies (i.e., how outcomes were measured, study populations and intervention details) precluded the use of meta-analyses. A qualitative synthesis was therefore deemed more appropriate, although it did not guarantee a definitive answer for decisionmakers. It also limited our ability to examine or compare subgroups of studies; for example, comparing results from pre-post studies with those from randomized trials.

To maintain a reasonable scope for both the authors and readers of the report, we limited our qualitative synthesis to four critical outcomes. Although these outcomes were chosen as those most important for making decisions, limiting our synthesis to these outcomes meant that we could not comment on the effectiveness of these interventions in improving other elements of asthma care (e.g., environmental control practices) or asthma outcomes (e.g., symptom-free days).

We did not include studies in which interventions specifically targeted both health care providers and patients for which we could not distinguish whether changes in outcomes were due to changes amongst the providers or patients. We did not evaluate patient adherence to health care provider prescribed treatment, which might moderate the clinical outcomes measured in our review. We suggest this review be considered along with the existing EPC report on patient adherence.[102]

Limitations of Evidence Base

There were relatively few published data available to evaluate the impact of interventions on most clinical outcomes (except for ED visits/hospitalizations), highlighting the need for more evidence for those seeking to implement evidence-based interventions targeting health care providers (Table 18). An important limitation is the fact that no studies answered our third Key Question (if changes in health care provider behavior (health care process outcomes) lead to changes in clinical outcomes). There is an implicit assumption that if health care providers carry out the appropriate health care process behaviors, then clinical outcomes will improve, but it would be important to know the strength of this association. Unfortunately, no studies provided data to answer this question.

There was no standardized definition for each type of intervention that was used by the authors of the studies we reviewed or for us to use in classifying studies. Therefore, there is the possibility of misclassification bias in assigning studies to an intervention type. It may be worthwhile for funding, regulatory and/or policymaking agencies to consider developing standardized definitions of these interventions. Such standardization would make it easier and more accurate to compare studies within an intervention type and between intervention types. In a similar way, standardization of baseline and outcome measures for intervention-based studies by these agencies would greatly enhance comparability between studies.

Arguably, most striking was the lack of measurement of potential negative consequences from implementing these interventions (e.g., longer patient visits, greater burden on office staff or increased financial cost). Conversely, there may be positive consequences (e.g., shorter patient visits, reduced burden on office staff, decreased cost) that were not captured in the studies we reviewed. For those considering whether to implement a given intervention, the current data will not allow them to fully evaluate the costs or benefits (financial and otherwise) and therefore the ability to make a fully informed and balanced decision is limited. There may be an opportunity for funding, regulatory and/or policymaking bodies to establish standardized measures to capture these potential negative or positive consequences.

Specific limitations in the evidence we identified is detailed using the PICOTS (Populations, Interventions, Comparator, Outcomes, Timing, and Setting) framework in the Future Research section.

Findings in Relationship to What Is Already Known

We conducted a search for relevant Cochrane reviews and excluded 63 of 86 at the title-search screening level for lack of relevance (e.g., not provider-focused interventions). Of the remaining 23 reviews, we identified 10 reviews as relevant to the topic of asthma and/or relevant to the types of interventions included in our study. Five of the ten studies we found had asthma-related outcomes relevant to and included in our review.[37,56,73,89,100] Of the five reviews that did not focus on asthma, but did evaluate relevant interventions, we observed similar modest effects among low quality intervention studies of education[103-107]; Pay-for-performance[108-110]; Reminder systems[111,112];and Feedback/Audit.[113,114] These findings suggest that additional evidence is needed to fully evaluate the effectiveness of these interventions in improving health care provider adherence to guidelines and, ultimately, clinical outcomes.

Future Research

Table 18. Future research

PICOT Framework	Observation	Recommendation for Future Research
Population	Inadequate clinical and sociodemographic descriptions of the patient population.	Measure asthma control/severity, race/ethnicity, gender, socioeconomic status, etc. in patient populations to more effectively compare effectiveness between studies of interventions. Test efficacy of multifaceted individualized interventions *targeting* a specific group of subjects (i.e., young or older age groups, high asthma severity, and high health care utilizers).
Intervention	Few studies utilized a randomized, controlled intervention approach.	Augment number of studies with RCT design, especially as reviewed RCTs tended to yield more equivocal results.
	The reported impact on healthcare provider behaviors (even when illustrating a beneficial effect) was modest, suggesting that certain barriers to provider adherence to asthma guidelines remained unaddressed.	Develop/incorporate new strategies or combinations of strategies to increase provider adherence to guidelines. Develop strategies to incorporate successful interventions into primary care practices that address time constraints, work flow issues and limited resources
	Relatively few computer-based interventions.	Computerized systems offer an opportunity to increase efficiency in the health care process, thereby potentially improving provider adherence to guidelines. If time constraints pose a barrier to adherence, electronic/ computer-based interventions may meaningfully improve delivery of asthma care.
	Strategies were generally "passive" (i.e., suggesting care to the provider; discussing asthma management generally, but not for specific patients).	Interventions should take a more *active* role in asthma care process (e.g., provide asthma action plans, patient education, environmental control practices), particularly processes associated with a low risk of harm and those inhibited by specific barriers such as time constraints, poor self-efficiency, lack of awareness. Focus on health care processes impeded by logistical barriers, rather than those barred by provider discord regarding recommendations or lack of outcome expectancy. This also suggests that systems-level interventions that address barriers external to the health care provider would be an important approach to effecting positive changes in health care provider behavior.

Table 18. Future research (continued)

	Observation	Recommendation for Future Research
Intervention (continued)	Interventions were often narrow in scope and failed to address the comprehensive and complex tasks health care providers must execute in order to be adherent to asthma guideline recommendations (as well as "competing" guidelines including well child care, chronic comorbidities).	Test interventions that address all of the elements of the asthma health care process (or as many as is feasible). For example, an intervention that would facilitate/expedite the following elements of care in a single visit might be beneficial: (1) Rx for controller medicine, (2) environmental control practice recommendations, (3) self-management education and asthma action plans, (4) documentation of asthma control/severity, (5) Rx of peak flow meter, (6) schedule of automatic follow-up visits within 3 months of visit. Specify *multifaceted interventions* to include provider education + feedback + decision support (or other combinations that seem most potent mixtures of interventions). Test similar multifaceted models. Multifaceted interventions are feasible because they are more translatable than interventions limited to one modality. Caveat: multifaceted interventions are more costly.
	Inadequate description or measure of dose.	Measure or address intervention "dose." For example, if only 50 percent of provider participate in intervention, dose is important.
	No examination of whether changes in health care provider behavior results in changes in clinical outcomes	Design studies that are more comprehensive in scope to capture changes in health care process measures and determine the strength of association with changes in clinical outcomes.
Comparisons	Pre/post designs common. Uncontrolled studies used.	Conduct more explicit comparisons of differing results between studies of different designs (i.e. direct comparisons of how results from pre-post studies differ from results from RCTs). Move beyond pre-post studies; use cluster RCTs; conduct studies with appropriate control groups.
Outcome	Heterogeneity in presentation of the outcome measures.	Develop minimum standards for presentation of outcomes (e.g., percent change in prescriptions for inhaled steroids). Other outcomes could be presented, but at minimum, one standard would facilitate comparisons between studies.
	Studies failed to link changes in health care process to clinical outcomes.	Develop studies that illustrate how specific changes in provision of care manifest improvements in patient outcomes.
	Subjectivity/variability in clinical outcome measures including: Hospitalizations, ED visits	Objective/reliable outcome measures: Administrative health care utilization data for verification of ED visits, hospitalizations; standardization of cut-points. Standardize timeframe for measurement of health care utilization outcomes, i.e. 12 months to account for seasonality effects.

Table 18. Future research (continued)

	Observation	Recommendation for Future Research
Outcome (continued)	Subjectivity/variability in health care process outcomes measures including: Lack of determination of appropriateness of controller medication prescriptions Lack of assessment of patient medication adherence as an outcome and/or a modifier of outcomes	Utilize pharmacy data or electronic monitoring of medication use to objectively measure controller medication adherence by patients as a clinical outcome. Consider additional metrics as indicators of appropriate care, e.g., Use of controller meds: >6 fills per 12 months. Controller-to-total asthma medication ratio: # controller fills in past 12 months/# controller fills + all other asthma med fills. (Cut-point: >0.5).
	Lack of use of significance tests	Develop standards for inclusion of significance testing of data presented (e.g., chi-squared for proportions)
	Cost	Develop standard measures of cost of intervention to determine feasibility for practices to implement
Timeframes		No new recommendations
Settings of care		No new recommendations

Implications for Clinical and Policy Decisionmaking

For health care providers and policy decisionmakers alike, there are strategies that can be implemented to improve the adherence of health care providers to asthma guideline recommendations. In particular, decision support, feedback/audit and clinical pharmacy support strategies more often were associated with improving provider adherence to guidelines than other interventions (e.g., education). With the exception of education interventions, these strategies were more often studied and more often improved provider adherence to guidelines. It is not clear from our review of the literature why some intervention types have been more studied than others. Given the multitude of tasks confronting the health care provider during an asthma care visit (e.g., provide self-management education and environmental control recommendations, prescribe controller medications or one of the three other health care process measures included in our study), it appears that no single type of intervention is capable of remediating all of the health care process outcomes to be addressed by health care providers. A combination of interventions may, however, allow simultaneous contribution to multiple elements of care. Computers, particularly electronic medical records (EMRs) may help to facilitate the need to intervene upon multiple components of asthma care, yet few studies in this review utilized the EMR as the vehicle for their intervention. With the increase in use of EMRs, interventions easily incorporated into an EMR environment may be appealing for providers seeking strategies that can be readily implemented into practice.

Further, organizational change interventions to enhance health care provider adherence to national guidelines were relatively understudied. This is important because organizational change is essentially the only systems-level type of intervention among those that we reviewed. Given the variety, complexity and barriers to completion of tasks confronting health care providers, systems-level (organizational change) interventions warrant further evaluation. An organizational change intervention may lend itself to being combined with other interventions (e.g., Decision Support and Feedback/Audit). Such "multicomponent" interventions would be expected to more likely meet the multiple care and treatment goals confronting health care providers caring for patients with asthma. It also appears that interventions that supplement or act independently of the health care provider's behavior (decision support; clinical pharmacy support) were effective in achieving the desired process outcomes (e.g., increased prescribing of

63

controller medications). Feedback/audit interventions, in specific, may be a useful strategy to incorporate into practice in that the feedback provides health care providers with insight into their own behaviors and performance and if provided on a regular basis may facilitate adherence to providing guideline-based care.

There were some promising findings, particularly among interventions that utilized decision support, feedback/audit or clinical pharmacy support strategies to improve health care provider adherence to guidelines. These intervention strategies tended to have higher levels of strength and larger magnitudes of effect in comparison with other intervention strategies (e.g., education or information only). However, heterogeneity within each intervention category such as variation in personnel delivering intervention, length of intervention, or multiple components makes it challenging to draw valid conclusions about the key components of each intervention. Consequently highlighting the key elements of a specific type of intervention such as decision support is an area of evaluation requiring further development.

Because educational–based interventions were most likely to show no benefit, this type of intervention warrants no further evaluation as an isolated strategy. Furthermore, most studies tested a single strategy, although there were some studies that utilized multiple strategies (Table 19) but too few to draw any definitive conclusions for evaluating whether "multimodal" are more successful than single-interventions.

In terms of outcomes (both health care process and clinical), there was significant variability in the frequency of outcome evaluation. Among the health care process measures, prescriptions of controller medicines were by far the most commonly evaluated, followed by asthma action plan/self-management education, then prescription of peak flow meters. Relatively understudied were processes related to documentation of asthma control/severity, environmental control practices and scheduling of followup visits. All of these are asthma care processes recommended in asthma guidelines, and known to be uncommonly practiced and documented. Therefore, future studies should focus more on how to improve these health care practices. In terms of clinical outcomes, we also observed unequal frequencies of study evaluation, with the most common outcomes being emergency department visits and hospitalizations, and infrequent evaluations of lung function, missed school/work, symptom-free days and quality of life. These understudied outcomes should be a focus of future studies of health care provider-targeted interventions.

Key Question 1 was the most completely addressed for the outcomes included in this report, particularly in terms of prescribing asthma controller medications. Key Question 2 was only partially addressed, as very few studies examined missed school or work as an outcome. Importantly, for Key Question 3, we found no studies that linked changes in health care provider behavior to changes in clinical outcomes among patients with asthma. More specifically, no studies measured the strength of association between behavior changes and clinical outcomes (e.g., percent predicted values; logistic regression). Having data on the associations between provider behavior and clinical outcomes would be important in understanding which changes in specific health care provider behaviors would be most beneficial in focusing on to improve patient outcomes. Standards of asthma care, such as guideline-based care based on national guidelines or health insurance payers, would be more meaningful if it was known to what extent given changes in health care provider behavior meaningfully effect changes in clinical outcomes. Future studies that examine this association between provider behavior and patient outcomes would be beneficial to a variety of stakeholders, including clinical experts creating future guidelines (to highlight best practices), funding agencies (to support unaddressed areas of research) and policymakers (who may also be interested in identifying the best evidence-based practices for providers to follow).

From a study design standpoint, approximately half of the studies used a nonrandomized design, weakening the strength of evidence for a number of interventions. If taken in the context of a need for more systems-level interventions, cluster randomized trials would be a suitable design to evaluate interventions while limiting the risk for contamination bias and improving the precision of the findings. Given the more costly nature of these study designs, funding agencies will need to appropriately support these types of intervention studies. Additionally, testing the efficacy of the more potent multifaceted interventions with targeted populations (i.e., adolescents, obese patients, high asthma severity, or high health care utilizers) may lead to identification of novel preventive and therapeutic strategies for high risk patients that would improve health care provider adherence to national asthma guidelines.

In terms of asthma guideline recommendations for care, we attempted to include all of the health care processes recommended in those documents. The National Asthma Education and Prevention Program (NAEPP) has promoted six specific elements of care through the Guideline Implementation Panel (GIP): use inhaled corticosteroids as the preferred controller medicine; use asthma action plans; determine asthma severity; determine asthma control; schedule follow-up visits; and control allergen and irritant exposures. In this report, we examined two of these six recommended areas of care including use of inhaled corticosteroids and use of asthma action plans. The remaining areas designated by GIP merit future research.

A number of studies were tested in busy primary care settings, suggesting that these interventions could be implementable by busy health care providers. However, harm was generally not measured in the studies we reviewed (only one study reported an unintended harm). Given that few studies reported on the frequency and intensity of exposure to the intervention, there is little evidence available to estimate the likelihood of sustainable implementation of these interventions into routine clinical practices. More specifically, issues of time constraints, work flow considerations and limited resources were not addressed in these studies, so we cannot be sure that these interventions can be translated into clinical practice without significant modification.

Many studies utilized a variety of health care providers, so generalizability of health care provider types is a strength. Although these studies included nurse practitioners and other mid-level/ancillary providers, there were few that were directed specifically at these providers necessitating additional interventions targeting these health care provider populations. In addition, cost implications of specific interventions may be associated with reduced use but was not addressed in this report. Lastly, relatively few studies targeted health care providers known to care for patient populations at risk for poor care and/or poor outcomes. Targeting such settings for future studies would be valuable, as there may be unique conditions to address in those settings, these patients may account for significant costs to the health care system, and these settings may be in the greatest need of assistance in improving asthma care outcomes.

Table 19. Primary and secondary interventions utilized by the included studies

Author, Year	Decision Support	Organizational Change	Feedback and Audit	Clinical Pharmacy Support	Education	Quality Improvement and Pay-for-Performance	Multicomponent	Information Only
Ables AZ, 2002[115]	N/A	N/A	N/A	N/A	P	N/A	N/A	N/A
Armour C., 2007[65]	N/A	N/A	N/A	P		N/A	N/A	N/A
Baker R., 2003[116]	N/A	N/A	N/A	N/A	P	N/A	N/A	N/A
Baker R., 2003[55]	N/A	N/A	P	N/A	S	N/A	N/A	N/A
Bell L.M., 2010[38]	P	N/A	N/A	N/A	S	N/A	N/A	N/A
Bender B. G., 2011[78]	N/A	N/A	N/A	N/A		N/A	P	N/A
Blackstien-Hirsch P., 2000[77]	S	N/A	N/A	N/A	P	N/A	N/A	N/A
Brown R, 2004[70]	N/A	N/A	N/A	N/A	P	N/A	N/A	N/A
Bryce FP, 1995[85]	N/A	N/A	S	N/A		N/A	N/A	P
Cabana M. D., 2006[100]	N/A	N/A	N/A	N/A	P	N/A	N/A	N/A
Cho S. H., 2010[41]	P	N/A	N/A	N/A	S	N/A	N/A	N/A
Clark NM, 1998[71]	N/A	N/A	N/A	N/A	P	N/A	N/A	N/A
Cloutier M. M., 2002[46]	P	N/A	N/A	N/A	S	N/A	N/A	N/A
Cloutier M. M., 2005[44]	P	N/A	N/A	N/A	S	N/A	N/A	N/A
Cloutier M.M., 2009[48]	P	N/A	N/A	N/A	S	N/A	N/A	N/A
Coleman C. I., 2003[60]	N/A	N/A	P	N/A	N/A	N/A	N/A	N/A
Cowie R. L., 2001[75]	N/A	N/A	N/A	N/A	P	N/A	N/A	N/A
Daniels E. C., 2005[80]	N/A	N/A	N/A	N/A	N/A	N/A	P	N/A
Davis AM, 2010[47]	P	N/A	N/A	N/A	N/A	N/A	N/A	N/A
Davis R. S., 2004[76]	N/A	N/A	N/A	N/A	P	N/A	N/A	N/A
de Vries T. W., 2010[66]	N/A	N/A	S	P	S	N/A	N/A	N/A
Eccles M., 2002[37]	P	N/A	N/A	N/A	S	N/A	N/A	N/A
Fairall L., 2010[33]	P	N/A	N/A	N/A	S	N/A	N/A	N/A
Feder G, 1995[56]	N/A	N/A	P	N/A	S	N/A	N/A	N/A
Finkelstein J. A., 2005[51]	N/A	P	S	N/A		N/A	N/A	N/A
Foster J. M., 2007[117]	N/A	N/A	P	N/A	S	N/A	N/A	N/A

66

Table 19. Primary and secondary interventions utilized by the included studies (continued)

Author, Year	Decision Support	Organizational Change	Feedback and Audit	Clinical Pharmacy Support	Education	Quality Improvement and Pay-for-Performance	Multicomponent	Information Only
Fox P., 2007[94]	N/A	S	N/A	N/A	N/A	P	N/A	N/A
Frankowski B. L., 2006[97]	N/A	N/A	N/A	N/A	N/A	N/A	P	N/A
Glasgow N. J., 2003[90]	N/A	P	N/A	N/A	N/A	N/A	N/A	N/A
Gorton T. A., 1995[118]	S	N/A	N/A	N/A	P	N/A	N/A	N/A
Hagmolen, W., 2008[79]	N/A	N/A	N/A	N/A	N/A	N/A	P	N/A
Halterman J. S., 2005[119]	P	N/A	N/A	N/A	N/A	N/A	N/A	N/A
Halterman J.S., 2006[87]	P	N/A	N/A	N/A	N/A	N/A	N/A	N/A
Herborg H., 2001[63] &[120]	N/A	N/A	P	S	N/A	N/A	N/A	N/A
Holton C., 2011[92]	N/A	N/A	N/A	N/A	P	N/A	N/A	N/A
Homer CJ., 2005[96]	N/A	N/A	N/A	N/A	N/A	P	N/A	N/A
Horswell R., 2008[43]	P	N/A	S	N/A	N/A	N/A	N/A	N/A
Hoskins G., 1997[59]	N/A	N/A	P	N/A	S	N/A	N/A	N/A
Kattan M., 2006[35]	P	N/A	S	N/A	N/A	N/A	N/A	N/A
Lesho E. P., 2005[45]	P	N/A	N/A	N/A	S	N/A	N/A	N/A
Liaw S. T., 2008[121]	N/A	N/A	N/A	N/A	P	N/A	N/A	N/A
Lozano P., 2004[122]	N/A	S	N/A	N/A	P	N/A	N/A	N/A
Lob, 2011[82]	N/A	N/A	N/A	N/A	N/A	N/A	P	N/A
Lundborg C. S., 1999[81]	N/A	N/A	N/A	N/A	N/A	N/A	P	N/A
Mahi-Taright S., 2004[74]	N/A	N/A	N/A	N/A	P	N/A	N/A	N/A
Mangione-Smith R., 2005[95]	N/A	S	N/A	N/A	N/A	P	N/A	N/A
Martens J. D., 2006[84]	N/A	N/A	N/A	N/A	N/A	N/A	N/A	P
Martens J. D., 2007[34]	P	N/A	N/A	N/A	N/A	N/A	N/A	N/A
Massie J., D., 2004[123]	N/A	N/A	N/A	N/A	N/A	N/A	P	N/A

Table 19. Primary and secondary interventions utilized by the included studies (continued)

Author, Year	Decision Support	Organizational Change	Feedback and Audit	Clinical Pharmacy Support	Education	Quality Improvement and Pay-for-Performance	Multicomponent	Information Only
McCowan C, 2001[89]	P	N/A	N/A	N/A	N/A	N/A	N/A	N/A
Mitchell E. A., 2005[36]	P	N/A	N/A	N/A	S	N/A	N/A	N/A
Newton W. P., 2010[42]	P	S	N/A	N/A	N/A	N/A	N/A	N/A
O'Laughlen MC, 2008[124]	P	N/A	N/A	N/A	S	N/A	N/A	N/A
Patel P. H., 2004[91]	N/A	P	N/A	N/A	N/A	N/A	N/A	N/A
Premaratne U. N., 1999[73]	N/A	N/A	N/A	N/A	P	N/A	N/A	N/A
Ragazzi H., 2011[49]	P	S	N/A	N/A	S	N/A	N/A	N/A
Rance K., 2011[39]	P	N/A	N/A	N/A	N/A	N/A	N/A	N/A
Renzi P. M., 2006[98]	P	N/A	N/A	N/A	N/A	N/A	N/A	N/A
Richman M. J., 2000[62]	N/A	N/A	P	N/A	S	N/A	N/A	N/A
Ruoff G., 2002[88]	P	N/A	N/A	N/A	N/A	N/A	N/A	N/A
Saini B, 2004[67]	N/A	N/A	S	P	N/A	N/A	N/A	N/A
Schneider A., 2008[57]	N/A	N/A	P	N/A	N/A	N/A	N/A	N/A
Shah S., 2011[68]	N/A	N/A	N/A	N/A	P	N/A	N/A	N/A
Shapiro A., 2011[40]	P	N/A	N/A	N/A	N/A	N/A	N/A	N/A
Shiffman R. N., 2000[50]	P	N/A	N/A	N/A	N/A	N/A	N/A	N/A
Smeele I. J., 1999[69]	N/A	N/A	N/A	N/A	P	N/A	N/A	N/A
Sondergaard J., 2002[54]	N/A	N/A	P	N/A	N/A	N/A	N/A	N/A
Stergachis A., 2002[72]	N/A	N/A	N/A	N/A	P	N/A	N/A	N/A
Suh D. C., 2001[61]	N/A	N/A	P	N/A	S	N/A	N/A	N/A
Sulaiman N. D., 2010[93]	N/A	N/A	N/A	N/A	P	N/A	N/A	N/A

Table 19. Primary and secondary interventions utilized by the included studies (continued)

Author, Year	Decision Support	Organizational Change	Feedback and Audit	Clinical Pharmacy Support	Education	Quality Improvement and Pay-for-Performance	Multicomponent	Information Only
Thyne S.M., 2007[52]	N/A	P	S	N/A	S	N/A	N/A	N/A
To T., 2008[86]	P	N/A	N/A	N/A	S	N/A	N/A	N/A
Veninga CCM, 1999[53]	N/A	N/A	P	N/A	N/A	S	N/A	N/A
Veninga CCM, 2000[58]	N/A	N/A	P	N/A	S	N/A	N/A	N/A
Weinberger M, 2002[99]	N/A	N/A	S	P	N/A	S	N/A	N/A
Yawn BP, 2008[64]	N/A	N/A	N/A	N/A	N/A	N/A	P	N/A

N/A = not applicable; P = primary intervention; S = secondary intervention(s)

Conclusions

In conclusion, there is some evidence to support the use of decision support tools, feedback and audit, and clinical pharmacy support interventions to improve the adherence of health care providers to prescribing asthma controller medicines and to reduce ED visits/hospitalizations. However, we found an insufficient level of evidence to evaluate the effectiveness of a number of interventions. This was attributable to a number of factors, including heterogeneity in interventions, variability in approaches to measuring outcomes, and a relative paucity of studies utilizing rigorous study designs (particularly randomized controlled trials). Therefore, there is a need to further evaluate other types of health care provider-targeted interventions (e.g., multimodal) and other health care process or clinical outcomes (e.g., missed days of work/school). There is also a significant need to focus on standardized measures of outcomes and more rigorous study designs.

References

1. Vital signs: asthma prevalence, disease characteristics, and self-management education: United States, 2001--2009. MMWR Morb Mortal Wkly Rep 2011; 60(17):547-52.

2. Expert Panel Report 3 (EPR-3): Guidelines for the Diagnosis and Management of Asthma-Summary Report 2007. J Allergy Clin Immunol. 2007; 120(5 Suppl):S94-138.

3. Evans R, Gergen PJ, Mitchell H et al. A randomized clinical trial to reduce asthma morbidity among inner-city children: results of the National Cooperative Inner-City Asthma Study. J Pediatr. 1999; 135(3):332-8.

4. Sulaiman ND, Barton CA, Liaw ST et al. Do small group workshops and locally adapted guidelines improve asthma patients' health outcomes? A cluster randomized controlled trial. Fam Pract. 2010; 27(3):246-54.

5. Szefler SJ, Mitchell H, Sorkness CA et al. Management of asthma based on exhaled nitric oxide in addition to guideline-based treatment for inner-city adolescents and young adults: a randomised controlled trial. Lancet. 2008; 372(9643):1065-72.

6. Wisnivesky JP, Lorenzo J, Lyn-Cook R et al. Barriers to adherence to asthma management guidelines among inner-city primary care providers. Ann Allergy Asthma Immunol. 2008; 101(3):264-70.

7. Halterman JS, Aligne CA, Auinger P et al. Inadequate therapy for asthma among children in the United States. Pediatrics. 2000; 105(1 Pt 3):272-6.

8. Halterman JS, Yoos HL, Kaczorowski JM et al. Providers underestimate symptom severity among urban children with asthma. Arch Pediatr Adolesc Med. 2002; 156(2):141-6.

9. Cabana MD, Slish KK, Nan B et al. Asking the correct questions to assess asthma symptoms. Clin Pediatr (Phila). 2005; 44(4):319-25.

10. Cabana MD, Bruckman D, Meister K et al. Documentation of asthma severity in pediatric outpatient clinics. Clin Pediatr. (Phila) 2003; 42(2):121-5.

11. Ortega AN, Gergen PJ, Paltiel AD et al. Impact of site of care, race, and Hispanic ethnicity on medication use for childhood asthma. Pediatrics. 2002; 109(1):E1.

12. Akinbami LJ, Moorman JE, Garbe PL, Sondik EJ. Status of childhood asthma in the United States, 1980-2007. Pediatrics. 2009; 123 Suppl 3:S131-45.

13. Flores G, Snowden-Bridon C, Torres S et al. Urban minority children with asthma: substantial morbidity, compromised quality and access to specialists, and the importance of poverty and specialty care. J Asthma. 2009; 46(4):392-8.

14. Akinbami L. The state of childhood asthma, United States, 1980-2005. Adv Data 2006; (381):1-24.

15. Cabana MD, Rand CS, Powe NR et al. Why don't physicians follow clinical practice guidelines? A framework for improvement. JAMA. 1999; 282(15):1458-65.

16. Bracha Y, Brottman G, Carlson A. Physicians, guidelines, and cognitive tasks. Eval Health Prof. 2011; 34(3):309-35.

17. Rastogi D, Shetty A, Neugebauer R et al. National Heart, Lung, and Blood Institute guidelines and asthma management practices among inner-city pediatric primary care providers. Chest. 2006; 129(3):619-23.

18. Bhogal SK, McGillivray D, Bourbeau J et al. Focusing the focus group: impact of the awareness of major factors contributing to non-adherence to acute paediatric asthma guidelines. J Eval Clin Pract. 2011; 17(1):160-7.

19. Corrigan SP, Cecillon DL, Sin DD et al. The costs of implementing the 1999 Canadian Asthma Consensus Guidelines recommendation of asthma education and spirometry for the family physician. Can Respir J. 2004; 11(5):349-53.

20. Butz AM, Eggleston P, Huss K et al. Children with asthma and nebulizer use: parental asthma self-care practices and beliefs. J Asthma. 2001; 38(7):565-73.

21. Coffman JM, Cabana MD, Yelin EH. Do school-based asthma education programs improve self-management and health outcomes? Pediatrics. 2009; 124(2):729-42.

22. Teach SJ, Crain EF, Quint DM et al. Improved asthma outcomes in a high-morbidity pediatric population: results of an emergency department-based randomized clinical trial. Arch Pediatr Adolesc Med. 2006; 160(5):535-41.

23. Wise RA, Bartlett SJ, Brown ED et al. Randomized trial of the effect of drug presentation on asthma outcomes: the American Lung Association Asthma Clinical Research Centers. J Allergy Clin Immunol. 2009; 124(3):436-44, 444e1-8.

24. Bratton SL, Cabana MD, Brown RW et al. Asthma educational seminar targeting Medicaid providers. Respir Care. 2006; 51(1):49-55.

25. Welsh EJ, Hasan M, Li P. Home-based educational interventions for children with asthma. Cochrane Database Syst Rev. 2011; (10):CD008469.

26. Bravata DM, Gienger AL, Holty JE et al. Quality improvement strategies for children with asthma: a systematic review. Arch Pediatr Adolesc Med. 2009; 163(6):572-81.

27. Bravata DM, Sundaram V, Lewis R et al. Closing the Quality Gap: A Critical Analysis of Quality Improvement Strategies: Volume 5Asthma Care. Evidence Report/Technology Assessment No. 9 (Prepared by Stanford University Evidence-based Practice Center under Contract No. 290-02-0017). Rockville, MD: Agency for Healthcare Research and Quality; January 2007. AHRQ Publication No. 04(07)-0051-5. 2007.

28. Higgins JPT, Green S (editors).Cochrane Handbook for Systematic Reviews of Interventions Version 5.0.2 [updated September 2009]. The Cochrane Collaboration, 2009. Available from www.cochrane-handbook.org.

29. Cochrane Effective Practice and Organisation of Care Group. Data collection checklist. 2002. Available at http://epoc.cochrane.org/sites/epoc.coc hrane.org/files/uploads/datacollectionc hecklist.pdf. (Accessed 2012).

30. Akinbami LJ, Sullivan SD, Campbell JD et al. Asthma outcomes: healthcare utilization and costs. J Allergy Clin Immunol. 2012; 129(3 suppl):s49-64.

31. Guyatt G, Oxman AD, Sultan S et al. GRADE guidelines 11-making an overall rating of confidence in effect estimates for a single outcome and for all outcomes. J Clin Epidemiol. 2012.

32. Owens DK, Lohr KN, Atkins D et al. AHRQ series paper 5: grading the strength of a body of evidence when comparing medical interventions-- agency for healthcare research and quality and the effective health-care program. J Clin Epidemiol, 2010. 63(5):513-23.

33. Fairall L, Bachmann MO, Zwarenstein M et al. Trop Med Int Health: Cost-effectiveness of educational outreach to primary care nurses to increase tuberculosis case detection and improve respiratory care: economic evaluation alongside a randomised trial. 2010; 15:277-86.

34. Martens JD, van der Weijden T, Severens JL et al. Effect of computer reminders on GPs' prescribing behaviour: a cluster-randomised trial. Int J Med Inform. 2007; 76 Suppl 3:S403-16.

35. Kattan M, Crain EF, Steinbach S et al. A randomized clinical trial of clinician feedback to improve quality of care for inner-city children with asthma. Pediatrics. 2006; 117:e1095-103.

36. Mitchell EA, Didsbury PB, Kruithof N et al. A randomized controlled trial of an asthma clinical pathway for children in general practice. Acta Paediatr. 2005; 94:226-33.

37. Eccles M, McColl E, Steen N *et al*. Effect of computerised evidence based guidelines on management of asthma and angina in adults in primary care: cluster randomised controlled trial. BMJ. 2002; 325:941.

38. Bell LM, Grundmeier R, Localio R et al. Electronic health record-based decision support to improve asthma care: a cluster-randomized trial. 2010; 125:e770-7.

39. Rance K, O'Laughlen M, Ting S.: Improving asthma care for African American children by increasing national asthma guideline adherence. J Pediatr Health Care. 2011; 25:235-49.

40. Shapiro A, Gracy D, Quinones W et al. Putting guidelines into practice: improving documentation of pediatric asthma management using a decision-making tool. Arch Pediatr Adolesc Med. 2011; 165:412-8.

41. Cho SH, Jeong JW, Park HW et al. Effectiveness of a computer-assisted asthma management program on physician adherence to guidelines J Asthma. 2010; 47:680-6.

42. Newton WP, Lefebvre A, Donahue KE et al Infrastructure for large-scale quality-improvement projects: early lessons from North Carolina Improving Performance in Practice. J Contin Educ Health Prof. 2010; 30:106-13.

43. Horswell R, Butler MK, Kaiser M et al. Disease management programs for the underserved. Dis Manag. 2008; 11:145-52.

44. Cloutier MM, Hall CB, Wakefield DB et al. Use of asthma guidelines by primary care providers to reduce hospitalizations and emergency department visits in poor, minority, urban children. Pediatrics. 2005; 146:591-7.

45. Lesho EP, Myers CP, Ott M et al. Do clinical practice guidelines improve processes or outcomes in primary care? Mil Med. 2005; 170:243-6.

46. Cloutier MM, Wakefield DB, Carlisle PS et al. The effect of Easy Breathing on asthma management and knowledge. Arch Pediatr Adolesc Med. 2002; 156:1045-51.

47. Davis AM, Cannon M, Ables AZ et al. Using the electronic medical record to improve asthma severity documentation and treatment among family medicine residents. Fam Med. 2010; 42:334-7.

48. Cloutier MM, Grosse SD, Wakefield DB et al. The economic impact of an urban asthma management program. Am J Manag Care. 2009; 15:345-51.

49. Ragazzi H, Keller A, Ehrensberger R et al. Evaluation of a practice-based intervention to improve the management of pediatric asthma. J Urban Health. 2011; 88 Suppl 1:38-48.

50. Shiffman RN, Freudigman M, Brandt CA et al. A guideline implementation system using handheld computers for office management of asthma: effects on adherence and patient outcomes. Pediatrics. 2000; 105:767-73.

51. Finkelstein JA, Lozano P, Fuhlbrigge AL et al. Practice-level effects of interventions to improve asthma care in primary care settings: the Pediatric Asthma Care Patient Outcomes Research Team. Health Serv Res. 2005; 40:1737-57.

52. Thyne SM, Marmor AK, Madden N et al. Comprehensive asthma management for underserved children. Paediatr Perinat Epidemiol. 2007; 21:29-34.

53. Veninga CCM, Lagerløv P, Wahlström R et al. Evaluating an educational intervention to improve the treatment of asthma in four European countries. Am J Respir Care Med. 1999; 160:1254-62.

54. Sondergaard J, Andersen M, Vach K et al. Detailed postal feedback about prescribing to asthma patients combined with a guideline statement showed no impact: a randomised controlled trial. Eur J Clin Pharmacol. 2002; 58:127-32.

55. Baker R, Fraser RC, Stone M et al. Randomised controlled trial of the impact of guidelines, prioritized review criteria and feedback on implementation of recommendations for angina and asthma. Br J Gen Pract. 2003; 53:284-91.

56. Feder G, Griffiths C, Highton C et al. clinical guidelines introduced with practice based education improve care of asthmatic and diabetic patients? A randomised controlled trial in general practices in east London. BMJ. 1995; 311:1473-8.

57. Schneider A, Wensing M, Biessecker K et al. Impact of quality circles for improvement of asthma care: results of a randomized controlled trial. J Eval Clin Pract. 2008; 14:185-90.

58. Veninga CCM, Denig P, Zwaagstra R . Journal of Clinical Epidemiology: Improving drug treatment in general practice. 2000; 53:762-72.

59. Hoskins G, Neville RG, Smith B et al. Does participation in distance learning and audit improve the care of patients with acute asthma attacks? The General Practitioners in Asthma Group. Health Bull (Edinb). 1997; 55:150-5.

60. Coleman CI, Reddy P, Laster-Bradley NM et al. Effect of practitioner education on adherence to asthma treatment guidelines. Ann Pharmacother. 2003; 37:956-61.

61. Suh DC, Shin SK, Okpara I et al. Impact of a targeted asthma intervention program on treatment costs in patients with asthma. Am J Manag Care. 2001; 7:897-906.

62. Richman MJ, Poltawsky JS. Partnership for excellence in asthma care: evidence-based disease management. Stud Health Technol Inform. 2000; 76:107-21.

63. Herborg H, Soendergaard B, Jorgensen T et al. Improving drug therapy for patients with asthma-part 2: Use of antiasthma medications. J Am Pharm Assoc (Wash). 2001; 41:551-9.

64. Yawn BP, Bertram S, Wollan P. Introduction of asthma APGAR tools improve asthma management in primary care practices. J Asthma Allergy. 2008; 1-10.

65. Armour C, Bosnic-Anticevich S, Brillant M et al. Pharmacy Asthma Care Program (PACP) improves outcomes for patients in the community. Thorax. 2007; 62:496-502.

66. De Vries TW, van den Berg PB, Duiverman EJ et al. Effect of a minimal pharmacy intervention on improvement of adherence to asthma guidelines. Arch Dis Child. 2010; 95:302-4.

67. Saini B, Krass I, Armour C. Development, implementation, and evaluation of a community pharmacy-based asthma care model. Ann Pharmacother. 2004; 38:1954-60.

68. Shah S, Sawyer SM, Toelle BG et al. Improving paediatric asthma outcomes in primary health care: a randomised controlled trial. Med J Aust. 2011; 195:405-9.

69. Smeele IJ, Grol RP, van Schayck CP et al. Can small group education and peer review improve care for patients with asthma/chronic obstructive pulmonary disease? Qual Health Care. 1999; 8:92-8.

70. Brown R, Bratton SL, Cabana MD, Kaciroti N, Clark NM. Chest: Physician asthma education program improves outcomes for children of low-income families. 2004; 126:369-74.

71. Clark NM, Gong M, Schork MA et al. Impact of education for physicians on patient outcomes. Pediatrics. 1998; 101(5):831-6.

72. Stergachis A, Gardner JS, Anderson MT et al. Improving pediatric asthma outcomes in the community setting: does pharmaceutical care make a difference? J Am Pharm Assoc (Wash). 2002; 42:743-52.

73. Premaratne UN, Sterne JA, Marks GB et al. Clustered randomised trial of an intervention to improve the management of asthma: Greenwich asthma study. BMJ. 1999; 318:1251-5.

74. Mahi-Taright S, Belhocine M, Ait-Khaled N. Can we improve the management of chronic obstructive respiratory disease? The example of asthma in adults. Int J Tuberc Lung Dis. 2004; 8:873-81.

75. Cowie RL, Underwood MF, Mack S. The impact of asthma management guideline dissemination on the control of asthma in the community. Can Respir J. 2001; 8 Suppl A:41A-5A.

76. Davis RS, Bukstein DA, Luskin AT et al. Changing physician prescribing patterns through problem-based learning: an interactive, teleconference case-based education program and review of problem-based learning. Ann Allergy Asthma Immunol. 2004; 93:237-42.

77. Blackstien-Hirsch P, Anderson G, Cicutto L et al.. Implementing continuing education strategies for family physicians to enhance asthma patients' quality of life. J Asthma. 2000; 37:247-57.

78. Bender BG, Dickinson P, Rankin A et al. The Colorado Asthma Toolkit Program: a practice coaching intervention from the High Plains Research Network. J Am Board Fam Med. 2011; 24:240-8.

79. Hagmolen of ten Have W, van den Berg NJ, van der Palen J et al. Implementation of an asthma guideline for the management of childhood asthma in general practice: a randomised controlled trial. Prim Care Respir J. 2008; 17:90-6.

80. Daniels EC, Bacon J, Denisio S et al. Translation squared: improving asthma care for high-disparity populations through a safety net practice-based research network. J Asthma. 2005; 42:499-505.

81. Lundborg CS, Wahlstrom R, Oke T et al. Influencing prescribing for urinary tract infection and asthma in primary care in Sweden: a randomized controlled trial of an interactive educational intervention. J Clin Epidemiol. 1999; 52:801-12.

82. Lob SH, Boer JH, Porter PG et al. Promoting Best-Care Practices in Childhood Asthma: Quality Improvement in Community Health Centers. Pediatrics 2011;128;20; Originally Published Online June 13, 2011; DOI: 10.1542/Peds.2010-1962 .

83. Cloutier MM, Tennen H, Wakefield DB et al. Improving clinician self-efficacy does not increase asthma guideline use by primary care clinicians. Acad Pediatr. 2012; 12(4):312-8.

84. Martens JD, Winkens RA, van der Weijden T et al. Does a joint development and dissemination of multidisciplinary guidelines improve prescribing behaviour: a pre/post study with concurrent control group and a randomised trial. BMC Health Serv Res. 2006; 6:145.

85. Bryce FP, Neville RG, Crombie IK et al. Controlled trial of an audit facilitator in diagnosis and treatment of childhood asthma in general practice. BMJ. 1995; 310:838-42.

86. To T, Cicutto L, Degani N et al. Can a community evidence-based asthma care program improve clinical outcomes?: a longitudinal study. J Med Care. 2008; 46:1257-66.

87. Halterman JS , Fisher S, Conn KM et al. Improved preventive care for asthma: a randomized trial of clinician prompting in pediatric offices. Arch Pediat Adolesc Med. 2006; 160.1018-25.

88. Ruoff G. Effects of flow sheet implementation on physician performance in the management of asthmatic patients. Fam Med. 2002; 34:514-7.

89. Mccowan C, Neville RG, Ricketts IW et al. Lessons from a randomized controlled trial designed to evaluate computer decision support software to improve the management of asthma. Med InformInternet Med. 2001; 26:191-201.

90. Glasgow NJ, Ponsonby AL, Yates R et al. Proactive asthma care in childhood: general practice based randomised controlled trial. BMJ. 2003; 327:659.

91. Patel PH, Welsh C, Foggs MB. Improved asthma outcomes using a coordinated care approach in a large medical group. Dis Manag. 2004; 7:102-11.

92. Holton C, Crockett A, Nelson M et al. Does spirometry training in general practice improve quality and outcomes of asthma care? Int J Qual Health Care. 2011; 23:545-53.

93. Sulaiman ND, Barton CA, Liaw ST et al. Do small group workshops and locally adapted guidelines improve asthma patients' health outcomes? A cluster randomized controlled trial. Fam Practice. 2010; 27:246-54.

94. Fox P, Porter PG, Lob SH, Boer JH, Rocha DA, Adelson JW. Pediatrics: Improving asthma-related health outcomes among low-income, multiethnic, school-aged children: Results of a demonstration project that combined continuous quality improvement and community health worker strategies. 2007; 120:e902-e911.

95. Mangione-Smith R, Schonlau M, Chan KS et al. Measuring the effectiveness of a collaborative for quality improvement in pediatric asthma care: Does implementing the chronic care model improve processes and outcomes of care? Ambul Pediatr. 2005; 5:75-82.

96. Homer CJ, Forbes P, Horvitz L et al. Impact of a quality improvement program on care and outcomes for children with asthma. Arch Pediatr Adolesc Med. 2005; 159:464-9.

97. Frankowski BL, Keating K, Rexroad A et al. Community collaboration: concurrent physician and school nurse education and cooperation increases the use of asthma action plans. J Sch Health. 2006; 76:303-6.

98. Renzi PM, Ghezzo H, Goulet S, Dorval E, Thivierge RL. Paper stamp checklist tool enhances asthma guidelines knowledge and implementation by primary care physicians. Can Respir J. 2006; 13:193-7.

99. Weinberger M , Murray MD, Marrero DG et al.. Effectiveness of pharmacist care for patients with reactive airways disease: A randomized controlled trial. JAMA. 2002; 288:1594-602.

100. Cabana MD, Slish KK, Evans D et al. Impact of physician asthma care education on patient outcomes. Pediatrics. 2006; 117:2149-57.

101. Terrin N, Schmid CH, Lau J . In an empirical evaluation of the funnel plot, researchers could not visually identify publication bias. J Clin Epidemiol. 2005; 58(9):894-901.

102. Viswanathan M, Golin CE, Jones CD, et al. Medication Adherence Interventions: Comparative Effectiveness. Closing the Quality Gap: Revisiting the State of the Science. Evidence Report No. 208. (Prepared by RTI internationaluniversity of North Carolina Evidence-based Practice Center under Contract No. 290-2007-10056-I.) AHRQ Publication No. 12-E010-EF. Rockville, MD: Agency for Healthcare Research and Quality. September 2012.

103. Akl EA, Sackett K, Pretorius R et al. Educational games for health professionals. Cochrane Database Syst Rev. 2008; (1):CD006411.

104. Forsetlund L, Bjorndal A, Rashidian A et al. Continuing education meetings and workshops: effects on professional practice and health care outcomes. Cochrane Database Syst Rev 2009; (2):CD003030.

105. Farmer AP, Legare F, Turcot L et al. Printed educational materials: effects on professional practice and health care outcomes. Cochrane Database Syst Rev. 2008; (3):CD004398.

106. Thomson O'Brien MA, Oxman AD, Davis DA et al. Educational outreach visits: effects on professional practice and health care outcomes. Cochrane Database Syst Rev. 2000; (2):CD000409.

107. Reeves S, Zwarenstein M, Goldman J et al. Interprofessional education: effects on professional practice and health care outcomes. Cochrane Database Syst Rev. 2008; (1):CD002213.

108. Gosden T, Forland F, Kristiansen IS et al. Capitation, salary, fee-for-service and mixed systems of payment: effects on the behaviour of primary care physicians. Cochrane Database Syst Rev. 2000; (3):CD002215.

109. Scott A, Sivey P, Ait Ouakrim D et al. The effect of financial incentives on the quality of health care provided by primary care physicians. Cochrane Database Syst Rev. 2011; (9):CD008451.

110. Sturm H, Austvoll-Dahlgren A, Aaserud M et al. Pharmaceutical policies: effects of financial incentives for prescribers. Cochrane Database Syst Rev. 2007; (3):CD006731.

111. Durieux P, Trinquart L, Colombet I et al. Computerized advice on drug dosage to improve prescribing practice. Cochrane Database Syst Rev. 2008; (3):CD002894.

112. Shojania KG, Jennings A, Mayhew A et al. The effects of on-screen, point of care computer reminders on processes and outcomes of care. Cochrane Database Syst Rev. 2009; (3):CD001096.

113. Ivers N, Jamtvedt G, Flottorp S et al. Audit and feedback: effects on professional practice and healthcare outcomes. Cochrane Database Syst Rev. 2012; 6:CD000259.

114. Flodgren G, Pomey MP, Taber SA, Eccles MP. Effectiveness of external inspection of compliance with standards in improving healthcare organisation behaviour, healthcare professional behaviour or patient outcomes. Cochrane Database Syst Rev. 2011; (11):CD008992.

115. Ables AZ, Godenick MT, Lipsitz SR. Improving family practice residents' compliance with asthma practice guidelines. Fam Med. 2002; 34:23-8.

116. Baker R, Fraser RC, Stone M. Evidence-based guidelines, prioritised review criteria and feedback have no effect on adherence to care recommendations for angina and asthma. Evidence-Based Healthcare. 7(3):157-8.

117. Foster JM, Hoskins G, Smith B et al. Practice development plans to improve the primary care management of acute asthma: randomised controlled trial. BMC Fam Pract. 2007; 8:23.

118. Gorton TA, Cranford CO, Golden WE et al. Primary care physicians' response to dissemination of practice guidelines. Arch Fam Med. 1995; 4:135-42.

119. Halterman JS, McConnochie KM, Conn KM et al. A randomized trial of primary care provider prompting to enhance preventive asthma therapy. Arch Pediatr Adolesc Med. 2005; 159:422-7.

120. Herborg H. Sbfbeal. Improving drug therapy for patients with asthma--part 1: Patient outcomes. J Am Pharm Assoc. 2001; (4):539-50.

121. Liaw ST, Sulaiman ND, Barton CA et al. An interactive workshop plus locally adapted guidelines can improve general practitioners asthma management and knowledge: a cluster randomised trial in the Australian setting. BMC Fam Pract. 2008; 9:22.

122. Lozano P, Finkelstein JA, Carey VJ et al. A multisite randomized trial of the effects of physician education and organizational change in chronic-asthma care: health outcomes of the Pediatric Asthma Care Patient Outcomes Research Team II Study. 2004; 158:875-83.

123. Massie J, Efron D, Cerritelli B et al. Archives of Disease in Childhood: Implementation of evidence based guidelines for paediatric asthma management in a teaching hospital. 2004; 89:660-4.

124. O'Laughlen MC, Hollen PJ, Rakes G et al. Improving pediatric asthma by the MSAGR algorithm: A multicolored, simplified, asthma guideline reminder. Pediatr Asthma, Allergy and Immunol. 2008; 21:119-27.

Appendix A. Acronyms and Abbreviations

A/P	Asian/Pacific Islander
AAP	Asthma action plan
BQC	benchmarking quality circle feedback intervention
CINAHL	Cumulative Index to Nursing and Allied Health Literature
CLIQ	Clinical Inquiry
CME	Continuing medical education
CON	Control
COPD	Chronic obstructive pulmonary disease
CPGs	clinical practice guidelines
DM	Diabetes mellitus
ED	emergency department
EMR	Electronic Medical Records
ENT	Ear nose throat
EPOC	Cochrane Effective Practice and Organisation of Care
EPR-3	Expert Panel Report 3
ERIC	Educational Resources Information Center
FEV	Forced Expiratory Volume
FVC	Forced Vital Capacity
GPs	General practitoner
HCSD	Health Care Services Division
HMO	Health maintenance organization
ICS	Inhaled Corticosteroids
INT	Intervention
MD	Medical Doctor
MSAGR	Multicolored, Simplified, Asthma Guideline Reminder
NAEPP	National Asthma Education and Prevention Program
NHLBI	National Heart, Lung, and Blood Institute
NYCHP	New York Children's Health Project
PACE	Practitioner Asthma Communication and Education
PCAPP	Primary Care Asthma Pilot Project
PDSA	Plan-do-study-act
PEFR	Peak Expiratory Flow Rate
PFR	Peak Flow Rate
PFT	Pulmonary Function Test
PLE	Peer Leader Education
PPO-FFS	Preferred provider organization – Fee for service
QC	quality circles
QOL	Quality of life
RCT	Randomized controlled trial
RDRB/CME	Research and Development Resource Base in Continuing Medical Education
SBHC	South Bronx Health Center
SOE	Strength of evidence
SP	Suburban practice
TOM	Therapeutic outcomes monitoring

TQC	traditional quality circle
UP	Urban practice
UTI	Urinary Tract Infection
WAAP	Written asthma action plan

Appendix B. Detailed Search Strategies

Search date –July 2012

Pubmed – 1160

(asthma[mh] OR asthma[tiab])
AND
(guideline[tiab] OR guidelines[tiab] OR practice guidelines as topic[mh] OR consensus conference[tiab] OR consensus statement[tiab] OR consensus statements[tiab] OR recommendation[tiab] OR recommendations[tiab]OR critical pathways[mh] OR critical pathways[tiab] OR critical pathway[tiab] OR clinical pathways[tiab] OR clinical pathway[tiab] OR primary health care/standards[mh])
AND
 (guideline adherence[mh] OR adherence[tiab] OR nurse's practice patterns[mh] OR Physician's Practice Patterns[mh] OR practice pattern[tiab] OR practice patterns[tiab] OR behavior[tiab] OR behaviour[tiab] OR Professional practice[mh] OR "outcome assessment (health care)"[mh] OR quality assurance[mh])
AND
(Physicians[mh] or physicians[tiab] OR physician[tiab] OR general practitioner[tiab] OR general practitioners[tiab] OR GPs[tiab] OR hospitalists[tiab] OR Primary health care[mh] OR Nurses[mh] OR nurses[tiab] OR nurse[tiab] OR physical therapy[tiab] or Physical therapy[mh] OR physical therapist[tiab] OR physical therapists[tiab] OR physiotherapist[tiab] OR physiotherapists[tiab] OR Respiratory therapy[mh] OR respiratory therapist[tiab] OR respiratory therapists[tiab] OR Pharmacists[mh] OR pharmacist[tiab] OR pharmacists[tiab] OR health professional[tiab] OR health professionals[tiab] OR health care provider[tiab] OR health care providers[tiab] OR healthcare provider[tiab] OR healthcare providers[tiab] OR pediatricians[tiab] OR pediatrician[tiab] OR paediatrician[tiab] OR paediatricians[tiab] OR specialist[tiab] OR specialists[tiab] OR pulmonologist[tiab] OR pulmonologists[tiab] OR doctor[tiab] OR doctors[tiab] OR allergist[tiab] OR allergists[tiab] OR internist[tiab] OR internists[tiab])

ERIC – 5
CINAHL =377
PsycINFO =80

(TX asthma) AND (TX guideline OR TX guidelines OR TX consensus conference OR TX consensus statement OR TX consensus statements OR TX recommendation OR TX recommendations OR TX critical pathways OR TX critical pathway OR TX clinical pathways OR TX clinical pathway OR TX primary health care) AND (TX adherence OR TX practice pattern OR TX practice patterns OR TX behavior OR TX behaviour OR TX Professional practice OR TX quality assurance OR TX outcome assessment) AND (TX Physicians OR TX physician OR TX general practitioner OR TX general practitioners OR TX hospitalists OR TX Primary health care OR TX Nurses OR TX nurse OR TX physical therapy OR TX physical therapist OR TX physical therapists OR TX physiotherapist OR TX physiotherapists OR TX respiratory therapist OR TX respiratory therapists OR TX Pharmacists OR TX pharmacist OR TX health professional OR TX health professionals OR TX health care provider OR TX health care providers OR TX healthcare provider OR TX healthcare providers OR TX pediatricians OR TX pediatrician OR TX paediatrician OR TX paediatricians OR TX specialist OR TX specialists OR TX pulmonologist OR TX pulmonologists OR TX doctor OR TX doctors OR TX allergist OR TX allergists OR TX internist OR TX internists)

EMBASE: 538

'asthma'/exp OR asthma:ab,ti

guideline:ab,ti OR guidelines:ab,ti OR 'practice guideline'/exp OR 'practice guideline':ab,ti OR 'consensus conference':ab,ti OR 'consensus statement':ab,ti OR 'consensus statements':ab,ti OR recommendation:ab,ti OR recommendations:ab,ti OR 'critical pathways':ab,ti OR 'critical pathway':ab,ti OR 'clinical pathways':ab,ti OR 'clinical pathway':ab,ti OR 'primary health care':ab,ti

adherence:ab,ti OR 'practice pattern':ab,ti OR 'practice patterns':ab,ti OR behavior:ab,ti OR behaviour:ab,ti OR 'professional practice':ab,ti OR 'quality assurance':ab,ti OR 'outcome assessment'/exp OR 'outcome assessment':ab,ti

'physician'/exp OR physicians:ab,ti OR physician:ab,ti OR 'general practitioner':ab,ti OR 'general practitioners':ab,ti OR hospitalists:ab,ti OR 'primary health care'/exp OR 'primary health care':ab,ti OR nurses:ab,ti OR nurse:ab,ti OR 'physical therapy':ab,ti OR 'physical therapist':ab,ti OR 'physical therapists':ab,ti OR physiotherapist:ab,ti OR physiotherapists:ab,ti OR 'respiratory therapist':ab,ti OR 'respiratory therapists':ab,ti OR pharmacists:ab,ti OR pharmacist:ab,ti OR 'health professional':ab,ti OR 'health professionals':ab,ti OR 'health care provider':ab,ti OR 'health care providers':ab,ti OR 'healthcare provider':ab,ti OR 'healthcare providers':ab,ti OR pediatricians:ab,ti OR pediatrician:ab,ti OR paediatrician:ab,ti OR paediatricians:ab,ti OR specialist:ab,ti OR specialists:ab,ti OR pulmonologist:ab,ti OR pulmonologists:ab,ti OR doctor:ab,ti OR doctors:ab,ti OR allergist:ab,ti OR allergists:ab,ti OR internist:ab,ti OR internists:ab,ti

Cochrane =92

asthma:ti,ab,kw OR MeSH descriptor Asthma explode all trees

guideline:ti,ab,kw OR guidelines:ti,ab,kw OR "practice guideline":ti,ab,kw OR "consensus conference":ti,ab,kw OR "consensus statement":ti,ab,kw OR "consensus statements":ti,ab,kw OR recommendation:ti,ab,kw OR recommendations:ti,ab,kw OR MeSH descriptor Critical Pathways explode all trees OR "critical pathways":ti,ab,kw OR "critical pathway":ti,ab,kw OR "clinical pathways":ti,ab,kw OR "clinical pathway":ti,ab,kw OR "primary health care":ti,ab,kw

MeSH descriptor Guideline Adherence explode all trees OR adherence:ti,ab,kw OR "practice pattern":ti,ab,kw OR "practice patterns":ti,ab,kw OR behavior:ti,ab,kw OR behaviour:ti,ab,kw OR "professional practice":ti,ab,kw OR "quality assurance":ti,ab,kw OR MeSH descriptor Outcome Assessment (Health Care) explode trees 2 and 3 OR "outcome assessment":ti,ab,kw

physicians:ti,ab,kw OR physician:ti,ab,kw OR "general practitioner":ti,ab,kw OR "general practitioners":ti,ab,kw OR hospitalists:ti,ab,kw OR MeSH descriptor Primary Health Care explode all trees OR "primary health care":ti,ab,kw OR nurses:ti,ab,kw OR nurse:ti,ab,kw OR "physical therapy":ti,ab,kw OR "physical therapist":ti,ab,kw OR "physical therapists":ti,ab,kw OR physiotherapist:ti,ab,kw OR physiotherapists:ti,ab,kw OR "respiratory therapist":ti,ab,kw OR "respiratory therapists":ti,ab,kw OR pharmacists:ti,ab,kw OR pharmacist:ti,ab,kw OR "health professional":ti,ab,kw OR "health professionals":ti,ab,kw OR "health care provider":ti,ab,kw OR "health care providers":ti,ab,kw OR "healthcare provider":ti,ab,kw OR "healthcare providers":ti,ab,kw OR pediatricians:ti,ab,kw OR pediatrician:ti,ab,kw OR paediatrician:ti,ab,kw OR paediatricians:ti,ab,kw OR specialist:ti,ab,kw OR specialists:ti,ab,kw OR pulmonologist:ti,ab,kw OR pulmonologists:ti,ab,kw OR doctor:ti,ab,kw OR doctors:ti,ab,kw OR allergist:ti,ab,kw OR allergists:ti,ab,kw OR internist:ti,ab,kw OR internists:ti,ab,kw

Research and Development Resource Base in Continuing Medical Education (RDRB/CME)
Asthma =60
Keywords: ("asthma")
AND
Keywords: ("guideline") OR ("guidelines")
AND
Keywords: ("adherence") OR ("pattern") OR ("patterns")
AND
Keywords: ("physicians") OR ("physician") OR ("practitioner")

Appendix C. Screening and Data Abstraction Forms

Title/Abstract Review
Selected – No

DistillerSR

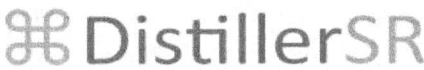 **DistillerSR**

Project   Meditation (Switch)   User   mreuben (My Settings)
Messages   4 new
Live Support Currently Unavailable   User Guide

Review   Datarama   Reports   References   Forms   Manage Levels   Users   Project   Logout

Refid: 12, Skateboards: Are they really perilous? A retrospective study from a district hospital.
Rethnam U, Yesupalan RS, Sinha A.

[Submit Form] and go to [ ] or Skip to Next

1. **Does this article POTENTIALLY apply to ANY of the key questions?**

   ⊙ NO, this article DOES NOT apply to any of the Key Questions (check all of the following reasons that apply)

   ☐ No original data (systematic reviews, editorial, commentary, letters, meta-analysis)
   ☐ Other meditation form - DBT, ACT, CBT, IMBT
   ☐ Study only includes children, adolescent(0-18years)
   ☐ No Control group
   ☐ Not Randomized
   ☐ Not relevant to key questions
   ☐ Other   [ ]

   ○ Yes, this article may apply to the key questions
   ○ Unclear-get it for article review

Please click below to see:
key questions

[Submit Form] and go to [ ] or Skip to Next

Title/Abstract Review
Selected- Yes

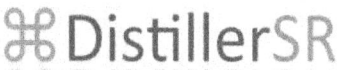 **DistillerSR**   ritu.sharma

Review   Datarama   Reports   References   Forms   Manage Levels   Users   Project   Logout

---

Refid: 12, Skateboards: Are they really perilous? A retrospective study from a district hospital.
Rethnam U, Yesupalan RS, Sinha A.

[Submit Form] and go to [   ] or Skip to Next

1. Does this article POTENTIALLY apply to ANY of the key questions?

○ No
◉ Yes

Include article for: (Check all that apply):
In the care of pediatric or adult patients with asthma, what is the evidence that interventions designed to improve health care provider adherence to guidelines:

☐ KQ1-Impact health care process outcomes (e.g., receiving appropriate treatment)
☐ KQ2-Impact clinical outcomes (e.g., hospitalizations, patient reported outcomes such as symptom control)
☐ KQ3-Impact health care process outcomes that then affect clinical outcomes

○ Unclear-No abstract or cannot tell from abstract alone --get it for full-text screen

Guidelines – Care path, Clinical pathway, recommendations, consensus statements, algorithm
Health care providers - Physicians, nurses, nurse practitioners, physiotherapists/physical therapists, respiratory therapists, pharmacists, and other health care providers

[Submit Form] and go to [   ] or Skip to Next

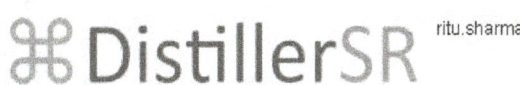
ritu.sharma

| Review | Datarama | Reports | References | Forms | Manage Levels | Users | Project | Logout |

Refid: 10, Clutchboards: Are they really perilous? A retrospective study from a district hospital.
Rethnam U, Yesupalan RS, Sinha A.

SubmitForm and go to [   ] or Skip to Next

1. Does this article POTENTIALLY apply to ANY of the key questions?

⦿ No
    NO, this article DOES NOT apply to any of the Key Questions (check only one reason)

    ○ Not conducted in humans
    ○ No original data (systematic reviews, meta-analysis, editorial, commentary)
    ○ Not in English and not able to determine eligibility
    ○ Does not address asthma
    ○ Addresses inpatient or emergency department care only
    ○ Does not target health care providers
    ○ Does not evaluate an intervention targeting adherence or behavior of health care provider
    ○ Does not provide any outcome of interest (e.g. provides only acceptability of intervention)
    ○ Other-please specify   [   ]

○ Yes
Clear Response

5. Comments:

[   ]

List of outcomes - Please click here to see the list of outcomes
Guidelines – Care path, Clinical pathway, recommendations, consensus statements, algorithm
Health care providers - Physicians, nurses, nurse practitioners, physiotherapists/physical therapists, respiratory therapists, pharmacists, and other health care providers

SubmitForm and go to [   ] or Skip to Next

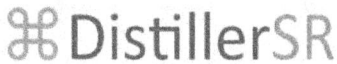 **DistillerSR**   ritu.sharma

Project	Asthma Guidelines (Switch) User mreuben (My Settings)
Messages	3 new

Live Support Currently Unavailable	User Guide

| Review | Datarama | Reports | References | Forms | Manage Levels | Users | Project | Logout |

Refid: 12, Skateboards: Are they really perilous? A retrospective study from a district hospital.
Rethnam U, Yesupalan RS, Sinha A.

[Submit Form] and go to [   ] or Skip to Next

1. Does this article POTENTIALLY apply to ANY of the key questions?

○ No
⊙ Yes

Include article for: (Check all that apply):
In the care of pediatric or adult patients with asthma, what is the evidence that interventions designed to improve health care provider adherence to guidelines:

☐ KQ1-Impact health care process outcomes (e.g., receiving appropriate treatment)
☐ KQ2-Impact clinical outcomes (e.g., hospitalizations, patient reported outcomes such as symptom control)
☐ KQ3-Impact health care process outcomes that then affect clinical outcomes

Clear Response

5. Comments:
[   ]

List of outcomes - Please click here to see the list of outcomes
Guidelines – Care path, Clinical pathway, recommendations, consensus statements, algorithm
Health care providers - Physicians, nurses, nurse practitioners, physiotherapists/physical therapists, respiratory therapists, pharmacists, and other health care providers

[Submit Form] and go to [   ] or Skip to Next

Study Characteristics

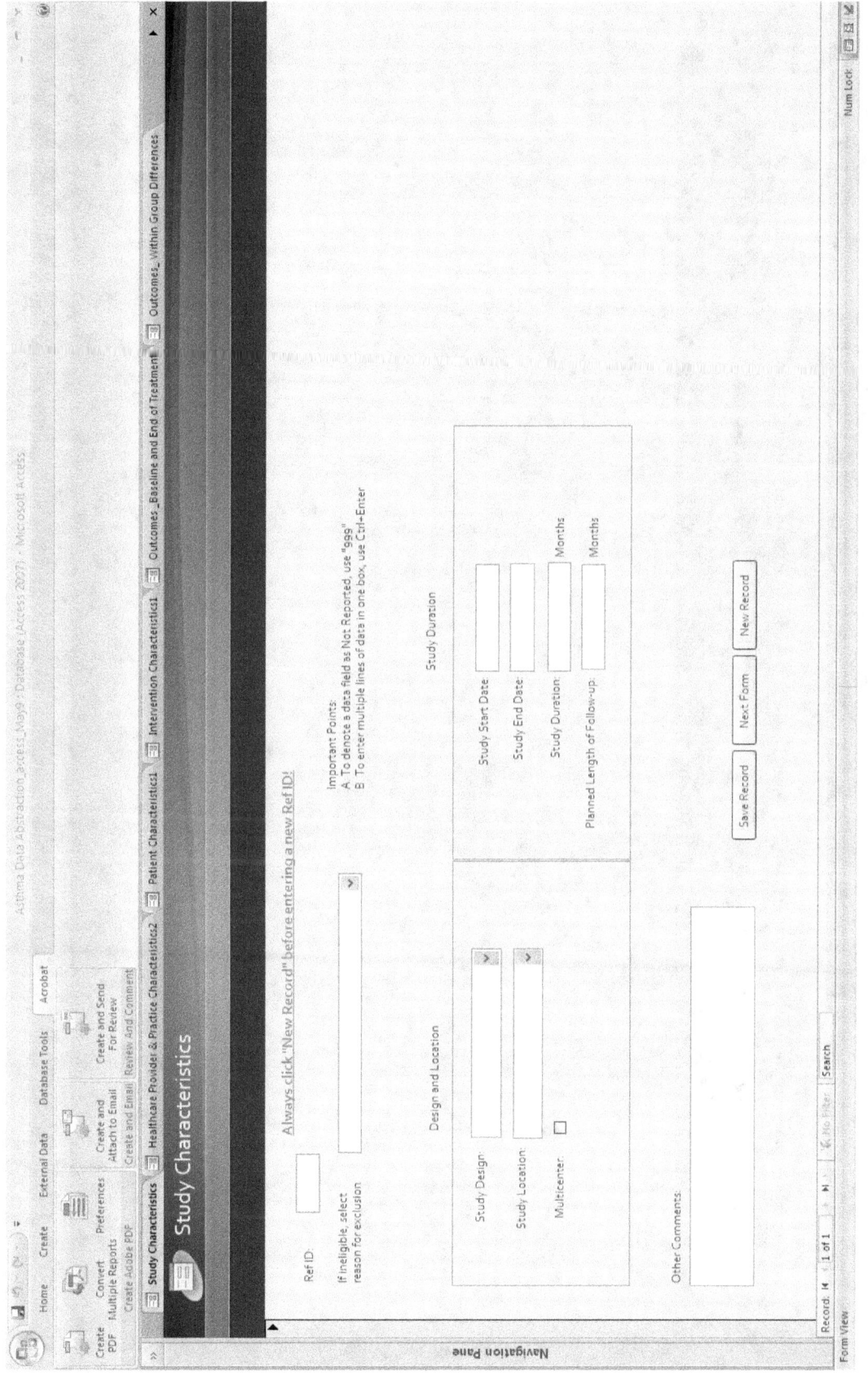

Healthcare Provider and Patient Characteristics (Arm D data fields are identical to A, B, and C)

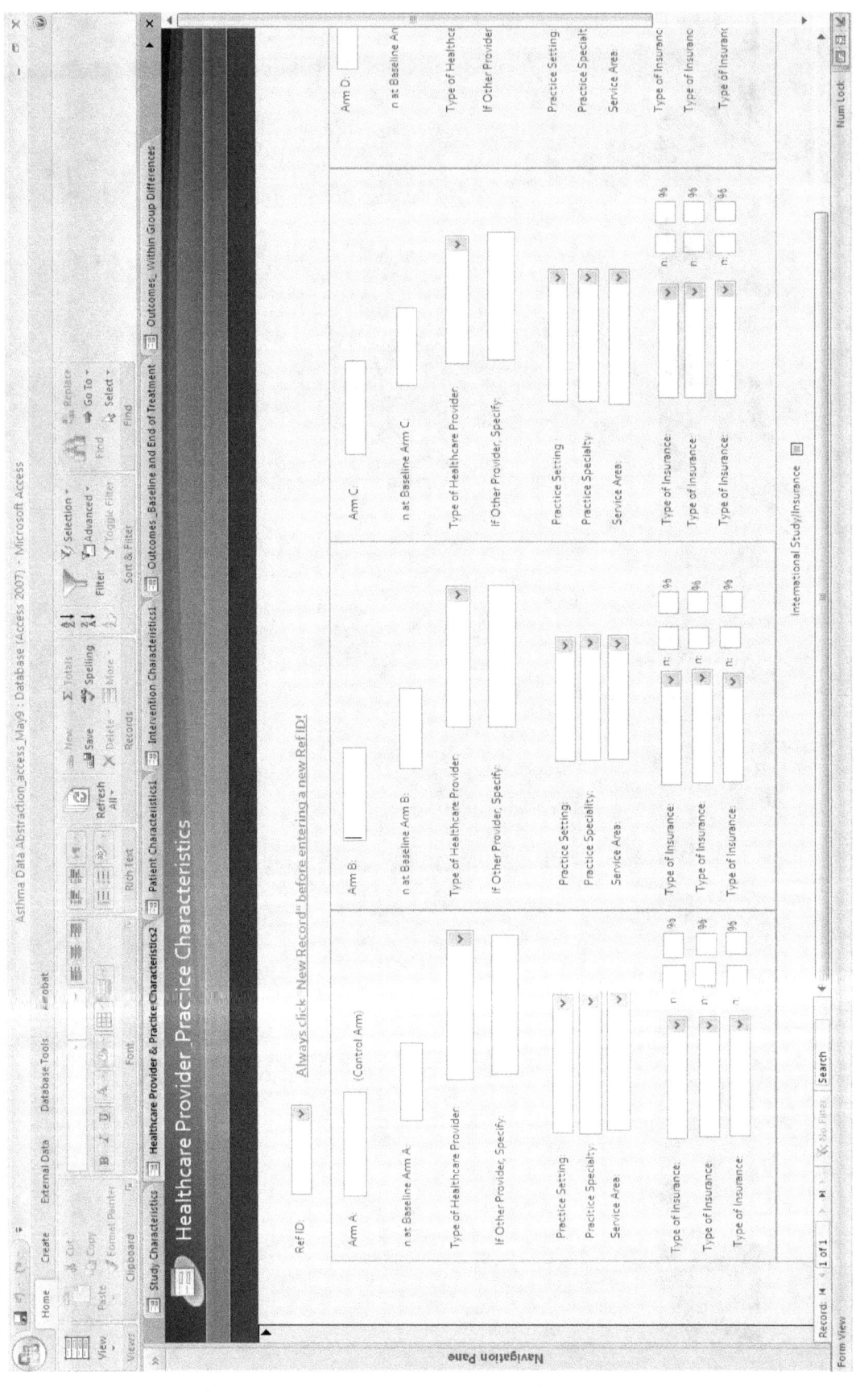

Healthcare Provider and Practice Characteristics – continued

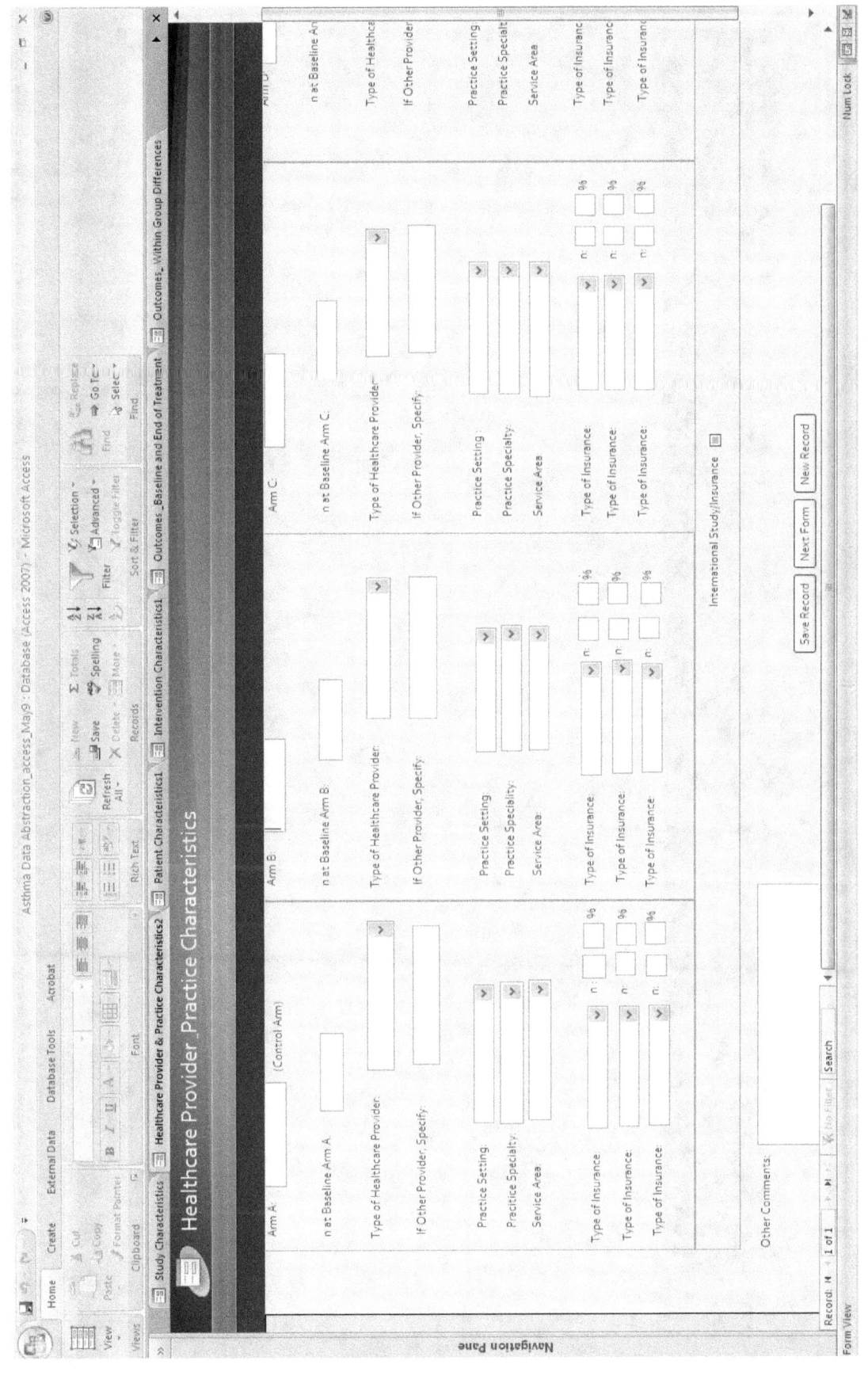

Patient Characteristics

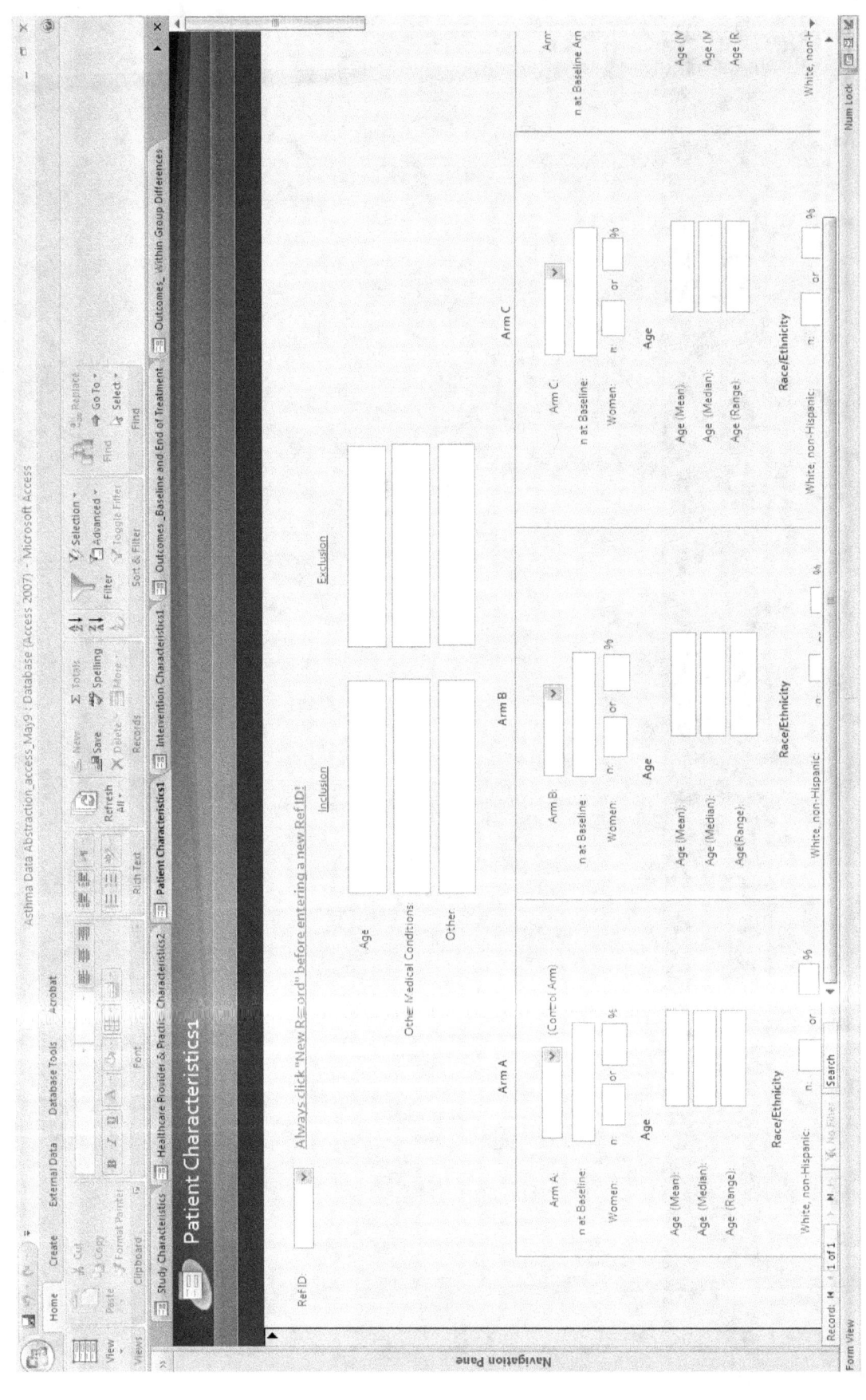

Patient Characteristics – Continued

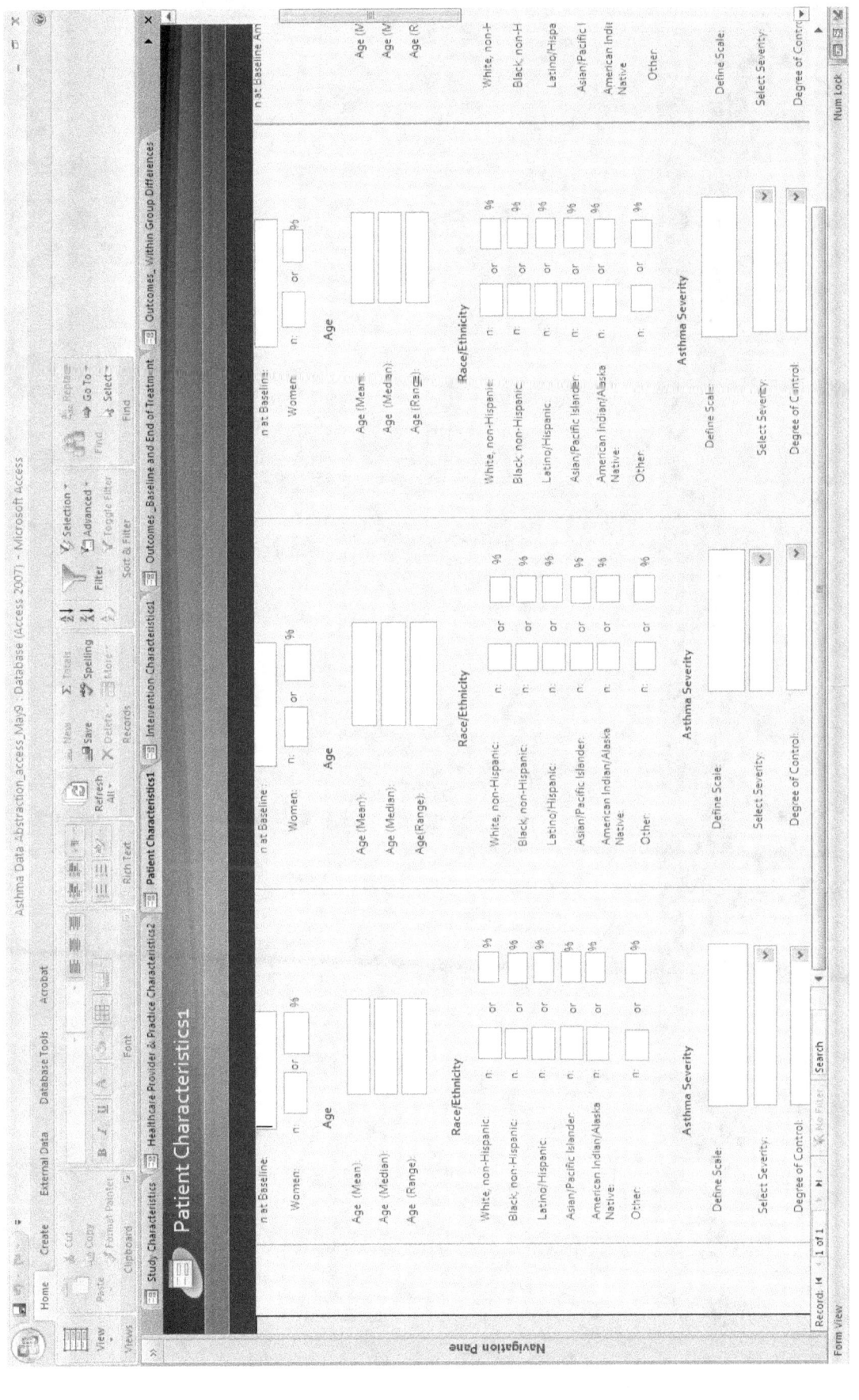

Patient Characteristics – Continued

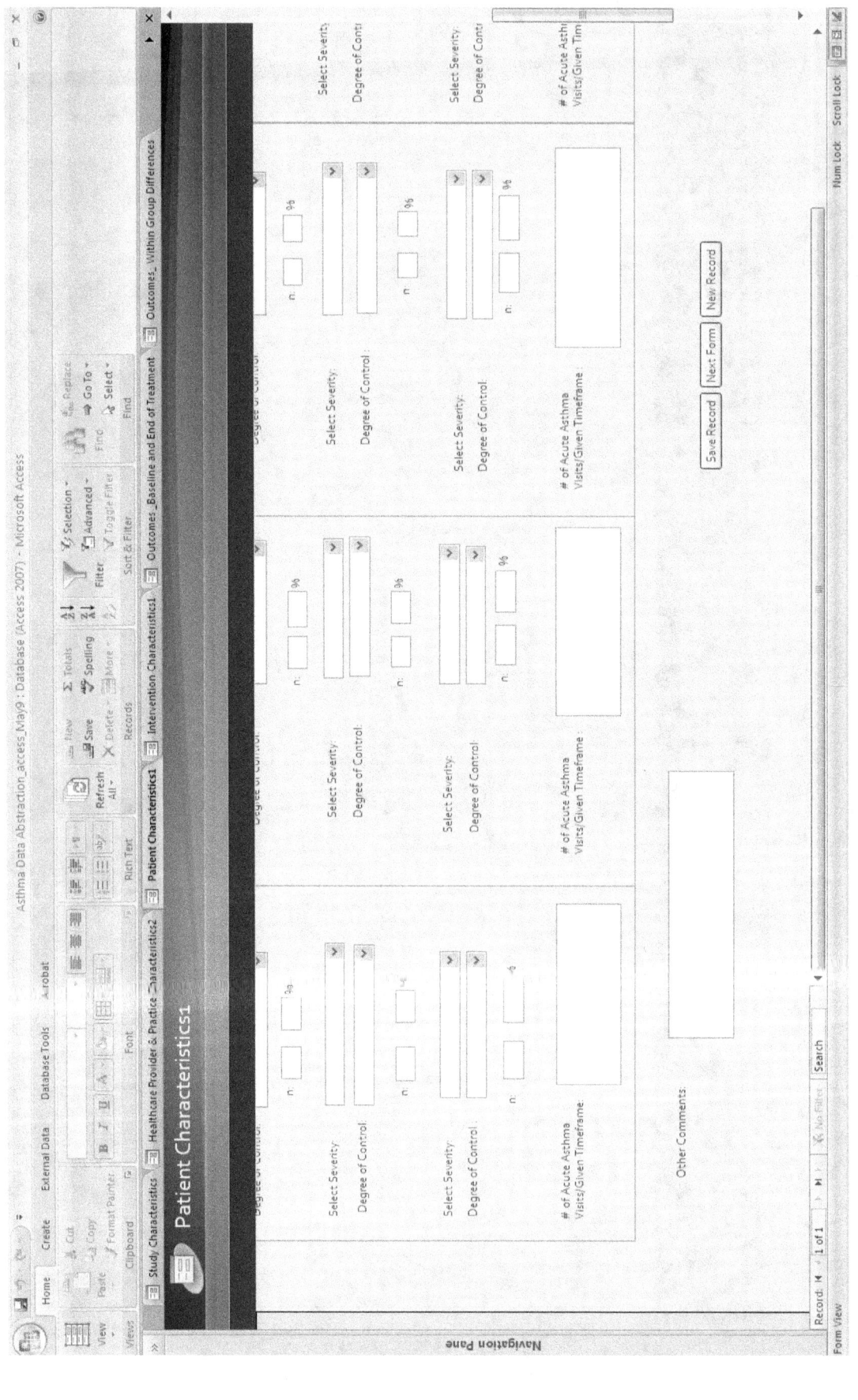

Intervention Characteristics

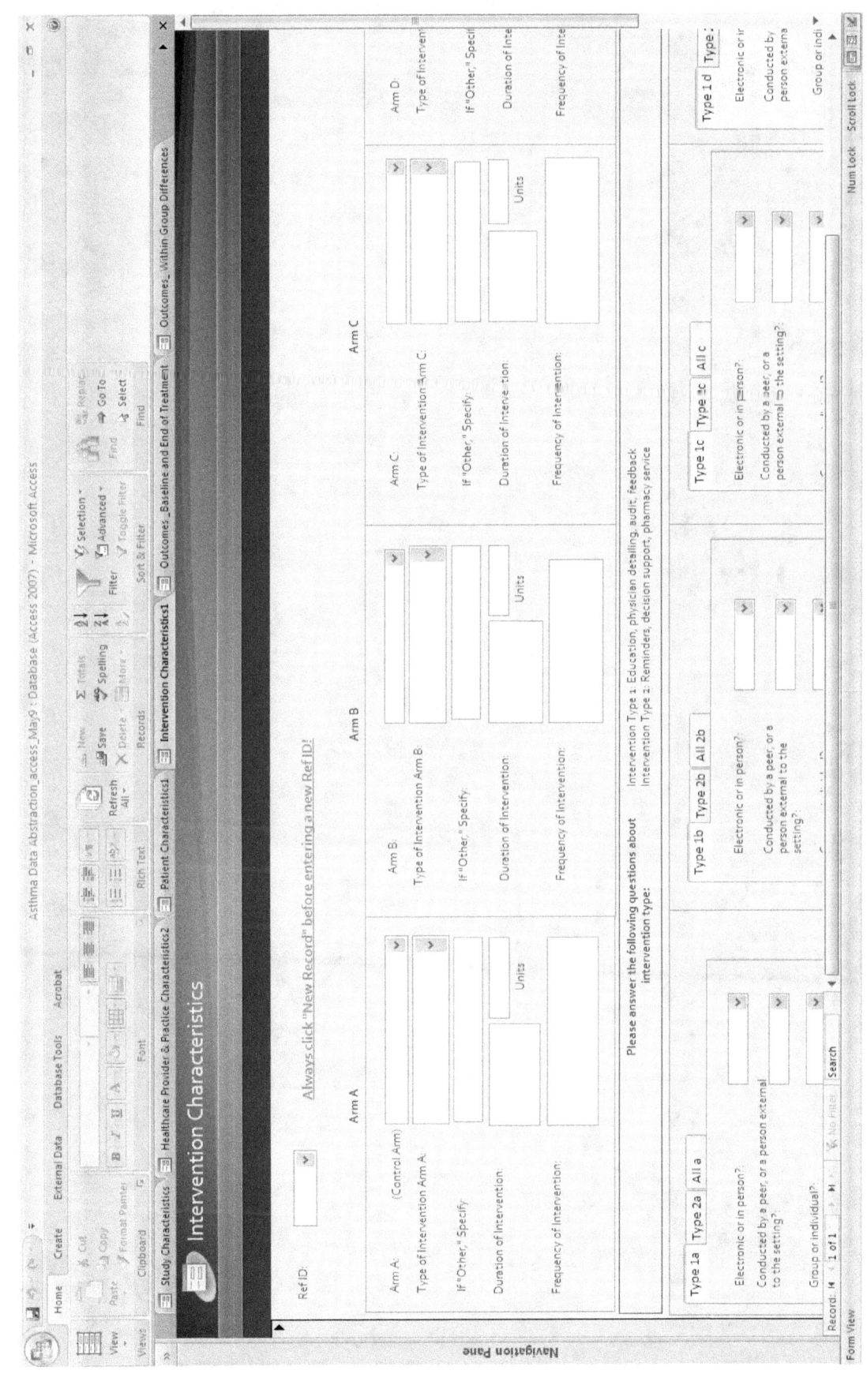

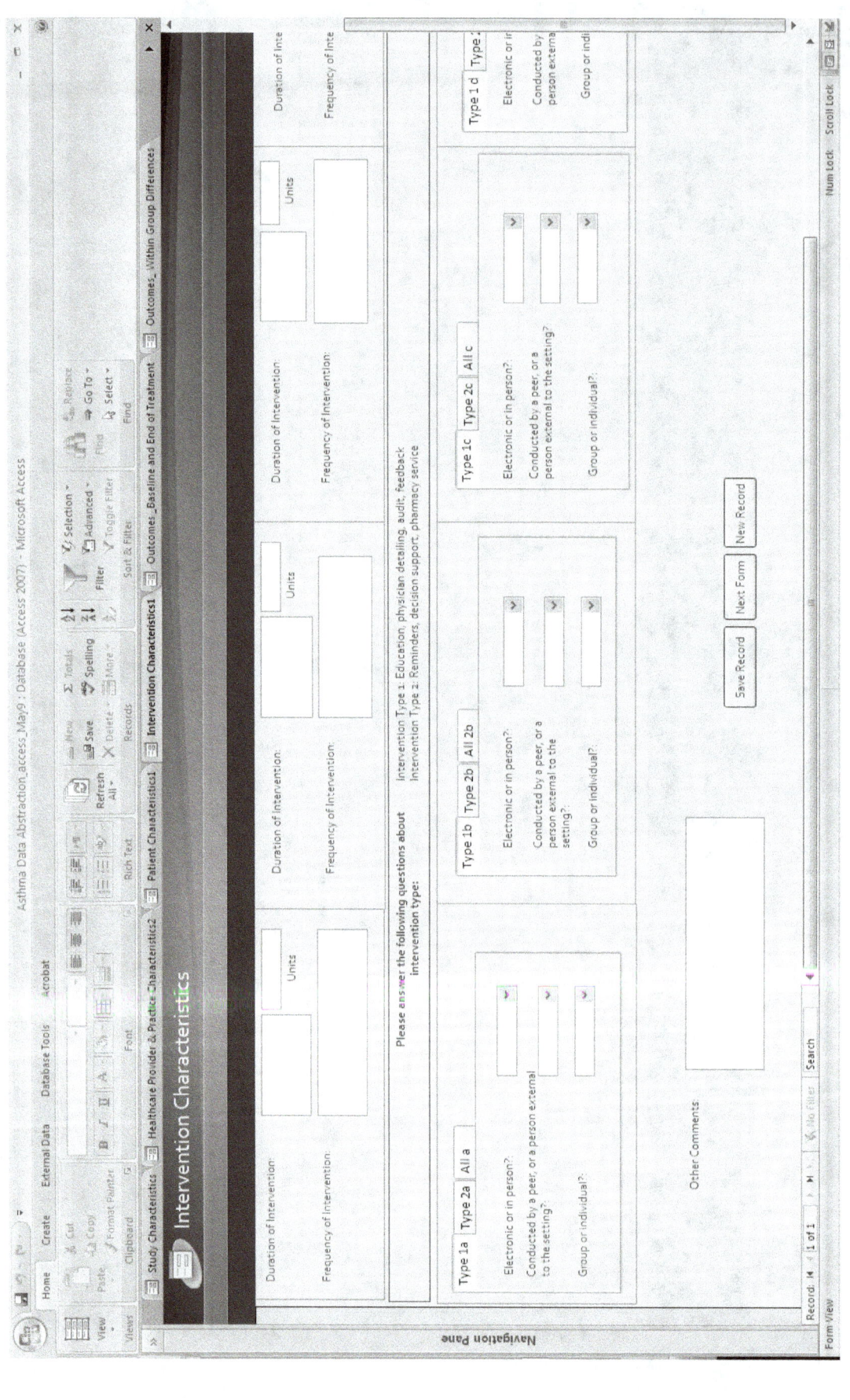

Outcomes – Baseline and End of Treatment

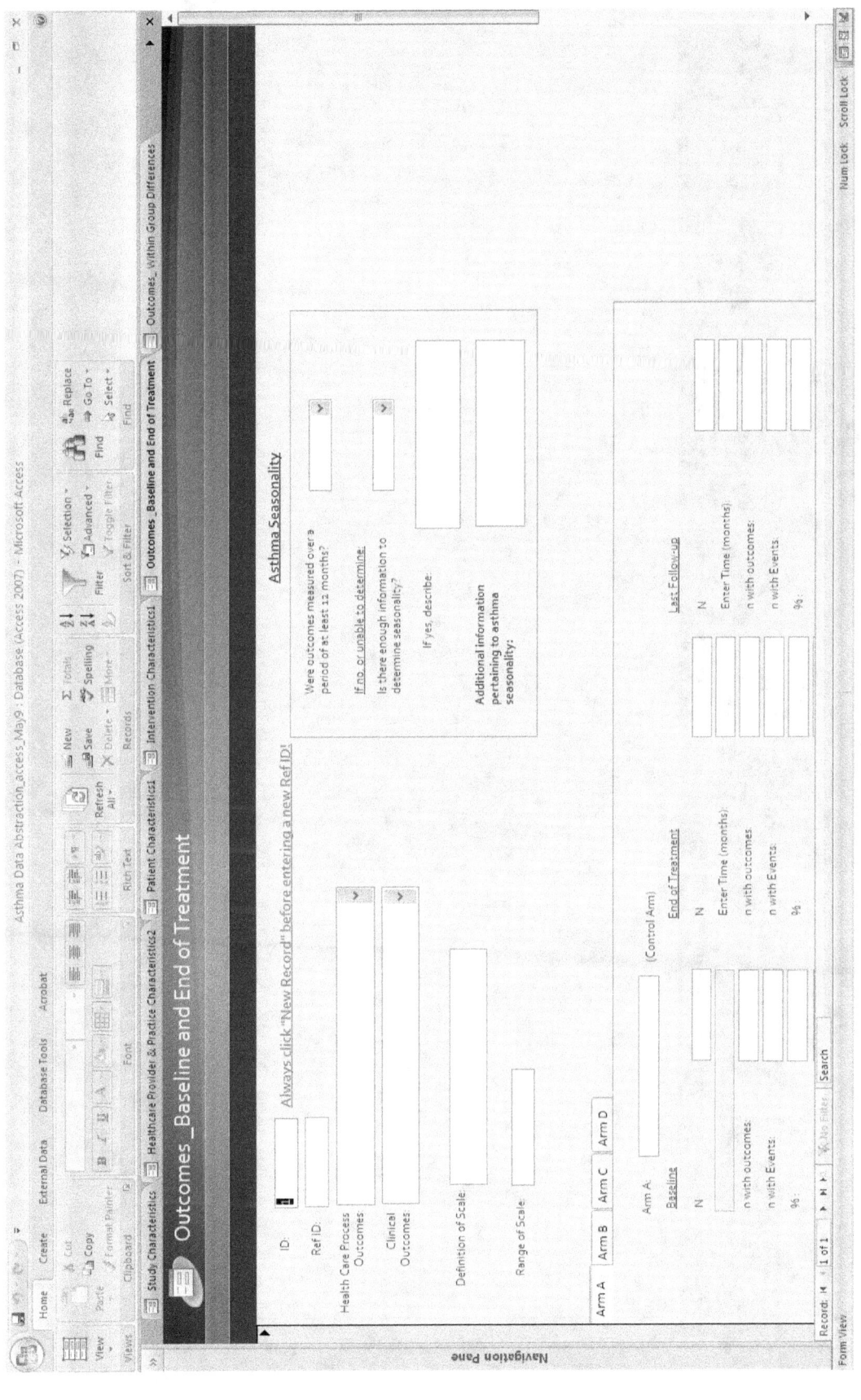

Outcomes – Baseline and End of Treatment – Continued

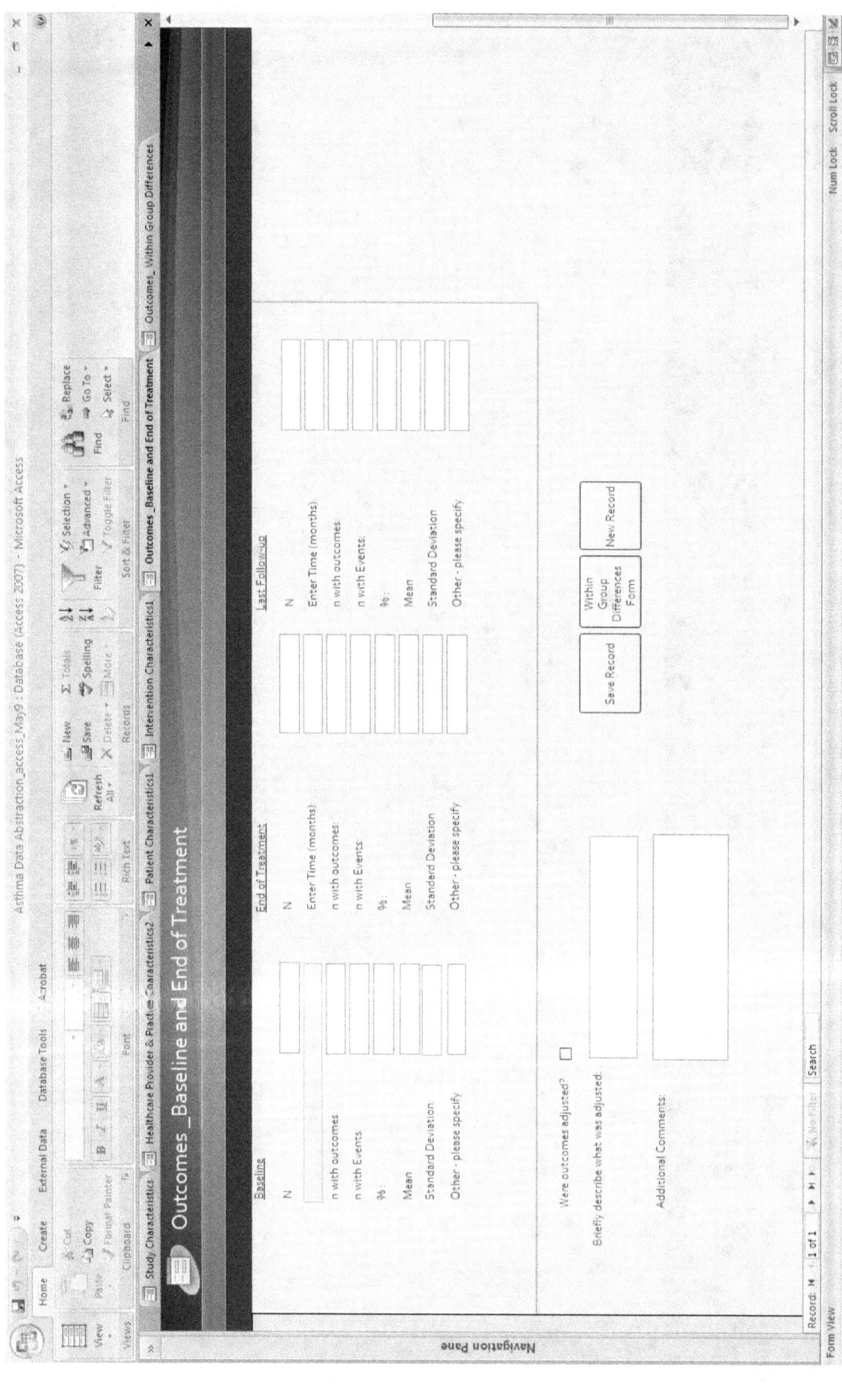

C-14

Outcomes – Within Group Differences

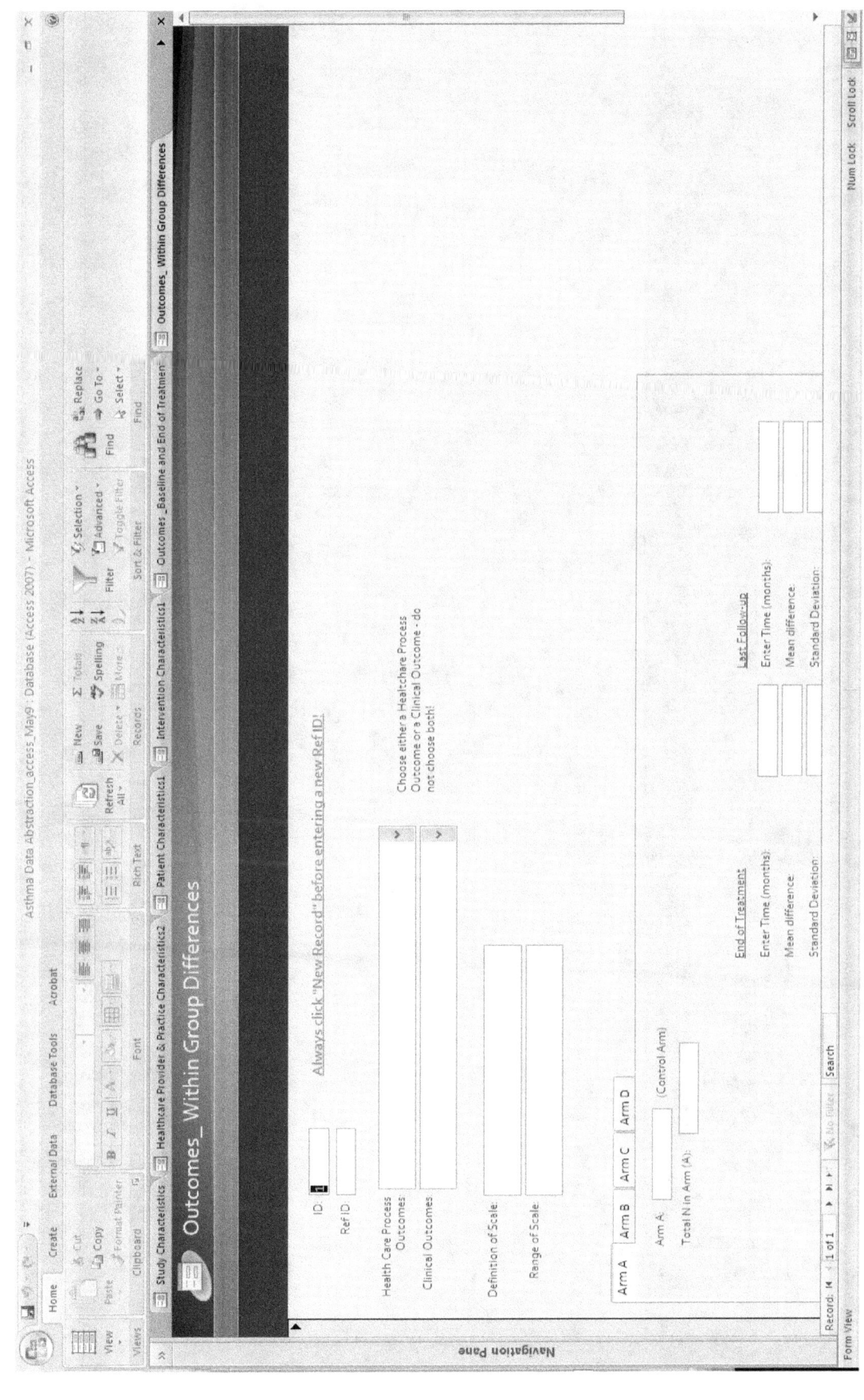

Outcomes – Within Group Differences

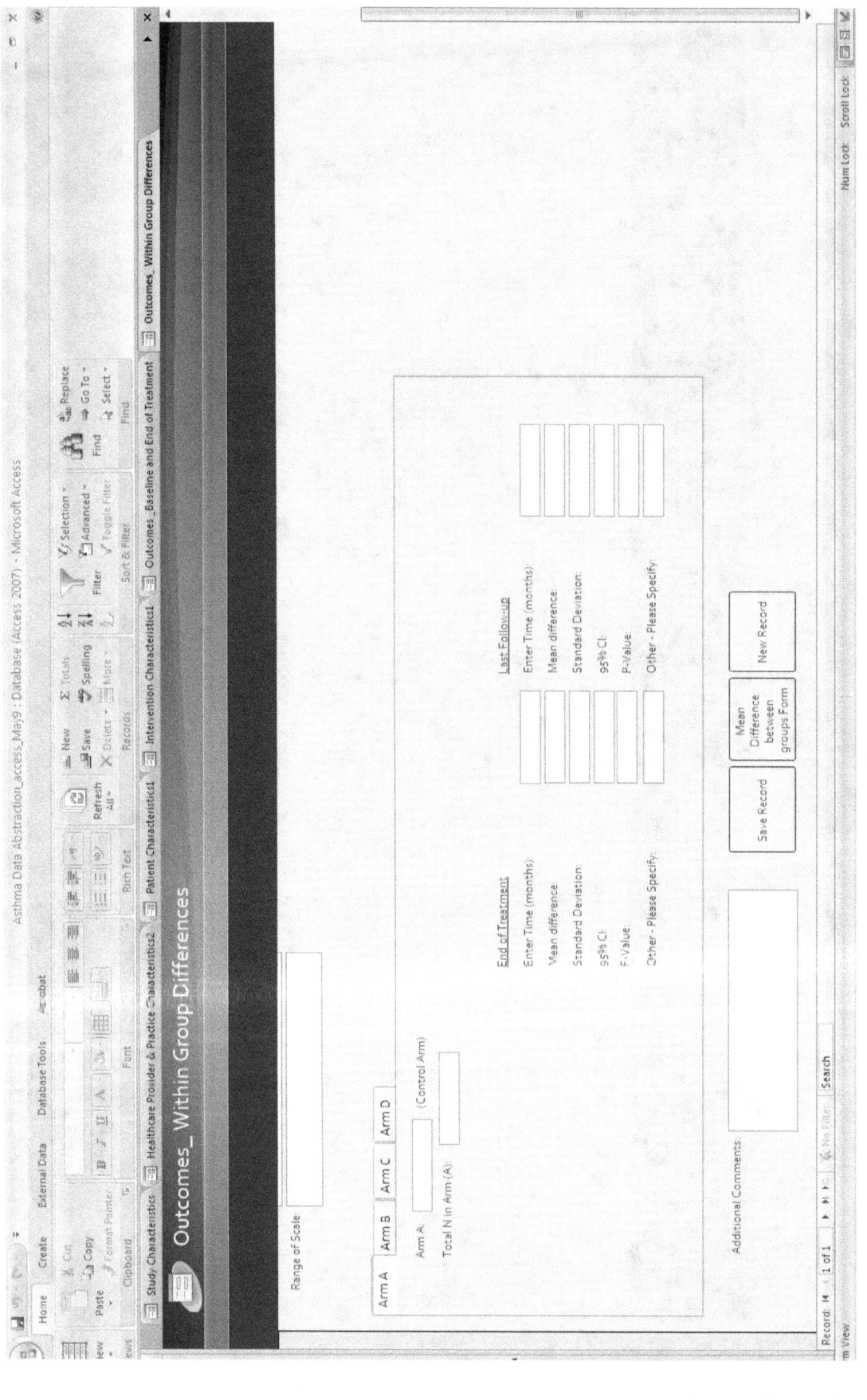

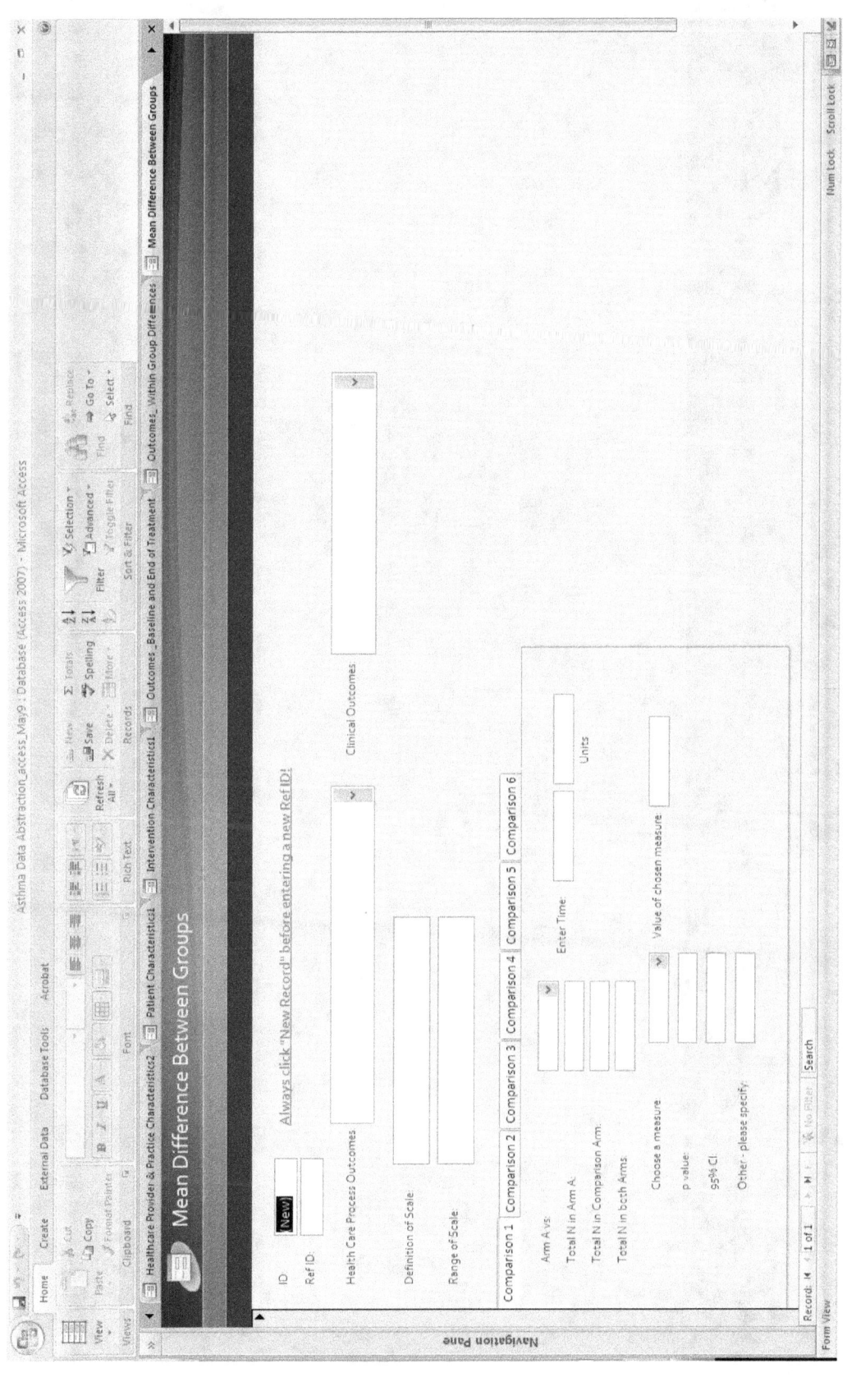

Outcomes – Mean Difference Between Groups – Continued

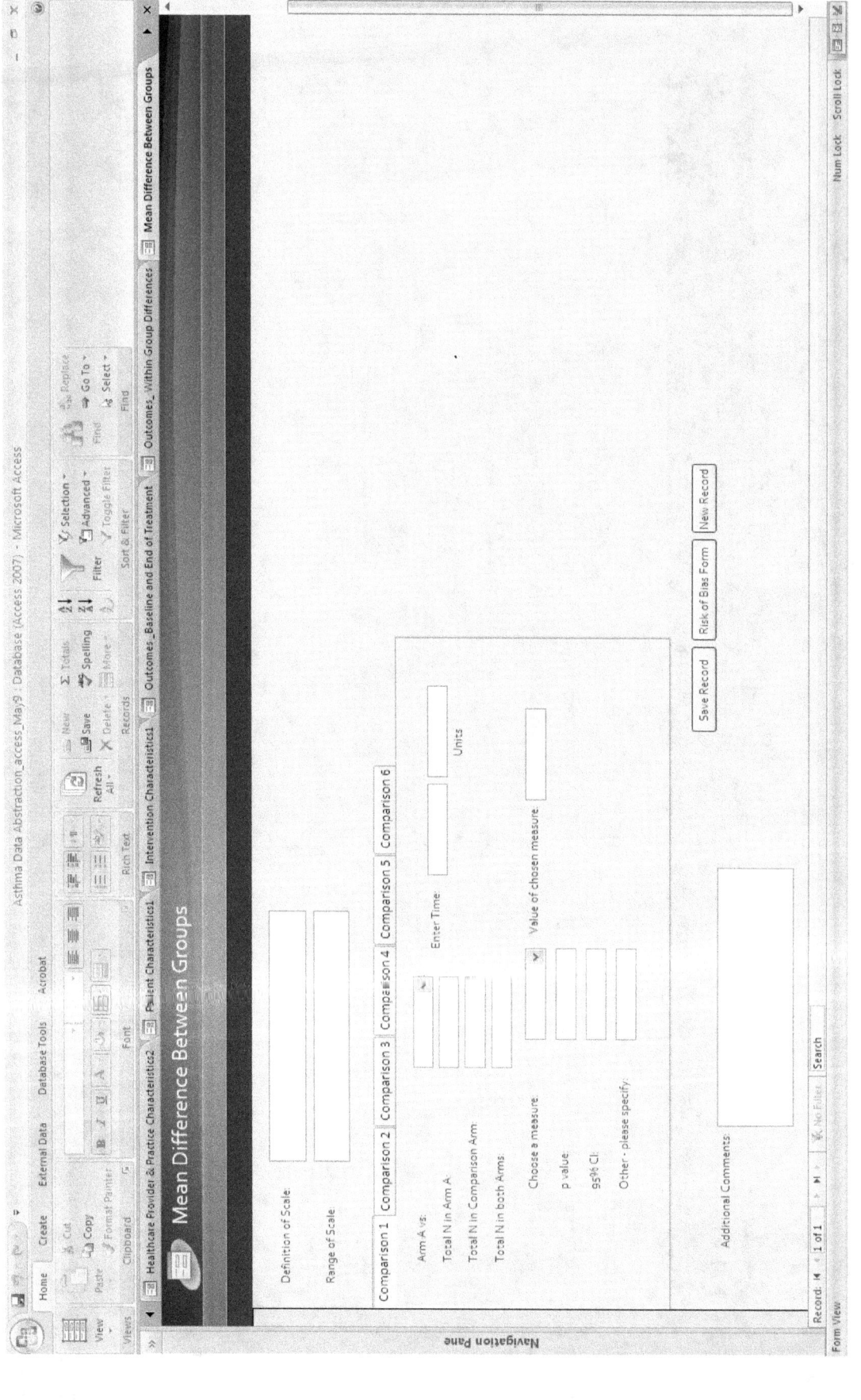

Risk of Bias

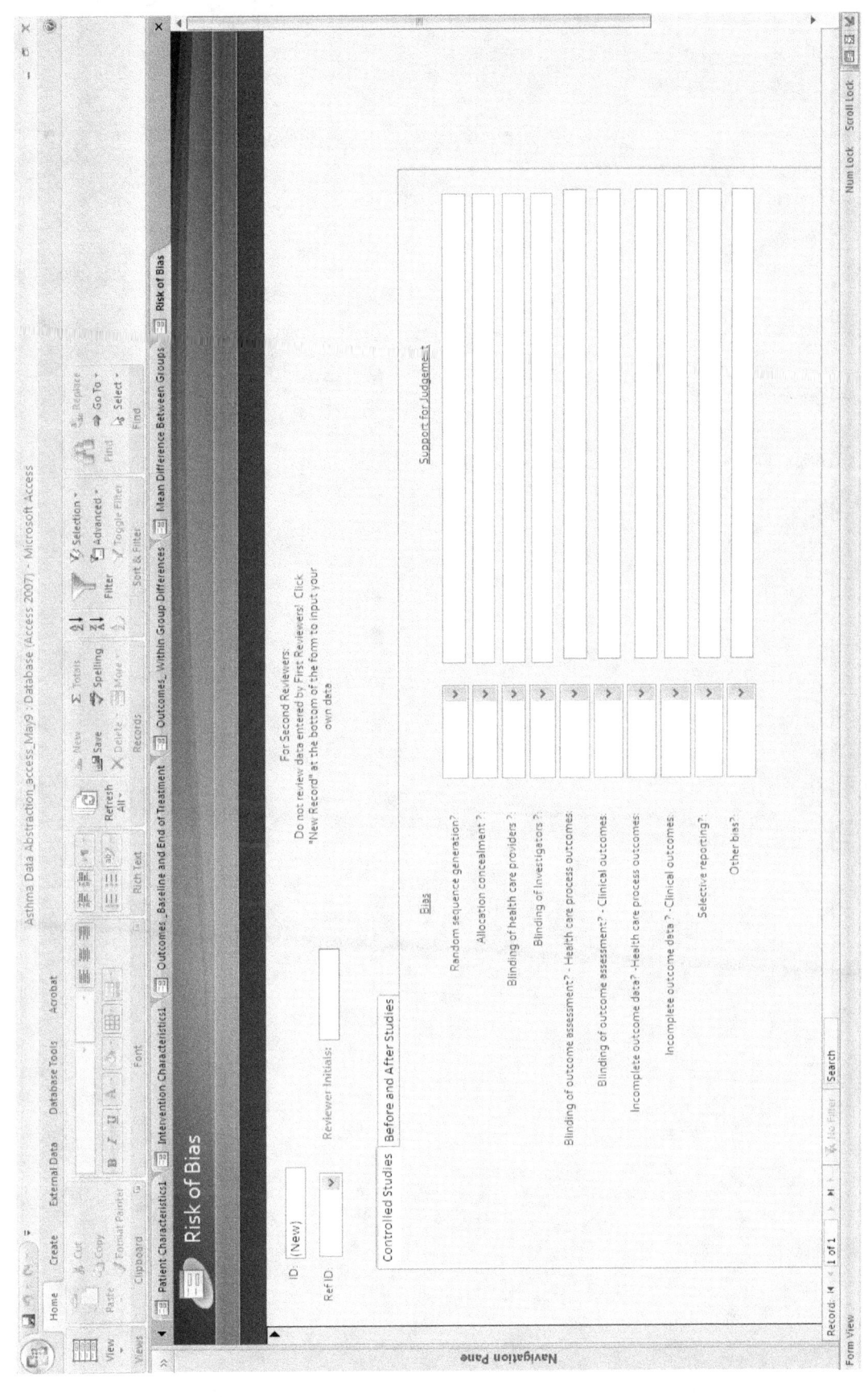

Appendix D. Excluded Studies

Appendix D lists studies that were excluded from this review, categorized by reason for exclusion and alphabetized.

No Original Data

Advocate's disease management program reduces readmissions for CHF and asthma Performance improvement advisor 2003; 7 (3): 44-47.

Al-Moamary M. Annals of Thoracic Medicine... a three-year journey Annals of Thoracic Medicine 2009; 4 (1): 1-2.

Al-Mobeireek A. and Dashash N.A. Prescribing for asthmatic children in primary care. Are we following the guidelines? (multiple letters) Saudi Medical Journal 2003; 24 (11): 1274.

Anhoj J. and Nielsen, L. Quantitative and qualitative usage data of an Internet-based asthma monitoring tool J Med Internet Res 2004; 6 (3): e23.

Anthonisen N. R. Database epidemiology Canadian Respiratory Journal 2009; 16 (6): 181-182.

Bai T. R. Do written self-management plans improve asthma control? The evidence is not conclusive Canadian Respiratory Journal 2003; 10 (3): 155-156.

Bauman A. E., Fardy H. J. and Harris P. G. Getting it right: Why bother with patient-centred care? Medical Journal of Australia 2003; 179 (5): 253-256.

Beilby J. J., Glasgow, N. J., and Fardy, H. J. The way forward: the International Primary Care Respiratory Group 2nd World Conference, Melbourne, 19-22 February 2004 Med J Aust 2004; 181 (2): 67-8.

Benchmarking children's hospitals improves asthma home management Healthcare Benchmarks Qual Improv 2009; 16 (10): 109-13.

Brown H. J. and Miles P. V. "Guidelines" for Guideline Implementation Journal of Pediatrics 2009; 154 (6): 784-785

Burrill R. and Carroll W. Towards evidence based medicine for paediatricians: Question 3 - Do written asthma action plans reduce hospital admissions? Archives of Disease in Childhood 2009; 94 (9): 742-743.

Cabana M. D. and Lewis T. C. Improving physician adherence to asthma guidelines J Clin Outcomes Manag 2001; 8 (3): 35-46.

Campbell, J., Campbell, S., and Woodward, G. Getting evidence into practice using an asthma desktop tool Aust Fam Physician 2006; 35 (1-2): 32-3.

Cartier A. Thanks to a plan of action, the general practitioner can better follow the evolution of asthma, a fluctuating disease, and the unforeseen recrudescences L'Union Médicale du Canada 1991; 120 (6): 491, 494-497.

Chang A. B. American College of Chest Physicians cough guidelines for children: Can its use improve outcomes? CHEST 2008; 134 (6): 1111-1112.

Chen S., Coffey S., Peisachovich E., et al. Implementing best practice guidelines onto personal digital assistants: Preliminary results and lessons learned Journal on Information Technology in Healthcare 2008; 6 (1): 33-41.

Cho S. H. How to organize cost-effective care for asthma patients Respirology 2009; 14 A104.

Chong E. Pharmacist-specific summary of adult asthma guidelines Canadian Pharmacists Journal 2007; 140 (SUPPL. 3): S12-S17.

Chrystyn H. Community care of asthma: The pharmacist as counsellor? Journal of Pharmacy and Pharmacology 1997; 49 (SUPPL. 3): 51-54.

Cicutto L. Supporting successful asthma management in schools: The role of asthma care providers Journal of Allergy and Clinical Immunology 2009; 124 (2): 390-393.

Corjulo M. T. Telephone triage for asthma medication refills Pediatric Nursing 2005; 31 (2): 116-120, 124.

Crockett A. and A. Leonard Local asthma guidelines can help reduce hospital admissions Asthma Journal 2001; 6 (1): 31-34.

Dean M. Implementing the 1998 Canadian asthma guidelines Canadian family physician M?decin de famille canadien 2000; 46 761-762, 768-770.

DiCenso A., Virani T., Bajnok I., et al. A toolkit to facilitate the implementation of clinical practice guidelines in healthcare settings Hospital quarterly 2002; 5 (3): 55-60.

D'Urzo A. D., Tamari I., Bouchard J., et al. Jugovic Limitations of a spirometry interpretation algorithm Canadian Family Physician 2011; 57 (10): 1153-1156.

Eccles M., J. Grimshaw, N. Steen, D. Parkin, I. Purves, E. McColl and N. Rousseau The design and analysis of a randomized controlled trial to evaluate computerized decision support in primary care: The COGENT study Family Practice 2000; 17 (2): 180-186.

Eccles M., McColl E., Steen N., et al. Computerised evidence-based guidelines may not improve asthma or angina management in primary care Evidence-Based Healthcare 2003; 7 (2): 81-82.

Einterz E. M. Apollo at the front Lancet 2005; 365 (9477): 2147-2148.

Emery J. D., Purves I. N., Beaumont R., et al. Parkin Effect of computerised evidence based guidelines [3] British Medical Journal 2003; 326 (7385): 394-396.

English, R. G., Fairall, L. R., and Bateman, E. D. Keeping allergy on the agenda: integrated guidelines for respiratory disease in developing countries Allergy 2007; 62 (3): 224-9.

Fardy, H. J. The 3+ plan for asthma management Aust Fam Physician 99; 28 (2): 95.

Feifer R. A., Verbrugge R. R., Khalid M., et al. Improvements in asthma pharmacotherapy and self-management: an example of a population-based disease management program Disease Management & Health Outcomes 2004; 12 (2): 93-102.

Global initiative for asthma: Global strategy for asthma management and prevention Global Initiative for Asthma 2002;

Hayes E., Djaferis M., Gattasso S., et al. Documenting to improve pediatric asthma outcomes: practical tools for nurse practitioners Advance for nurse practitioners 2004; 12 (9): 51-53, 55-56.

Heale J., Davis D., Norman G., et al. A randomized controlled trial assessing the impact of problem-based versus didactic teaching methods in CME Proceedings of the . Annual Conference on Research in Medical Education. Conference on Research in Medical Education 1988; 27 72-77.

Lack of self-efficacy keeps inner-city primary care providers from following national asthma management guidelines AHRQ Research Activities 2009; (345): 15-15.

Li J. T., Oppenheimer J., Bernstein I. L., et al. Attaining optimal asthma control: A practice parameter Journal of Allergy and Clinical Immunology 2005; 116 (5): S3-S11.

Loymans R., ter Riet G. and Sterk P. J. Assessing primary care physicians' beliefs and attitudes of asthma exacerbation treatment and follow-up Open Respiratory Medicine Journal 2011; 5 (1): 10.

Mansour, M. E. How do we support follow-up with the primary care provider after an emergency department visit for asthma? Pediatrics 2009; 124 (4): 1206-7.

Marshik, P. L. Pharmacologic treatment of pediatric asthma. Consider disease severity as well as delivery method Adv Nurse Pract 2004; 12 (3): 35-6, 41-6.

McDermott M. F., Walter J., Catrambone C., et al. The Chicago Emergency Department Asthma Collaborative CHEST 1999; 116 (4 SUPPL. 1): 196S-197S.

McIvor, A. and Hodder, R. Canadian Adult Asthma Update 2008 key messages: a focus on translating knowledge into action in primary care Can Respir J 2008; 15 (3): 121-2.

McLean W. M. and L. D. MacKeigan When does pharmaceutical care impact health outcomes? A comparison of community pharmacy-based studies of pharmaceutical care for patients with asthma Annals of Pharmacotherapy 2005; 39 (4): 625-631.

Meadows M. Breathing better: action plans keep asthma in check FDA Consumer 2003; 37 (2): 20-27.

Metzger W. J. The asthma guidelines: Implications for the practicing physician American Family Physician 1992; 46 (4): 1060-1062.

Meyer H. Targeted Care Improvements Show Promising Results For Treating Children With Asthma Health Affairs 2011; 30 (3): 404-407.

Mihaltan, F. [Asthma--between "control" and "severity"] Pneumologia 2008; 57 (4): 192-3.

Modell, M., Iliffe, S., Austin, A., and Leaning, M. S. From guidelines to decision support in the management of asthma Stud Health Technol Inform 95; 16 105-13.

Oppedisano, R. and Kavuru, M. S. Asthma patient education: a primer for the primary care physician Compr Ther 96; 22 (11): 695-702.

Partridge, M. R. Introduction to the Global Initiative for Asthma and the new guidelines West Indian Med J 2003; 52 Suppl 7 6-9.

Partridge, M. R. The implementation of asthma guidelines in general practice Respir Med 97; 91 (10): 575-7.

Philpot E. E. and Kwasnicki J. M. The impact of the NHLBI guidelines on asthma management in the prescribing habits of physicians at two community hospitals J Allergy Clin Immunol 1993; 91

Rance, K. and Trent, C. Broccoli and pixie stix. Profile of a pediatric asthma program Adv Nurse Pract 2004; 12 (3): 47-8.

Reed, C. E. Inhaled corticosteroids: why do physicians and patients fail to comply with guidelines for managing asthma? Mayo Clin Proc 2004; 79 (4): 453-5.

Roberts D. H., Gilmartin G. S., Neeman N., et al. Design and measurement of quality improvement indicators in ambulatory pulmonary care: Creating a "culture of quality" in an academic pulmonary division CHEST 2009; 136 (4): 1134-1140.

Schonberger H. J. A. M. and Van Schayck C. P. Prevention of asthma in genetically predisposed children in primary care - From clinical efficacy to a feasible intervention programme Clinical and Experimental Allergy 1998; 28 (11): 1325-1331.

Scullion J. E. A specialist nurse led liaison model of care reduced unscheduled care for acute asthma in a deprived multiethnic area Evidence Based Nursing 2004; 7 (3): 77-77.

Self T. H., Kelso T. M., Abou-Shala N., et al. Clinical pharmacist initiated programs for improving outcomes in adult, African American asthmatics 1992;

Sladek, K. [Education program in asthma] Pneumonol Alergol Pol 2002; 70 Suppl 1 87-90.

Soumerai S. B., Majumdar S. R. and Lipton H. L. Evaluating and improving physician prescribing Pharmacoepidemiology 2000; 483-503.

Specialized asthma unit improves care, cuts costs Health Care Cost Reengineering Rep 98; 3 (7): 97-101.

Thomson M. A., O'Brien A. D. Oxman D. A., et al. Educational outreach visits: Effects on professional practice and health care outcomes Educational Outreach Visits: Effects on Professional Practice and Health Care Outcomes 2000;

Two approaches toward systematic change boost asthma care Dis Manag Advis 2005; 11 (1): 4-8, 1.

Van Rees-Wortelboer M. M. The Stimulation Program
Health Examination. VII. Evaluation of the part on 'General
Practice and CARA' Nederlands Tijdschrift voor
Geneeskunde 1996; 140 (12): 672-675.

Weinberger, M. M. What is the problem with asthma care
for children? Arch Pediatr Adolesc Med 2011; 165 (5):
473-5.

Weir, S. S. Disease management in primary care: rapid
cycle quality improvement of asthma care N C Med J 2005;
66 (3): 221-2.

Williams, D., Portnoy, J. M., and Meyerson, K. Strategies
for improving asthma outcomes: a case-based review of
successes and pitfalls J Manag Care Pharm 2010; 16 (1
Suppl C): S3-14; quiz S16-7.

Wroth T. H. and Boals J. C. 4th Application of quality-
improvement methods in a community practice: the
Sandhills Pediatrics Asthma Initiative North Carolina
medical journal 2005; 66 (3): 218-220.

Yawn, B. P. Participatory research in rural primary care
Minn Med 2004; 87 (9): 52-4.

Zeitz H. J., Davis W. J., Kniker W. T., et al. Problem-based
learning (PBL) for asthma continuing medical education
(CME) Ann Allergy Asthma Immunol 1996; 76 121.

Non-English

Andersen, M., Kragstrup, J., and Sorensen, J. [How
participation in a clinical trial affects doctors' choice of
treatment] Ugeskr Laeger 2006; 168 (46): 3987-91.

Eimers M., A. Van Der Aalst, B. Pelzer, M. Teichert and
H. De Wit Does a good PTAM lead to improved
prescribing? Huisarts en Wetenschap 2008; 51 (7): 340-
345.

Geijer RMM., Van Hensbergen W., Bottema BJAM, et al.
Standard for the treatment of asthma in adults of the Dutch
Association for General Practitioners Huisarts en
Wetenschap 2001; 44 (4): 153-164.

Geraedts, M., Selbmann, H. K., and Meisner, C. [Effects of
a regional intervention to promote asthma guidelines
implementation] Gesundheitswesen 2002; 64 (5): 235-41.

Gillissen, A. and Worth, H. [New paradigm in asthma
management] MMW Fortschr Med 2010; 152 (11): 33-4.

Kaufmann-Kolle P., J. Szecsenyi, B. Broge, W. E. Haefeli
and A. Schneider Does implementation of benchmarking in
quality circles improve the quality of care of patients with
asthma and reduce drug interaction? Zeitschrift fur Evidenz
Fortbildung und Qualitat im Gesundheitswesen 2011; 105
(5): 389-395.

Kull, I., Johansson, G. S., Lisspers, K., Jagorstrand, B.,
Romberg, K., Tilling, B., and Stallberg, B. [Efficient care
in asthma/COPD primary health care clinics]
Lakartidningen 2008; 105 (42): 2937-40.

Launois R, A. C. Megnigbeto, V. Perez, M. Roy, A.
Camus, M. Gailhardou, F. Lancon and M. Queniart A
disease management program in France: Lessons from the
RESALIS experiment before and after public health
interventions Journal d'Economie Medicale 2002; 20 (6):
333-352.

Plaza, V., Cobos, A., Ignacio-Garcia, J. M., Molina, J.,
Bergonon, S., Garcia-Alonso, F., and Espinosa, C. [Cost-
effectiveness of an intervention based on the Global
INitiative for Asthma (GINA) recommendations using a
computerized clinical decision support system: a physicians
randomized trial] Med Clin (Barc) 2005; 124 (6): 201-6.

Ruiz Espiricueta, J. E., Gonzalez Diaz, S. N., Rodriguez, G.
G., Cruz, A. A., Canseco Villarreal, C., and Valdez
Ramirez, M. A. [Assessment of an educational course on
asthma for primary care physicians] Rev Alerg Mex 2005;
52 (2): 83-9.

Schauerte G., O. Laub, H. Hohre, S. Schwab, M.
Unverdorben, C. Bredl, M. Schober and J. Lecheler
Healthcare program for children with bronchial asthma
Atemwegs- und Lungenkrankheiten 2009; 35 (9): 379-387.

Scriba P. C. and C. Fuchs Health services research: Trend-
setting promotional initiative Deutsches Arzteblatt 2010;
107 (17): A812-A816.

Segura Mendez, N. H., Herrera, S., Hernandez Martinez, E., Torres Salazar, A., Espinola Reyna, G., and del Rivero Hernandez, L. [Application of the International Guide for the Diagnosis and Treatment of Asthma using first-contact physicians, before and after an educational strategy] Rev Alerg Mex 2003; 50 (3): 83-5.

Sladek, K. [Education program in asthma] Pneumonol Alergol Pol 2002; 70 Suppl 1 87-90.

Van Rees-Wortelboer M. M. The Stimulation Program Health Examination. VII. Evaluation of the part on 'General Practice and CARA' Nederlands Tijdschrift voor Geneeskunde 1996; 140 (12): 672-675.

Warlies F. and M. Saladin The outcome of the train-the-trainer seminars arranged by the "Work Team Patients Education" for instructing adult patients with chronic obstructive pulmonary diseases (asthma and COPD) Atemwegs- und Lungenkrankheiten 2005; 31 (10): 510-522.

Does not Address Asthma

Camacho M., Nogales, MR. Manjon, M. Del Granado, A. Pio and S. Ottmani Results of PAL feasibility test in primary health care facilities in four regions of Bolivia International Journal of Tuberculosis and Lung Disease 2007; 11 (11): 1246-1252.

Jans, M. P., Schellevis, F. G., Van Hensbergen, W., and van Eijk, J. T. Improving general practice care of patients with asthma or chronic obstructive pulmonary disease: evaluation of a quality system Eff Clin Pract 2000; 3 (1): 16-24.

Jiwa M, Hughes J, Sriram D et al. Piloting and validating an innovation to triage patients presenting with cough to community pharmacies in Western Australia. Quality in Primary Care 2012; 20(2):83-91.

Jones RCM, Copper S. Does implementing COPD guidelines improve patient care and save money in practice? Asthma in General Practice 1999; 7 (1): 12-15.

Kuilboer, M. M., van Wijk, M. A., Mosseveld, M., van der Does, E., de Jongste, J. C., Overbeek, S. E., Ponsioen, B., and van der Lei, J. Computed critiquing integrated into daily clinical practice affects physicians' behavior--a randomized clinical trial with AsthmaCritic Methods Inf Med 2006; 45 (4): 447-54.

Levac, K. A. Putting outcomes into practice in physician offices J Nurs Care Qual 2002; 17 (1): 51-62; quiz 90.

Meulepas, M. A., Jacobs J. F, Smeenk, F. W., Smeele, I., Lucas, A. E., Bottema, B. J., and Grol, R. P. Effect of an integrated primary care model on the management of middle-aged and old patients with obstructive lung diseases Scand J Prim Health Care 2007; 25 (3): 186-92.

Newton-Syms F. A. O., Dawson P. H., Cooke J., et al. The influence of an academic representative on prescribing by general practitioners British Journal of Clinical Pharmacology 1992; 33 (1): 69-73.

Ornstein, S. M., Jenkins, R. G., MacFarlane, L., Glaser, A., Snyder, K., and Gundrum, T. Electronic medical records as tools for quality improvement in ambulatory practice: theory and a case study Top Health Inf Manage 98; 19 (2): 35-43.

Rascati KL, Okano GJ, Burch C. Evaluation of Physician Intervention Letters Medical Care 1996; 34 (8): 760-766.

Roberts D. H., Gilmartin G. S., Neeman N., et al. Design and measurement of quality improvement indicators in ambulatory pulmonary care: Creating a "culture of quality" in an academic pulmonary division CHEST 2009; 136 (4): 1134-1140.

Stange K. C., Goodwin M. A., Zyzanski S. J., et al. Dietrich Sustainability of a practice-individualized preventive service delivery intervention American Journal of Preventive Medicine 2003; 25 (4): 296-300.

Tierney, W. M., Overhage, J. M., Murray, M. D., Harris, L. E., Zhou, X. H., Eckert, G. J., Smith, F. E., Nienaber, N., McDonald, C. J., and Wolinsky, F. D. Can computer-generated evidence-based care suggestions enhance evidence-based management of asthma and chronic obstructive pulmonary disease? A randomized, controlled trial Health Serv Res 2005; 40 (2): 477-97.

Addressed Inpatient or Emergency Care Only

Benchmarking children's hospitals improves asthma home management Healthcare Benchmarks Qual Improv 2009; 16 (10): 109-13.

Chandler, T. Reducing re-admission for asthma: impact of a nurse-led service Paediatr Nurs 2007; 19 (10): 19-21.

Davies, B., Edwards, N., Ploeg, J., and Virani, T. Insights about the process and impact of implementing nursing guidelines on delivery of care in hospitals and community settings BMC Health Serv Res 2008; 8 29.

Doherty S. R. and Jones P. D. Use of an 'evidence-based implementation' strategy to implement evidence-based care of asthma into rural district hospital emergency departments Rural and remote health 2006; (1): 529.

Hadjianastassiou VG., Karadaglis D. and Gavalas M. A comparison between different formats of educational feedback to junior doctors: A prospective pilot intervention study Journal of the Royal College of Surgeons of Edinburgh 2001; 46 (6): 354-357.

Higuchi, K. S., Davies, B. L., Edwards, N., Ploeg, J., and Virani, T. Implementation of clinical guidelines for adults with asthma and diabetes: a three-year follow-up evaluation of nursing care J Clin Nurs 2011; 20 (9-10): 1329-38.

Kwok, R., Dinh, M., Dinh, D., and Chu, M. Improving adherence to asthma clinical guidelines and discharge documentation from emergency departments: implementation of a dynamic and integrated electronic decision support system Emerg Med Australas 2009; 21 (1): 31-7.

Mackey, D., Myles, M., Spooner, C. H., Lari, H., Tyler, L., Blitz, S., Senthilselvan, A., and Rowe, B. H. Changing the process of care and practice in acute asthma in the emergency department: experience with an asthma care map in a regional hospital CJEM 2007; 9 (5): 353-65.

Mason, N., Roberts, N., Yard, N., and Partridge, M. R. Nebulisers or spacers for the administration of bronchodilators to those with asthma attending emergency departments? Respir Med 2008; 102 (7): 993-8.

Masters, G., Hall, S. E., Phillips, M., and Boldy, D. Outcomes measurement for asthma following acute presentation to an emergency department Aust Health Rev 2001; 24 (3): 53-60.

Specialized asthma unit improves care, cuts costs Health Care Cost Reengineering Rep 98; 3 (7): 97-101.

Wazeka, A., Valacer, D. J., Cooper, M., Caplan, D. W., and DiMaio, M. Impact of a pediatric asthma clinical pathway on hospital cost and length of stay Pediatr Pulmonol 2001; 32 (3): 211-6.

Webb, L. Z., Kuykendall, D. H., Zeiger, R. S., Berquist, S. L., Lischio, D., Wilson, T., and Freedman, C. The impact of status asthmaticus practice guidelines on patient outcome and physician behavior QRB Qual Rev Bull 92; 18 (12): 471-6.

Wright, S. W., Trott, A., Lindsell, C. J., Smith, C., and Gibler, W. B. Evidence-based emergency medicine. Creating a system to facilitate translation of evidence into standardized clinical practice: a preliminary report Ann Emerg Med 2008; 51 (1): 80-6, 86.e1-8.

Does not Target Health Care Providers

Baker, D., Middleton, E., and Campbell, S. The impact of chronic disease management in primary care on inequality in asthma severity J Public Health Med 2003; 25 (3): 258-60.

Blenkinsopp A., J. Holmes, G. Mitra and M. Pringle Joining up self-care: Evaluation of a PCT-wide programme of support for self-care Primary Health Care Research and Development 2009; 10 (2): 83-97.

Bunting B. A. and C. W. Cranor The Asheville Project: Long-term clinical, humanistic, and economic outcomes of a community-based medication therapy management program for asthma Journal of the American Pharmacists Association 2006; 46 (2): 133-147.

Cabana M. D., D. C. Chaffin, L. G. Jarlsberg, S. M.Thyne and N. M. Clark Selective provision of asthma self-management tools to families Pediatrics 2008; 121 (4): e900-e905.

Chamnan, P., Boonlert, K., Pasi, W., Yodsiri, S., Pong-on, S., Khansa, B., and Yongkulwanitchanan, P. Implementation of a 12-week disease management program improved clinical outcomes and quality of life in adults with asthma in a rural district hospital: pre- and post-intervention study Asian Pac J Allergy Immunol 2010; 28 (1): 15-21.

Delaronde S., D. L. Peruccio and B. J. Bauer Improving asthma treatment in a managed care population American Journal of Managed Care 2005; 11 (6): 361-368.

Dickinson J., S. Hutton and A. Atkin Implementing the British Thoracic Society's guidelines: The effect of a nurse-run asthma clinic on prescribed treatment in an English general practice Respiratory Medicine 1998; 92 (2): 264-267.

D'Urzo A. D., I. Tamari, J. Bouchard, R. Jhirad and P. Jugovic Limitations of a spirometry interpretation algorithm Canadian Family Physician 2011; 57 (10): 1153-1156.

Hartmann C. W., C. N. Sciamanna, D. C. Blanch, S. Mui, H. Lawless, M. Manocchia, R. K. Rosen and A. Pietropaoli A website to improve asthma care by suggesting patient questions for physicians: Qualitative analysis of user experiences Journal of Medical Internet Research 2007; 9 (1): 1-12.

Higgins, J. C., Kiser, W. R., McClenathan, S., and Tynan, N. L. Influence of an interventional program on resource use and cost in pediatric asthma Am J Manag Care 98; 4 (10): 1465-9.

Lind A., L. Kaplan and G. D. Berg Evaluation of an asthma disease management program in a medicaid population Disease Management and Health Outcomes 2006; 14 (3): 151-161.

Lougheed M. D., D. Moosa, S. Finlayson, W. M. Hopman, M. Quinn, K. Szpiro and J. Reisman Impact of a provincial asthma guidelines continuing medical education project: The Ontario Asthma Plan of Action's Provider Education in Asthma Care Project Canadian Respiratory Journal 2007; 14 (2): 111-117.

Morell, F., Genover, T., Reyes, L., Benaque, E., Roger, A., and Ferrer, J. [Monitoring of asthma outpatients after adapting treatment to meet international guidelines] Arch Bronconeumol 2007; 43 (1): 29-35.

Pinnock, H., Adlem, L., Gaskin, S., Harris, J., Snellgrove, C., and Sheikh, A. Accessibility, clinical effectiveness, and practice costs of providing a telephone option for routine asthma reviews: phase IV controlled implementation study Br J Gen Pract 2007; 57 (542): 714-22.

Rimington, L. D. and Pearson, M. G. Asthma management in primary care: does increasing patient medication improve symptoms? Clin Respir J 2008; 2 (2): 92-7.

Ruoff, G. Effects of flow sheet implementation on physician performance in the management of asthmatic patients Fam Med 2002; 34 (7): 514-7.

Schauerte, G., Fendel, T., Schwab, S., and Bredl, C. [Children with bronchial asthma: effects of an integrated health-care programme] Pneumologie 2010; 64 (2): 73-80.

Windt R. and G. Glaeske Effects of a German asthma disease management program using sickness fund claims data Journal of Asthma 2010; 47 (6): 674-679.

Intervention does not Address Adherence or Behavior of Health Care Providers

Abramson M. J., R. L. Schattner, N. D. Sulaiman, K. E. Birch, P. P. Simpson, E. A. Del Colle, R. A. Aroni, R. Wolfe and F. C. K. Thien Do spirometry and regular follow-up improve health outcomes in general practice patients with asthma or COPD? A cluster randomised controlled trial Medical Journal of Australia 2010; 193 (2): 104-109.

Adler, R. N. and McBride, J. Tools and strategies for improving asthma management Fam Pract Manag 2010; 17 (1): 16-21.

Advocate's disease management program reduces readmissions for CHF and asthma Performance improvement advisor 2003; 7 (3): 44-47.

Andersen, M., Kragstrup, J., and Sondergaard, J. How conducting a clinical trial affects physicians' guideline adherence and drug preferences JAMA 2006; 295 (23): 2759-64.

Andrews T. and J. R. Banks Achieving and Maintaining asthma control in an urban pediatric disease management program: The breathmobile program Pediatrics 2008; 122 (SUPPL. 4): S209-S210.

Anthonisen N. R. Database epidemiology Canadian Respiratory Journal 2009; 16 (6): 181-182.

Barbanel D., S. Eldridge and C. Griffiths Can a self-management programme delivered by a community pharmacist improve asthma control? A randomised trial Thorax 2003; 58 (10): 851-854.

Barnes, N. C., Douglas, G., and Higgins, B. Intermittent use of inhaled corticosteroids for the treatment of mild asthma is not recommended Prim Care Respir J 2009; 18 (4): 341-2; author reply 342.

Bunting B. A. and C. W. Cranor The Asheville Project: Long-term clinical, humanistic, and economic outcomes of a community-based medication therapy management program for asthma Journal of the American Pharmacists Association 2006; 46 (2): 133-147.

Cabana M. D., D. C. Chaffin, L. G. Jarlsberg, S. M.Thyne and N. M. Clark Selective provision of asthma self-management tools to families Pediatrics 2008; 121 (4): e900-e905.

Campbell, J., Campbell, S., and Woodward, G. Getting evidence into practice using an asthma desktop tool Aust Fam Physician 2006; 35 (1-2): 32-3.

Capen C. L. and J. M. Sherman Fatal asthma in children: a nurse managed model for prevention Journal of pediatric nursing 1998; 13 (6): 367-375.

Chandler, T. Reducing re-admission for asthma: impact of a nurse-led service Paediatr Nurs 2007; 19 (10): 19-21.

Clark, N. M., Gong, M., Schork, M. A., Kaciroti, N., Evans, D., Roloff, D., Hurwitz, M., Maiman, L. A., and Mellins, R. B. Long-term effects of asthma education for physicians on patient satisfaction and use of health services Eur Respir J 2000; 16 (1): 15-21.

Cloutier M. M., C. B. Hall and T. Rowe Easy Breathing: An asthma management program for inner city children Am J Resp Crit Care Med 2000; 161

Cloutier M. M., D. B. Wakefield, J. Tsimikas, C. B. Hall, H. Tennen and K. Brazil Organizational Attributes of Practices Successful at a Disease Management Program Journal of Pediatrics 2009; 154 (2): 290-295.

Cloutier M. M., D. B. Wakefield, P. Sangeloty-Higgins, S. Delaronde and C. B. Hall Asthma guideline use by pediatricians in private practices and asthma morbidity Pediatrics 2006; 118 (5): 1880-1887.

Cloutier, M. M., Wakefield, D. B., Sangeloty-Higgins, P., Delaronde, S., and Hall, C. B. Asthma guideline use by pediatricians in private practices and asthma morbidity Pediatrics 2006; 118 (5): 1880-7.

Cockcroft D. W. and V. A. Swystun Asthma control versus asthma severity Journal of Allergy and Clinical Immunology 1996; 98 (6 I): 1016-1018.

Coleman C. I., P. Reddy, N. M. Laster-Bradley, S. Dorval, B. Munagala and C. M. White Prescriber and pharmacist responses to intervention letters for Connecticut Medicaid beneficiaries with asthma American Journal of Health-System Pharmacy 2003; 60 (11): 1142-1144.

Collins T. M., D. A. Mott, W. E. Bigelow and D. R. Zimmerman A controlled letter intervention to change prescribing behavior: Results of a dual-targeted approach Health Services Research 1997; 32 (4): 471-489.

Crockett A. and A. Leonard Local asthma guidelines can help reduce hospital admissions Asthma Journal 2001; 6 (1): 31-34.

Dales R. E., K. L. Vandemheen, J. Clinch and S. D. Aaron Spirometry in the primary care setting: Influence on clinical diagnosis and management of airflow obstruction CHEST 2005; 128 (4): 2443-2447.

Dean M. Implementing the 1998 Canadian asthma guidelines Canadian family physician M?decin de famille canadien 2000; 46 761-762, 768-770.

Del Colle E., J. Green, A. Adikari, R. Schattner, P. Simpson, R. Wolfe, N. Sulaiman, M. Abramson and F. Thien Regular spirometry with medical review is not associated with improvement in lung function in general practice Respirology 2010; 15 A9.

Delaronde S., D. L. Peruccio and B. J. Bauer Improving asthma treatment in a managed care population American Journal of Managed Care 2005; 11 (6): 361-368.

Emmerton L., J. Shaw and N. Kheir Asthma management by New Zealand pharmacists: A pharmaceutical care demonstration project Journal of Clinical Pharmacy and Therapeutics 2003; 28 (5): 395-402.

English, R. G., Fairall, L. R., and Bateman, E. D. Keeping allergy on the agenda: integrated guidelines for respiratory disease in developing countries Allergy 2007; 62 (3): 224-9.

Feifer RA., Verbrugge RR, Khalid M, et al. Improvements in asthma pharmacotherapy and self-management: an example of a population-based disease management program Disease Management & Health Outcomes 2004; 12 (2): 93-102.

Gallagher, C. Initiating a pediatric office-based quality improvement program J Healthc Qual 2001; 23 (2): 4-9; quiz 9-10, 52.

Goyder E. C., L. Blank, E. Ellis, A. Furber, J. Peters, K. Sartain and C. Massey Reducing inequalities in access to health care: Developing a toolkit through action research Quality and Safety in Health Care 2005; 14 (5): 336-339.

Grainger-Rousseau T. J. and J. C. Mc Elnay A model for community pharmacist involvement with general practitioners in the management of asthma patients Journal of Applied Therapeutics 1996; 1 (2): 145-161.

Grainger-Rousseau, T. J., Miralles, M. A., Hepler, C. D., Segal, R., Doty, R. E., and Ben-Joseph, R. Therapeutic outcomes monitoring: application of pharmaceutical care guidelines to community pharmacy J Am Pharm Assoc (Wash) 97; NS37 (6): 647-61.

Grant, R., Bowen, S. K., Neidell, M., Prinz, T., and Redlener, I. E. Health care savings attributable to integrating guidelines-based asthma care in the pediatric medical home J Health Care Poor Underserved 2010; 21 (2 Suppl): 82-92.

Guarnaccia, S., Lombardi, A., Gaffurini, A., Chiarini, M., Domenighini, S., D'Agata, E., Schumacher, R. F., Spiazzi, R., and Notarangelo, L. D. Application and implementation of the GINA asthma guidelines by specialist and primary care physicians: a longitudinal follow-up study on 264 children Prim Care Respir J 2007; 16 (6): 357-62.

Hayes E., M. Djaferis, S. Gattasso, T. Hosmer and K. Williamson Documenting to improve pediatric asthma outcomes: practical tools for nurse practitioners Advance for nurse practitioners 2004; 12 (9): 51-53, 55-56.

Heale J., D. Davis, G. Norman, C. Woodward, V. Neufeld and P. Dodd A randomized controlled trial assessing the impact of problem-based versus didactic teaching methods in CME Proceedings of the . Annual Conference on Research in Medical Education. Conference on Research in Medical Education 1988; 27 72-77.

Higuchi, K. S., Davies, B. L., Edwards, N., Ploeg, J., and Virani, T. Implementation of clinical guidelines for adults with asthma and diabetes: a three-year follow-up evaluation of nursing care J Clin Nurs 2011; 20 (9-10): 1329-38.

Holt, E. W., Tan, J., and Hosgood, H. D. The impact of spirometry on pediatric asthma diagnosis and treatment J Asthma 2006; 43 (7): 489-93.

Ingemansson M., M. Jonsson and Hedlin G. Improving quality of care for children with asthma by learning with an interactive approach: A prospective randomized controlled study in 14 Swedish primary health care centers Allergy, Asthma and Clinical Immunology 2010; 6 9.

Jans, M. P., Schellevis, F. G., Van Hensbergen, W., and van Eijk, J. T. Improving general practice care of patients with asthma or chronic obstructive pulmonary disease: evaluation of a quality system Eff Clin Pract 2000; 3 (1): 16-24.

Jiwa M, Hughes J, Sriram D et al. Piloting and validating an innovation to triage patients presenting with cough to community pharmacies in Western Australia. Quality in Primary Care 2012; 20(2):83-91.

Kasiar J., C. L. Bonsignore and B. H. Dennis Assessment of inhaled steroids for asthma patients overusing inhaled albuterol Hospital Pharmacy 1998; 33 (12): 1507-1511.

Lack of self-efficacy keeps inner-city primary care providers from following national asthma management guidelines AHRQ Research Activities 2009; (345): 15-15.

Lagerlov P., Veninga C. C. M., Muskova M., et al. Asthma management in five European countries: Doctors' knowledge, attitudes and prescribing behaviour European Respiratory Journal 2000; 15 (1): 25-29.

Laurence, C. O., Beilby, J., Campbell, S., Campbell, J., Ponte, L., and Woodward, G. Process for improving the integration of care across the primary and acute care settings in rural South Australia: asthma as a case study Aust J Rural Health 2004; 12 (6): 264-8.

Le, T. T., Rait, M. A., Jarlsberg, L. G., Eid, N. S., and Cabana, M. D. A randomized controlled trial to evaluate the effectiveness of a distance asthma learning program for pediatricians J Asthma 2010; 47 (3): 245-50.

Levac, K. A. Putting outcomes into practice in physician offices J Nurs Care Qual 2002; 17 (1): 51-62; quiz 90.

Lind A., L. Kaplan and G. D. Berg Evaluation of an asthma disease management program in a medicaid population Disease Management and Health Outcomes 2006; 14 (3): 151-161.

Loymans R., G. ter Riet and P. J. Sterk Assessing primary care physicians' beliefs and attitudes of asthma exacerbation treatment and follow-up Open Respiratory Medicine Journal 2011; 5 (1): 10.

Ma, J. and Stafford, R. S. US physician adherence to standards in asthma pharmacotherapy varies by patient and physician characteristics J Allergy Clin Immunol 2003; 112 (3): 633-5.

Magzamen S., D. Van Sickle, L. D. Rose and C. Cronk Environmental pediatrics Pediatric Annals 2011; 40 (3): 144-151.

Majak, P., Bak-Walczak, E., Stelmach, I., Jerzynska, J., Krakowiak, J., and Stelmach, W. An increasing trend of the delay in asthma diagnosis after the discontinuation of a population-based intervention J Asthma 2011; 48 (4): 414-8.

Maslennikova G. Y., L. M. Shmarova, J. A. Lapidus and R. G. Oganov Asthma education in Russia: Effectiveness of a training programme for primary-care doctors Asthma Journal 2001; 6 (3): 134-138.

McCowan C. The facilitator effect: Results from a four-year follow-up of children with asthma British Journal of General Practice 1997; 47 (416): 156-160.

McIvor, A. and Hodder, R. Canadian Adult Asthma Update 2008 key messages: a focus on translating knowledge into action in primary care Can Respir J 2008; 15 (3): 121-2.

McLean, W., Gillis, J., and Waller, R. The BC Community Pharmacy Asthma Study: A study of clinical, economic and holistic outcomes influenced by an asthma care protocol provided by specially trained community pharmacists in British Columbia Can Respir J 2003; 10 (4): 195-202.

Meadows M. Breathing better: action plans keep asthma in check FDA Consumer 2003; 37 (2): 20-27.

Mihaltan, F. [Asthma--between "control" and "severity"] Pneumologia 2008; 57 (4): 192-3.

Morrow, R., Fletcher, J., Mulvihill, M., and Park, H. The asthma dialogues: a model of interactive education for skills J Contin Educ Health Prof 2007; 27 (1): 49-58.

Murphy K. R., Hopp R. J., Kittelson E. B., G. Hansen, M. L. Windle and J. N. Walburn Life-threatening asthma and anaphylaxis in schools: A treatment model for school-based programs Annals of Allergy, Asthma and Immunology 2006; 96 (3): 398-405.

Naish, J., Eldridge, S., Moser, K., and Sturdy, P. Did the London Initiative Zone investment programme affect general practice structure and performance in East London? A time series analysis of cervical screening coverage and asthma prescribing Public Health 2002; 116 (6): 361-7.

Najada, A., Abu-Hasan, M., and Weinberger, M. Outcome of asthma in children and adolescents at a specialty-based care program Ann Allergy Asthma Immunol 2001; 87 (4): 335-43.

Neville R. G., G. Hoskins, C. McCowan and B. Smith Pragmatic 'real world' study of the effect of audit of asthma on clinical outcome Primary Care Respiratory Journal 2004; 13 (4): 198-204.

Newcomb, P. Results of an asthma disease management program in an urban pediatric community clinic J Spec Pediatr Nurs 2006; 11 (3): 178-88.

Newton-Syms F. A. O., Dawson P. H., Cooke J., et al. The influence of an academic representative on prescribing by general practitioners British Journal of Clinical Pharmacology 1992; 33 (1): 69-73.

Ogundele M. Challenge of introducing evidence based medicine into clinical practice: An example of local initiatives in paediatrics Clinical Governance: An International Journal 2011; 16 (3): 231-249.

O'Laughlen, M. C., Hollen, P., and Ting, S. An intervention to change clinician behavior: Conceptual framework for the multicolored simplified asthma guideline reminder (MSAGR) J Am Acad Nurse Pract 2009; 21 (8): 417-22.

Partridge, M. R. Introduction to the Global Initiative for Asthma and the new guidelines West Indian Med J 2003; 52 Suppl 7 6-9.

Pastor-Sanchez R., C. A. Gomez-Escolar, F. A. De Toledo Saavedra, N. F. De Cano Martin and A. D. Martinez Medafar: A coordination strategy study Pharmacy World and Science 2009; 31 (4): 505.

Pilotto L. S., B. J. Smith, A. R. Heard, H. J. McElroy, J. Weekley and P. Bennett Trial of nurse-run asthma clinics based in general practice versus usual medical care Respirology (Carlton, Vic.) 2004; (3): 356-62.

Plaza, V., Cobos, A., Ignacio-Garcia, J. M., Molina, J., Bergonon, S., Garcia-Alonso, F., and Espinosa, C. [Cost-effectiveness of an intervention based on the Global INitiative for Asthma (GINA) recommendations using a computerized clinical decision support system: a physicians randomized trial] Med Clin (Barc) 2005; 124 (6): 201-6.

Rascati K. L., G. J. Okano and C. Burch Evaluation of Physician Intervention Letters Medical Care 1996; 34 (8): 760-766.

Reed, C. E. Inhaled corticosteroids: why do physicians and patients fail to comply with guidelines for managing asthma? Mayo Clin Proc 2004; 79 (4): 453-5.

Rimington, L. D. and Pearson, M. G. Asthma management in primary care: does increasing patient medication improve symptoms? Clin Respir J 2008; 2 (2): 92-7.

Ruiz Espiricueta, J. E., Gonzalez Diaz, S. N., Rodriguez, G. G., Cruz, A. A., Canseco Villarreal, C., and Valdez Ramirez, M. A. [Assessment of an educational course on asthma for primary care physicians] Rev Alerg Mex 2005; 52 (2): 83-9.

Ruoff, G. Effects of flow sheet implementation on physician performance in the management of asthmatic patients Fam Med 2002; 34 (7): 514-7.

Saini, B., Filipovska, J., Bosnic-Anticevich, S., Taylor, S., Krass, I., and Armour, C. An evaluation of a community pharmacy-based rural asthma management service Aust J Rural Health 2008; 16 (2): 100-8.

Schaffner W., W. A. Ray, C. F. Federspiel and W. O. Miller Improving antibiotic prescribing in office practice. A controlled trial of three educational methods Journal of the American Medical Association 1983; 250 (13): 1728-1732.

Schatz M., C. Gibbons, C. Nelle, K. Harden and R. S. Zeiger Impact of a care manager on the outcomes of higher risk asthmatic patients: A randomized controlled trial Journal of Asthma 2006; 43 (3): 225-229.

Schneider A., K. Biessecker, R. Quinzler, P. Kaufmann-Kolle, F. J. Meyer, M. Wensing and J. Szecsenyi Asthma patients with low perceived burden of illness: A challenge for guideline adherence Journal of Evaluation in Clinical Practice 2006;

Self T. H., T. M. Kelso, N. Abou-Shala and M. J. Rumbak Clinical pharmacist initiated programs for improving outcomes in adult, African American asthmatics 1992;

Simpson M. D., D. L. Burton, M. A. Burton, P. M. Gissing and S. L. Bowman Pharmaceutical Care: Impact on Asthma Medication Use Journal of Pharmacy Practice and Research 2004; 34 (1): 26-29.

Sin, D. D., Bell, N. R., and Man, S. F. Effects of increased primary care access on process of care and health outcomes among patients with asthma who frequent emergency departments Am J Med 2004; 117 (7): 479-83.

Splett, P. L., Erickson, C. D., Belseth, S. B., and Jensen, C. Evaluation and sustainability of the healthy learners asthma initiative J Sch Health 2006; 76 (6): 276-82.

Tennen H., Cloutier M. M., Wakefield D. B., et al. The buffering effect of hope on clinician's behavior: A test in pediatric primary care Journal of Social and Clinical Psychology 2009; 28 (5): 554-576.

Ting, S. Multicolored simplified asthma guideline reminder (MSAGR) for better adherence to national/global asthma guidelines Ann Allergy Asthma Immunol 2002; 88 (3): 326-30.

Tschopp, J. M., Frey, J. G., Pernet, R., Burrus, C., Jordan, B., Morin, A., Garrone, S., Imhof, K., Besse, F., Marty, S., Uldry, C., and Assal, J. P. Bronchial asthma and self-management education: implementation of Guidelines by an interdisciplinary programme in health network Swiss Med Wkly 2002; 132 (7-8): 92-7.

Walter E. B., A. S. Hellkamp, K. C. Goldberg, D. Montgomery, B. Patterson and R. J. Dolor Improving influenza vaccine coverage among asthmatics: a practice-based research network study Journal of Clinical Outcomes Management 2008; 15 (5): 229-234.

Wanich N. H. and M. S. Kaplan Management of asthma based on exhaled nitric oxide in addition to guideline-based treatment for inner-city adolescents and young adults: A randomised controlled trial Pediatrics 2009; 124 (SUPPL. 2): S147.

Weinberger, M. M. What is the problem with asthma care for children? Arch Pediatr Adolesc Med 2011; 165 (5): 473-5.

Weiss K. B., P. Lozano and J. A. Finkelstein A randomized controlled clinical trial to improve asthma care for children through provider education and health systems change: A description of the Pediatric Asthma Care Patient Outcomes Research Team (PAC-PORT II) Study Design Health Serv Outcomes Res Methodology

White P. T., C. A. Pharoah, H. R. Anderson and P. Freeling Randomized controlled trial of small group education on the outcome of chronic asthma in general practice Journal of the Royal College of General Practitioners 1989; 39 (322): 182-186.

White P., A. Atherton, G. Hewett and K. Howells Using information from asthma patients: A trial of information feedback in primary care British Medical Journal 1995; 311 (7012): 1065-1069.

Williams, D., Portnoy, J. M., and Meyerson, K. Strategies for improving asthma outcomes: a case-based review of successes and pitfalls J Manag Care Pharm 2010; 16 (1 Suppl C): S3-14; quiz S16-7.

Wright, J., Warren, E., Reeves, J., Bibby, J., Harrison, S., Dowswell, G., Russell, I., and Russell, D. Effectiveness of multifaceted implementation of guidelines in primary care J Health Serv Res Policy 2003; 8 (3): 142-8.

Wright, S. W., Trott, A., Lindsell, C. J., Smith, C., and Gibler, W. B. Evidence-based emergency medicine. Creating a system to facilitate translation of evidence into standardized clinical practice: a preliminary report Ann Emerg Med 2008; 51 (1): 80-6, 86.e1-8.

Wroth, T. H. and Boals, J. C. 4th Application of quality-improvement methods in a community practice: the Sandhills Pediatrics Asthma Initiative N C Med J 2005; 66 (3): 218-20.

Yawn, B. P., Enright, P. L., Lemanske, R. F. Jr, Israel, E., Pace, W., Wollan, P., and Boushey, H. Spirometry can be done in family physicians' offices and alters clinical decisions in management of asthma and COPD Chest 2007; 132 (4): 1162-8.

Zeiger R. S., S. Heller and M. H. Mellon Facilitated referral to asthma specialist reduces relapses in asthma emergency department visits J Allergy Clin Immunol 1991; 87 1161-1168.

No Outcomes of Interest

Andersen, M., Kragstrup, J., and Sorensen, J. [How participation in a clinical trial affects doctors' choice of treatment] Ugeskr Laeger 2006; 168 (46): 3987-91.

Anhoj, J. and Nielsen, L. Quantitative and qualitative usage data of an Internet-based asthma monitoring tool J Med Internet Res 2004; 6 (3): e23.

Blais, R., Laurier, C., and Pare, M. Effect of feedback letters to physicians and pharmacists on the appropriate use of medication in the treatment of asthma J Asthma 2008; 45 (3): 227-31.

Blenkinsopp A., J. Holmes, G. Mitra and M. Pringle Joining up self-care: Evaluation of a PCT-wide programme of support for self-care Primary Health Care Research and Development 2009; 10 (2): 83-97.

Boulet, L. P., Dorval, E., Labrecque, M., Turgeon, M., Montague, T., and Thivierge, R. L. Towards Excellence in Asthma Management: final report of an eight-year program aimed at reducing care gaps in asthma management in Quebec Can Respir J 2008; 15 (6): 302-10.

Bratton, S. L., Cabana, M. D., Brown, R. W., White, D. F., Wang, Y., Lang, S. W., and Clark, N. M. Asthma educational seminar targeting Medicaid providers Respir Care 2006; 51 (1): 49-55.

Brimkulov N., S. E. Ottmani, A. Pio, T. Chubakov, A. Sultanova, N. Davletalieva, A. Kalieva, J. Rittman, M. Erhola, R. Cholurova and L. Blanc Feasibility test results of the practical approach to lung health in Bishkek, Kyrgyzstan International Journal of Tuberculosis and Lung Disease 2009; 13 (4): 533-539.

Carlton, B. G., Lucas, D. O., Ellis, E. F., Conboy-Ellis, K., Shoheiber, O., and Stempel, D. A. The status of asthma control and asthma prescribing practices in the United States: results of a large prospective asthma control survey of primary care practices J Asthma 2005; 42 (7): 529-35.

De Vries T. W., P. B. Van Den Berg, E. J. Duiverman and L. T. W. De Jong-van Den Berg Effect of a minimal pharmacy Intervention on adherence to asthma medication guidelines for children Pharmaceutisch Weekblad 2010; 145 (50): 195-197.

Doran T., C. Fullwood, H. Gravelle, D. Reeves, E. Kontopantelis, U. Hiroeh and M. Roland Pay-for-performance programs in family practices in the United Kingdom New England Journal of Medicine 2006; 355 (4): 375-384.

Fang X., S. Li, L. Gao, N. Zhao, X. Wang and C. Bai Quality of care for copd and asthma in China: Clinicians' adherence to guidelines and the effects of a short term training course Respirology 2011; 16 252-253.

Fifield J., J. McQuillan, M. Martin-Peele, V. Nazarov, A. J. Apter, T. Babor, J. Burleson, R. Cushman, J. Hepworth, E. Jackson, S. Reisine, J. Sheehan and J. Twiggs Improving pediatric asthma control among minority children participating in medicaid: providing practice redesign support to deliver a chronic care model J Asthma 2010; 47 (7): 718-27.

Gallagher, C. Initiating a pediatric office-based quality improvement program J Healthc Qual 2001; 23 (2): 4-9; quiz 9-10, 52.

Grainger-Rousseau T. J. and J. C. Mc Elnay A model for community pharmacist involvement with general practitioners in the management of asthma patients Journal of Applied Therapeutics 1996; 1 (2): 145-161.

Grant, R., Bowen, S. K., Neidell, M., Prinz, T., and Redlener, I. E. Health care savings attributable to integrating guidelines-based asthma care in the pediatric medical home J Health Care Poor Underserved 2010; 21 (2 Suppl): 82-92.

Harrison, S., Dowswell, G., Wright, J., and Russell, I. General practitioners' uptake of clinical practice guidelines: a qualitative study J Health Serv Res Policy 2003; 8 (3): 149-53.

Hartmann C. W., C. N. Sciamanna, D. C. Blanch, S. Mui, H. Lawless, M. Manocchia, R. K. Rosen and A. Pietropaoli A website to improve asthma care by suggesting patient questions for physicians: Qualitative analysis of user experiences Journal of Medical Internet Research 2007; 9 (1): 1-12.

Hartmann, C. W., Sciamanna, C. N., Blanch, D. C., Mui, S., Lawless, H., Manocchia, M., Rosen, R. K., and Pietropaoli, A. A website to improve asthma care by suggesting patient questions for physicians: qualitative analysis of user experiences J Med Internet Res 2007; 9 (1): e3.

Hendricson, W. D., Wood, P. R., Hidalgo, H. A., Kromer, M. E., Parcel, G. S., and Ramirez, A. G. Implementation of a physician education intervention. The Childhood Asthma Project Arch Pediatr Adolesc Med 94; 148 (6): 595-601.

Herrick D. E., C. R. Lowe, J. G. Micalizzi and G. S. Kerby The impact of an evidence-based continuing education course on participant self-efficacy and asthma educator-certified (AE-C) accreditation Journal of Allergy and Clinical Immunology 2011; 127 (2): AB67.

Hoskins, G., Neville, R. G., McCowan, C., Smith, B., Clark, R. A., and Ricketts, I. W. Scottish Asthma Management Initiative Health Bull (Edinb) 2000; 58 (6): 478-88.

Howard R., A. Avery and J. Cantrill How pharmacists working on the PINCER trial helped reduce hazardous prescribing International Journal of Pharmacy Practice 2010; 18 5-6.

Jans M. P., F. G. Schellevis, E. M. L. E. Coq, P. D. Bezemer and J. T. M. Van Eijk Health outcomes of asthma and COPD patients: The evaluation of a project to implement guidelines in general practice International Journal for Quality in Health Care 2001; 13 (1): 17-25.

Kasiar J., C. L. Bonsignore and B. H. Dennis Assessment of inhaled steroids for asthma patients overusing inhaled albuterol Hospital Pharmacy 1998; 33 (12): 1507-1511.

Kryj-Radziszewska, E., Windak, A., Margas, G., Wizner, B., and Grodzicki, T. [The influence of guidelines of asthma management in adults in reference to family physicians knowledge in the field of treatment] Przegl Lek 2008; 65 (4): 166-71.

Kuilboer M. M., M. A. M. Van Wijk, M. Mosseveld, E. Van Der Does, J. C. De Jongste, S. E. Overbeek, B. Ponsioen and J. Van Der Lei Computed critiquing integrated into daily clinical practice affects physicians' behavior: A randomized clinical trial with asthma critic Methods of Information in Medicine 2006; 45 (4): 447-454.

Labelle, M., Beaulieu, M., Renzi, P., Rahme, E., and Thivierge, R. L. Integrating clinical practice guidelines into daily practice: impact of an interactive workshop on drafting of a written action plan for asthma patients J Contin Educ Health Prof 2004; 24 (1): 39-49.

Lee, E., McNally, D. L., and Zuckerman, I. H. Evaluation of a physician-focused educational intervention on medicaid children with asthma Ann Pharmacother 2004; 38 (6): 961-6.

Lomotan EA, Hoeksema LJ, Edmonds DE, Ramirez-Garnica G, Shiffman RN, Horwitz LI. Evaluating the use of a computerized clinical decision support system for asthma by pediatric pulmonologists. Int. J. Med. Informatics 2012; 81(3):157-65.

Lougheed M. D., D. Moosa, S. Finlayson, W. M. Hopman, M. Quinn, K. Szpiro and J. Reisman Impact of a provincial asthma guidelines continuing medical education project: The Ontario Asthma Plan of Action's Provider Education in Asthma Care Project Canadian Respiratory Journal 2007; 14 (2): 111-117.

Lougheed, M. D., Moosa, D., Finlayson, S., Hopman, W. M., Quinn, M., Szpiro, K., and Reisman, J. Impacts of a provincial asthma guidelines continuing medical education project: The Ontario Asthma Plan of Action's Provider Education in Asthma Care Project Can Respir J 2007; 14 (2): 111-7.

Lundborg C. S., G. Tomson, R. Wahlstrom, T. Oke and V. K. Diwan GPs' knowledge and attitudes regarding treatment of UTI and asthma in Sweden: A randomised controlled educational trial on guideline implementation European Journal of Public Health 2000; 10 (4): 241-246.

Martens, J. D., van der Weijden, T., Winkens, R. A., Kester, A. D., Geerts, P. J., Evers, S. M., and Severens, J. L. Feasibility and acceptability of a computerised system with automated reminders for prescribing behaviour in primary care Int J Med Inform 2008; 77 (3): 199-207.

Mash B., Rhode H., Pather M., et al. Evaluation of the asthma guideline implementation project in the Western Cape, South Africa Current Allergy and Clinical Immunology 2010; 23 (4): 154-161.

Modell, M., Iliffe, S., Austin, A., and Leaning, M. S. From guidelines to decision support in the management of asthma Stud Health Technol Inform 95; 16 105-13.

Moonie, S. A., Strunk, R. C., Crocker, S., Curtis, V., Schechtman, K., and Castro, M. Community Asthma Program improves appropriate prescribing in moderate to severe asthma J Asthma 2005; 42 (4): 281-9.

Murphy K. R., R. J. Hopp, E. B. Kittelson, G. Hansen, M. L. Windle and J. N. Walburn Life-threatening asthma and anaphylaxis in schools: A treatment model for school-based programs Annals of Allergy, Asthma and Immunology 2006; 96 (3): 398-405.

O'Laughlen, M. C., Hollen, P., and Ting, S. An intervention to change clinician behavior: Conceptual framework for the multicolored simplified asthma guideline reminder (MSAGR) J Am Acad Nurse Pract 2009; 21 (8): 417-22.

Pinnock H., G. Hoskins, B. Smith, T. Weller and D. Price A pilot study to assess the feasibility and acceptability of undertaking acute asthma professional development in three different UK primary care settings Primary Care Respiratory Journal 2003; 12 (1): 7-11.

Roberts, N. J., Evans, G., Blenkhorn, P., and Partridge, M. R. Development of an electronic pictorial asthma action plan and its use in primary care Patient Educ Couns 2010; 80 (1): 141-6.

Schaffner W., W. A. Ray, C. F. Federspiel and W. O. Miller Improving antibiotic prescribing in office practice. A controlled trial of three educational methods Journal of the American Medical Association 1983; 250 (13): 1728-1732.

Shegog R., L. K. Bartholomew, M. M. Sockrider, D. I. Czyzewski, S. Pilney, P. D. Mullen and S. L. Abramson Computer-based decision support for pediatric asthma management: Description and feasibility of the Stop Asthma Clinical System Health Informatics Journal 2006; 12 (4): 259-273.

Steiner, R. M. and Walsworth, D. T. Using quality experts from manufacturing to transform primary care J Contin Educ Health Prof 2010; 30 (2): 95-105.

Sullivan, S. D., Lee, T. A., Blough, D. K., Finkelstein, J. A., Lozano, P., Inui, T. S., Fuhlbrigge, A. L., Carey, V. J., Wagner, E., and Weiss, K. B. A multisite randomized trial of the effects of physician education and organizational change in chronic asthma care: cost-effectiveness analysis of the Pediatric Asthma Care Patient Outcomes Research Team II (PAC-PORT II) Arch Pediatr Adolesc Med 2005; 159 (5): 428-34.

Tai, S. S., Nazareth, I., Donegan, C., and Haines, A. Evaluation of general practice computer templates. Lessons from a pilot randomised controlled trial Methods Inf Med 99; 38 (3): 177-81.

Thomas K. W., C. S. Dayton and M. W. Peterson Evaluation of internet-based clinical decision support systems Journal of Medical Internet Research 1999; 1 (2): 5-13.

Thomas, K. W., Dayton, C. S., and Peterson, M. W. Evaluation of internet-based clinical decision support systems J Med Internet Res 99; 1 (2): E6.

Ting, S. Multicolored simplified asthma guideline reminder (MSAGR) for better adherence to national/global asthma guidelines Ann Allergy Asthma Immunol 2002; 88 (3): 326-30.

To T., S. McLimont, C. Wang and L. Cicutto How much do health care providers value a community-based asthma care program?-survey to collect their opinions on the utilities of and barriers to its uptake BMC Health Services Research 2009; 9

Tomson Y., J. Hasselstram, G. Tomson and H. Ã…berg Asthma education for Swedish primary care physicians - A study on the effects of 'academic detailing' on practice and patient knowledge European Journal of Clinical Pharmacology 1997; 53 (3-4): 191-196.

Treweek S. The potential of electronic medical record systems to support quality improvement work and research in Norwegian general practice BMC Health Services Research 2003; 3 1-9.

Tuomisto L. E., M. Kaila and M. Erhola Asthma Programme in Finland: Comparison of adult asthma referral letters in 1994 and 2001 Respiratory Medicine 2007; 101 (3): 595-600.

Twiggs J. E., J. Fifield, E. Jackson, R. Cushman and A. Apter Treating asthma by the guidelines: Developing a medication management information system for use in primary care Disease Management 2004; 7 (3): 244-260.

Van Sickle, D. and Singh, R. B. A video-simulation study of the management of asthma exacerbations by physicians in India Clin Respir J 2008; 2 (2): 98-105.

Veninga, C. C., Lagerlov, P., Wahlstrom, R., Muskova, M., Denig, P., Berkhof, J., Kochen, M. M., and Haaijer-Ruskamp, F. M. Evaluating an educational intervention to improve the treatment of asthma in four European countries. Drug Education Project Group Am J Respir Crit Care Med 99; 160 (4): 1254-62.

Wazeka A, Valacer D J, Cooper M, et al. Impact of a pediatric asthma clinical pathway on hospital cost and length of stay Pediatr Pulmonol 2001; 32 (3): 211-6.

White P, Atherton A, Hewett G, et al. Using information from asthma patients: A trial of information feedback in primary care British Medical Journal 1995; 311 (7012): 1065-1069.

White, M., Michaud, G., Pachev, et al. Randomized trial of problem-based versus didactic seminars for disseminating evidence-based guidelines on asthma management to primary care physicians J Contin Educ Health Prof 2004; 24 (4): 237-43.

Witt K, Knudsen E, Ditlevsen S, et al. Academic detailing has no effect on prescribing of asthma medication in Danish general practice: a 3-year randomized controlled trial with 12-monthly follow-ups Fam Pract 2004; 21 (3): 248-53.

Yeh KW, Chao SY, Chiang LC, et al. Increasing asthma care knowledge and competence of public health nurses after a national asthma education program in Taiwan Asian Pacific Journal of Allergy and Immunology 2006; 24 (4): 183-189.

Other

Adler, R. N. and McBride, J. Tools and strategies for improving asthma management Fam Pract Manag 2010; 17 (1): 16-21.

Baddar, S., Worthing, E. A., Al-Rawas, O. A., Osman, Y., and Al-Riyami, B. M. Compliance of physicians with documentation of an asthma management protocol Respir Care 2006; 51 (12): 1432-40.

Baldacci S, Maio S, Simoni M et al. The ARGA study with general practitioners: Impact of medical education on asthma/rhinitis management. Respir. Med. 2012; 106(6):777-85.

Borkgren-Okonek M., C. Gronkiewicz and E. J. Diamond Underutilization of disease-specific electronic medical record templates limits adherence to evidence-based guidelines in outpatient asthma management CHEST 2010; 138 (4):

Boulet, L. P., Dorval, E., Labrecque, M., Turgeon, M., Montague, T., and Thivierge, R. L. Towards Excellence in Asthma Management: final report of an eight-year program aimed at reducing care gaps in asthma management in Quebec Can Respir J 2008; 15 (6): 302-10.

Brimkulov N., S. E. Ottmani, A. Pio, T. Chubakov, A. Sultanova, N. Davletalieva, A. Kalieva, J. Rittman, M. Erhola, R. Cholurova and L. Blanc Feasibility test results of the practical approach to lung health in Bishkek, Kyrgyzstan International Journal of Tuberculosis and Lung Disease 2009; 13 (4): 533-539.

Cho S. H. How to organize cost-effective care for asthma patients Respirology 2009; 14 A104.

Dales R. E., K. L. Vandemheen, J. Clinch and S. D. Aaron Spirometry in the primary care setting: Influence on clinical diagnosis and management of airflow obstruction CHEST 2005; 128 (4): 2443-2447.

Davies, B., Edwards, N., Ploeg, J., and Virani, T. Insights about the process and impact of implementing nursing guidelines on delivery of care in hospitals and community settings BMC Health Serv Res 2008; 8 29.

Eccles M., E. McColl, N. Steen and S. T. Liaw Computerised evidence-based guidelines may not improve asthma or angina management in primary care Evidence-Based Healthcare 2003; 7 (2): 81-82.

Emmerton L., J. Shaw and N. Kheir Asthma management by New Zealand pharmacists: A pharmaceutical care demonstration project Journal of Clinical Pharmacy and Therapeutics 2003; 28 (5): 395-402.

Fang X., S. Li, L. Gao, N. Zhao, X. Wang and C. Bai Quality of care for copd and asthma in China: Clinicians' adherence to guidelines and the effects of a short term training course Respirology 2011; 16 252-253.

Global initiative for asthma: Global strategy for asthma management and prevention Global Initiative for Asthma 2002;

Howard R., A. Avery and J. Cantrill How pharmacists working on the PINCER trial helped reduce hazardous prescribing International Journal of Pharmacy Practice 2010; 18 5-6.

Jones, E. M. and Portnoy, J. M. Modification of provider behavior to achieve improved asthma outcomes Curr Allergy Asthma Rep 2003; 3 (6): 484-90.

Kallenbach, A., Ludwig-Beymer, P., Welsh, C., Norris, J., and Giloth, B. Process improvement for asthma. An integrated approach J Nurs Care Qual 2003; 18 (4): 245-56; quiz 257-8.

Lagerlov, P., Loeb, M., Andrew, M., and Hjortdahl, P. Improving doctors' prescribing behaviour through reflection on guidelines and prescription feedback: a randomised controlled study Qual Health Care 2000; 9 (3): 159-65.

Lasley M. V. Adherence to follow-up recommendations in asthma Pediatrics 2008; 122 (SUPPL. 4): S211-S212.

Lukacs, S. L., France, E. K., Baron, A. E., and Crane, L. A. Effectiveness of an asthma management program for pediatric members of a large health maintenance organization Arch Pediatr Adolesc Med 2002; 156 (9): 872-6.

Lundborg C. S., R. Wahlström, T. Oke, G. Tomson and V. K. Diwan Influencing prescribing for urinary tract infection and asthma in primary care in Sweden: A randomized controlled trial of an interactive educational intervention Journal of Clinical Epidemiology 1999; 52 (8): 801-812.

Majak, P., Bak-Walczak, E., Stelmach, I., Jerzynska, J., Krakowiak, J., and Stelmach, W. An increasing trend of the delay in asthma diagnosis after the discontinuation of a population-based intervention J Asthma 2011; 48 (4): 414-8.

Martens, J. D., van der Aa, A., Panis, B., van der Weijden, T., Winkens, R. A., and Severens, J. L. Design and evaluation of a computer reminder system to improve prescribing behaviour of GPs Stud Health Technol Inform 2006; 124 617-23.

McDermott M. F., J. Walter, C. Catrambone and K. B. Weiss The Chicago Emergency Department Asthma Collaborative CHEST 1999; 116 (4 SUPPL. 1): 196S-197S.

Roberts N. J., K. Boyd, A. Briggs, A. L Caress and M. R. Partridge Is it cost-effective to replace nurses with lay asthma educators in primary care? Thorax 2010; 65 A8.

Roberts, N. J., Evans, G., Blenkhorn, P., and Partridge, M. R. Development of an electronic pictorial asthma action plan and its use in primary care Patient Educ Couns 2010; 80 (1): 141-6.

Schauerte, G., Fendel, T., Schwab, S., and Bredl, C. [Children with bronchial asthma: effects of an integrated health-care programme] Pneumologie 2010; 64 (2): 73-80.

Smith J. R., M. J. Noble, S. D. Musgrave, J. Murdoch, G. Price, A. Martin, J. Windley, R. Holland, B. D. W. Harrison, D. Price, A. Howe, I. Harvey and A. M. Wilson The at-risk registers in severe asthma (ARRISA) study: A cluster-randomised controlled trial in primary care Thorax 2010; 65 A62.

Steiner, R. M. and Walsworth, D. T. Using quality experts from manufacturing to transform primary care J Contin Educ Health Prof 2010; 30 (2): 95-105.

Verstappen, W. H., van der Weijden, T., Sijbrandij, J., Smeele, I., Hermsen, J., Grimshaw, J., and Grol, R. P. Effect of a practice-based strategy on test ordering performance of primary care physicians: a randomized trial JAMA 2003; 289 (18): 2407-12.

Yawn, B. P., Enright, P. L., Lemanske, R. F. Jr, Israel, E., Pace, W., Wollan, P., and Boushey, H. Spirometry can be done in family physicians' offices and alters clinical decisions in management of asthma and COPD Chest 2007; 132 (4): 1162-8.

Appendix E. Evidence Tables

The following studies were grouped together: Haymore 2005 & Herborg 2011; Lozano 2004 & Finkelstein 2005; Cloutier 2005 & Cloutier 2009

Evidence Table 1. Study characteristics of all included studies

Author, Year RefID	Study Design	Study location	Multicenter	Study Start/End Date	Study Duration	Planned length of followup	Intervention
Ables AZ, 2002[1]	Pre-post	United States	NO	10/01/1998 - 03/31/2000	18 months	NR	Education
Armour C., 2007[2]	Randomized	Australia	YES	11/2004 - 07/2005	9 months	NR	Clinical Pharmacy Service
Baker R., 2003[3]	Randomized	Europe	NO	08/1998 - 01/2000	15 months	12 months	Audit and Feedback
Bell L.M., 2010[4]	Randomized	United States	YES	12/01/2005 - 04/15/2008	29 months	NR	Decision Support
Bender B. G., 2011[5]	Pre-post	United States	YES	NR	NR	NR	Multicomponent
Blackstien-Hirsch P., 2000[6]	Pre-post	Canada	NO	NR	NR	6 months	Education
Brown R, 2004[7]	Randomized	United States	YES	NR	NR	24 months	Education
Bryce FP, 1995[8]	Randomized	Europe	YES	1990 - 1993	36 months	12 months	Information Only
Cabana M. D., 2006[9]	Randomized	United States	YES	07/2001 -	NR	12 months	Education
Cho S. H., 2010[10]	Pre-post	Asia	YES	03/2004 - 12/2004	9 months	3 months	Decision Support
Clark NM, 1998[11]	Randomized	United States	YES	NR	NR	22 months	Education
Cloutier M. M., 2002[12]	Pre-post	United States	YES	07/01/1997 - 12/31	24 months	NR	Decision Support
Cloutier M. M., 2005[13]	Pre-post	United States	YES	06/01/1998 - 08/31/2002	50 months	NR	Decision Support
Cloutier M.M., 2009[14]	Pre post	United States	YES	06/01/1998 - 07/01/2002	36 months	NR	Decision Support
Cloutier M.M., 2012[15]	Cluster-randomized (practice is the unit of randomization)	United States	NO	NR	36	NR	Multicomponent.
Coleman C. I., 2003[16]	Pre post	United States	NO	04/2001 - 06/2001	3 months	6 months	Audit and Feedback
Cowie R. L.,	Pre-post	Canada	YES	NR	NR	12 months	Education

Author, Year RefID 2001[17]	Study Design	Study location	Multicenter	Study Start/End Date	Study Duration	Planned length of followup	Intervention
Daniels E. C., 2005[18]	Cluster Randomized	United States	YES	NR	NR	NR	Multicomponent
Davis AM, 2010[19]	Pre-post	United States	NO	07/01/2007 - 12/31/2008	18 months	NR	Decision Support
Davis R. S., 2004[20]	Pre-post	United States	NO	NR	NR	6 months	Education
de Vries T. W., 2010[21]	Non-randomized pre-post	Europe	NO	07/01/2006 - 06/30/2007	12 months	NR	Clinical Pharmacy Service
Eccles M., 2002[22]	Randomized	Europe	YES	NR	24 months	12 months	Decision Support
Fairall L., 2010[23]	Randomized	Africa	NO	05/2003 - 11/2003	6 months	3 months	Decision Support
Feder G, 1995[24]	Randomized	Europe	YES	1/93	6 months	12 months	Audit and Feedback
Finkelstein J. A., 2005[25]	Randomized	United States	YES	NR	NR	24 months	Organizational Change
Foster J. M., 2007[26]	Randomized	Europe	YES	2002	NR	12 months	Audit and Feedback
Fox P., 2007[27]	Pre-post	United States	YES	2001 - 2004	36 months	12 and 24 months	Quality Improvement
Frankowski B. L., 2006[28]	Pre-post	United States	YES	04/2003 - 03/2005	11 months	NR	Multicomponent
Glasgow N. J., 2003[29]	Randomized	Australia	YES	02/2000	NR	12 months	Decision Support
Gorton T. A., 1995[30]	Controlled before after	United States	NO	NR	4 months	4 months	Education
Hagmolen, W., 2008[31]	Randomized	Europe	YES	12/2000 - 08/2003	33 months	12 months	Multicomponent
Halterman J. S., 2005[32]	Randomized	United States	NO	NR	NR	6 months	Decision Support
Halterman J.S., 2006[33]	Randomized	United States	YES	11/20/2003 - 09/14/2004	NR	NR	Decision Support
Herborg H., 2001[34,35]	Non-randomized controlled	Europe	YES	08/1994 - 07/1995	NR	12 months	Audit and Feedback
Holton C., 2011[36]	Randomized	Australia	YES	2006 - 2007	12 months	12 months	Education
Homer CJ, 2005[37]	Randomized	United States	YES	01/2001 - 2002	12 months	12 months	Quality Improvement
Horswell R., 2008[38]	Pre-post	United States	NO	2000 - 2006	84 months	84 months	Decision Support

E-2

Author, Year RefID	Study Design	Study location	Multicenter	Study Start/End Date	Study Duration	Planned length of followup	Intervention
Hoskins G., 1997[39]	Pre-post	Europe	NO	1991 - 1993	24 months	NR	Audit and Feedback
Kattan M., 2006[40]	Randomized	United States	YES	10/1998 - 08/2000	12 months	NR	Decision Support
Lesho E. P., 2005[41]	Pre-post	Europe	NO	NR	NR	12 months	Decision Support
Liaw S. T., 2008[42]	Cluster Randomized	Australia	NO	02/2001 - 11/2001	9 months	6 months	Education
Lob S. H., 2011[43]	Quasi-experimental (longitudinal at clinic level and cross-sectional at patient level)	United States	YES	2006-2008	28 months	12 and 21 months	Multicomponent Multimodal
Lozano P., 2004[44]	Randomized	United States	YES	NR	24 months	24 months	Education
Lundborg C. S., 1999[45]	Cluster Randomized	Europe	NO	NR	19 months	NR	Multimodal
Mahi-Taright S., 2004[46]	Pre-post	Africa	YES	1992	NR	NR	Education
Mangione-Smith R., 2005[47]	Controlled Before-After	United States	YES	02/15/2000 - 03/01/2001	12 months	16 months	Quality Improvement
Martens J. D., 2006[48]	Randomized	Europe	YES	2001 - 2004	NR	NR	Information Only
Martens J. D., 2007[49]	Randomized	Europe	YES	10/2003	NR	12 months	Decision Support
McCowan C, 2001[50]	Randomized	Europe	YES	NR	6 months	6 months	Decision Support
Mitchell E. A., 2005[51]	Randomized	Australia	YES	01/1999 - 12/2000	9 months	NR	Decision Support
Newton W. P., 2010[52]	Pre-post	United States	YES	09/2006 - 2008	24 months	24 months	Decision Support
O'Laughlen MC, 2008[53]	Pre-post	United States	YES	NR	7 months	4 months	Decision Support
Patel P. H., 2004[54]	Pre-post	United States	NO	06/01/1998 - 12/31/2000	30 months	13 months	Organizational Change
Premaratne U. N., 1999[55]	Randomized	Europe	YES	09/1993 - 09/1996	36 months	36 months	Education
Ragazzi H., 2011[56]	Pre-post	United States	YES	2004 - 2004	12 months	12 months	Decision Support
Rance K., 2011[57]	Pre-post	United States	NO	06/2009 - 08/2009	1.5 months	NR	Decision Support

Author, Year RefID	Study Design	Study location	Multicenter	Study Start/End Date	Study Duration	Planned length of followup	Intervention
Renzi P. M., 2006[58]	Randomized	Canada	NO	08/2002 - 2003	12 months	12 months	Decision Support
Richman M. J., 2000[59]	Pre-post	United States	YES	NR	NR	12 months	Audit and Feedback
Ruoff G., 2002[60]	Pre-post	United States	NO	2000 - 2000	NR	6 months	Decision Support
Saini B, 2004[61]	Controlled pre-post	Australia	YES	11/1997 - 05/2001	42 months	6 months	Clinical Pharmacy Service
Schneider A., 2008[62]	Randomized	Europe	YES	05/2005	NR	12 months	Audit and Feedback
Shah S., 2011[63]	Randomized	Australia	YES	2006 - 2008	NR	12 months	Education
Shapiro A., 2011[64]	Pre-post	United States	YES	11/01/2004 - 05/31/2009	54 months	NR	Decision Support
Shiffman R. N., 2000[65]	Pre-post	United States	YES	09/30/1996 - 10/01/1998	24 months	NR	Decision Support
Smeele I. J., 1999[66]	Randomized	Europe	YES	NR	12 months	12 months	Education
Sondergaard J., 2002[67]	Randomized	Europe	YES	06/01/1998 - 06/01/1999	12 months	12 months	Audit and Feedback
Stergachis A., 2002[68]	Randomized	United States	YES	NR	24 months	12 months	Education
Suh D. C., 2001[69]	Pre-post	United States	YES	01/1997 - 09/1998	21 months	9 months	Audit and Feedback
Sulaiman N. D., 2010[70]	Randomized	Australia	YES	02/2001 - 11/2001	10 months	6 months	Education
Thyne S.M., 2007[71]	Pre-post	United States	NO	NR	NR	NR	Organizational Change
To T., 2008[72]	Pre-post	Canada	YES	NR	12 months	12 months	Decision Support
Veninga CCM, 1999[73]	Randomized	Europe	YES	03/1995 - 11/1996	NR	12 months	Audit and Feedback
Veninga CCM, 2000[74]	Randomized	Europe	YES	NR	NR	NR	Audit and Feedback
Weinberger M, 2002[75]	Randomized	United States	YES	07/1998 - 12/1999	18 months	12 months	Clinical Pharmacy Service
Yawn BP, 2008[76]	Pre-post	United States	YES	NR	NR	9 months	Audit and Feedback

NR= Not reported

References

1. Ables AZ, Godenick MT, Lipsitz SR. Family Medicine: Improving family practice residents' compliance with asthma practice guidelines. 2002; 34:23-8.

2. Armour C, Bosnic-Anticevich S, Brillant M et al. Thorax: Pharmacy Asthma Care Program (PACP) improves outcomes for patients in the community. 2007; 62:496-502.

3. Baker R, Fraser RC, Stone M, Lambert P, Stevenson K, Shiels C. Br J Gen Pract: Randomised controlled trial of the impact of guidelines, prioritized review criteria and feedback on implementation of recommendations for angina and asthma. 2003; 53:284-91.

4. Bell LM, Grundmeier R, Localio R et al. Pediatrics: Electronic health record-based decision support to improve asthma care: a cluster-randomized trial. 2010; 125:e770-7.

5. Bender BG, Dickinson P, Rankin A, Wamboldt FS, Zittleman L, Westfall JM. J Am Board Fam Med: The Colorado Asthma Toolkit Program: a practice coaching intervention from the High Plains Research Network. 2011; 24 :240-8.

6. Blackstien-Hirsch P, Anderson G, Cicutto L, McIvor A, Norton P. Journal of Asthma: Implementing continuing education strategies for family physicians to enhance asthma patients' quality of life. 2000; 37:247-57.

7. Brown R, Bratton SL, Cabana MD, Kaciroti N, Clark NM. Chest: Physician asthma education program improves outcomes for children of low-income families. 2004; 126:369-74.

8. Bryce FP, Neville RG, Crombie IK, Clark RA, McKenzie P. British Medical Journal: Controlled trial of an audit facilitator in diagnosis and treatment of childhood asthma in general practice. 1995; 310:838-42.

9. Cabana MD, Slish KK, Evans D et al. Pediatrics: Impact of physician asthma care education on patient outcomes. 2006; 117:2149-57.

10. Cho SH, Jeong JW, Park HW et al. J Asthma: Effectiveness of a computer-assisted asthma management program on physician adherence to guidelines. 2010; 47:680-6.

11. Clark N, Gong M, Schork, M, et al. Impact of education for physicians on patient outcomes. Pediatrics 1998; 101(5):831-6.

12. Cloutier MM , Wakefield DB, Carlisle PS, Bailit HL, Hall CB. Arch Pediatr Adolesc Med: The effect of Easy Breathing on asthma management and knowledge. 2002; 156:1045-51.

13. Cloutier MM , Hall CB, Wakefield DB, Bailit H. J Pediatr: Use of asthma guidelines by primary care providers to reduce hospitalizations and emergency department visits in poor, minority, urban children. 2005; 146:591-7.

14. Cloutier MM , Grosse SD, Wakefield DB, Nurmagambetov TA, Brown CM. American Journal of Managed Care: The economic impact of an urban asthma management program. 2009; 15:345-51.

15. Cloutier MM , Tennen H, Wakefield DB, Brazil K, Hall CB. Improving clinician self-efficacy does not increase asthma guideline use by primary care clinicians. Acad Pediatr. 2012; 12(4):312-8.

16. Coleman CI, Reddy P, Laster-Bradley NM, Dorval S, Munagala B, White CM. Ann Pharmacother: Effect of practitioner education on adherence to asthma treatment guidelines. 2003; 37:956-61.

17. Cowie RL, Underwood MF, Mack S. Can Respir J: The impact of asthma management guideline dissemination on the control of asthma in the community. 2001; 8 Suppl A:41A-5A.

18. Daniels EC, Bacon J, Denisio S et al. J Asthma: Translation squared: improving asthma care for high-disparity populations through a safety net practice-based research network. 2005; 42:499-505.

19. Davis AM, Cannon M, Ables AZ, Bendyk H. Family Medicine: Using

Pediatrics: Improving asthma-related health outcomes among low-income, multiethnic, school-aged children: Results of a demonstration project that combined continuous quality improvement and community health worker strategies. 2007; 120:e902-e911.

28 Frankowski BL, Keating K, Rexroad A *et al.* J Sch Health: Community collaboration: concurrent physician and school nurse education and cooperation increases the use of asthma action plans. 2006; 76:303-6.

29 Glasgow NJ, Ponsonby AL, Yates R, Beilby J, Dugdale P. BMJ: Proactive asthma care in childhood: general practice based randomised controlled trial. 2003; 327:659.

30 Gorton TA, Cranford CO, Golden WE, Walls RC, Pawelak JE. Arch Fam Med: Primary care physicians' response to dissemination of practice guidelines. 1995; 4:135-42.

31 Hagmolen of ten Have W, van den Berg NJ, van der Palen J, van Aalderen WM, Bindels PJ. Prim Care Respir J: Implementation of an asthma guideline for the management of childhood asthma in general practice: a randomised controlled trial. 2008; 17:90-6.

32 Halterman JS, McConnochie KM, Conn KM *et al.* Archives of Pediatrics and Adolescent Medicine: A randomized trial of primary care provider prompting to enhance preventive asthma therapy. 2005; 159:422-7.

33 Halterman JS, Fisher S, Conn KM *et al.* Archives of Pediatrics & Adolescent Medicine: Improved preventive care for asthma: a randomized trial of clinician prompting in pediatric offices. 2006; 160:1018-25.

34 Herborg H, Soendergaard B, Jorgensen T *et al.* J Am Pharm Assoc (Wash): Improving drug therapy for patients with asthma-part 2: Use of antiasthma medications. 2001; 41:551-9.

35 Herborg H. SBFBeal. Improving drug therapy for patients with asthma-part 1: Patient outcomes. J Am Pharm Assoc (Wash) 2001; (4):539-50.

the electronic medical record to improve asthma severity documentation and treatment among family medicine residents. 2010; 42:334-7.

20 Davis RS, Bukstein DA, Luskin AT, Kailin JA, Goodenow G. Ann Allergy Asthma Immunol: Changing physician prescribing patterns through problem-based learning: an interactive, teleconference case-based education program and review of problem-based learning. 2004; 93:237-42.

21 de Vries TW , van den Berg PB, Duiverman EJ, de Jong-van den Berg LT. Arch Dis Child: Effect of a minimal pharmacy intervention on improvement of adherence to asthma guidelines. 2010; 95:302-4.

22 Eccles M, McColl E, Steen N *et al.* BMJ: Effect of computerised evidence based guidelines on management of asthma and angina in adults in primary care: cluster randomised controlled trial. 2002; 325:941.

23 Fairall L, Bachmann MO, Zwarenstein M *et al.* Trop Med Int Health: Cost-effectiveness of educational outreach to primary care nurses to increase tuberculosis case detection and improve respiratory care: economic evaluation alongside a randomised trial. 2010; 15:277-86.

24 Feder G, Griffiths C, Highton C, Eldridge S, Spence M, Southgate L. British Medical Journal: Do clinical guidelines introduced with practice based education improve care of asthmatic and diabetic patients? A randomised controlled trial in general practices in east London. 1995; 311:1473-8.

25 Finkelstein JA, Lozano P, Fuhlbrigge AL *et al.* Health Serv Res: Practice-level effects of interventions to improve asthma care in primary care settings: the Pediatric Asthma Care Patient Outcomes Research Team. 2005; 40:1737-57.

26 Foster JM, Hoskins G, Smith B, Lee AJ, Price D, Pinnock H. BMC Fam Pract: Practice development plans to improve the primary care management of acute asthma: randomised controlled trial. 2007; 8:23.

27 Fox P, Porter PG, Lob SH, Boer JH, Rocha DA, Adelson JW.

36 Holton C, Crockett A, Nelson M *et al.* International Journal for Quality in Health Care: Does spirometry training in general practice improve quality and outcomes of asthma care? 2011; 23:545-53.

37 Homer CJ, Forbes P, Horvitz L, Peterson LE, Wypij D, Heinrich P. Archives of Pediatrics and Adolescent Medicine: Impact of a quality improvement program on care and outcomes for children with asthma. 2005; 159:464-9.

38 Horswell R, Butler MK, Kaiser M *et al.* Dis Manag: Disease management programs for the underserved. 2008; 11:145-52.

39 Hoskins G, Neville RG, Smith B, Clark RA. Health Bull (Edinb): Does participation in distance learning and audit improve the care of patients with acute asthma attacks? The General Practitioners in Asthma Group. 1997; 55:150-5.

40 Kattan M, Crain EF, Steinbach S *et al.* Pediatrics: A randomized clinical trial of clinician feedback to improve quality of care for inner-city children with asthma. 2006; 117:e1095-103.

41 Lesho EP, Myers CP, Ott M, Winslow C, Brown JE. Mil Med: Do clinical practice guidelines improve processes or outcomes in primary care? 2005; 170:243-6.

42 Liaw ST, Sulaiman ND, Barton CA *et al.* BMC Fam Pract: An interactive workshop plus locally adapted guidelines can improve general practitioners asthma management and knowledge: a cluster randomised trial in the Australian setting. 2008; 9:22.

43 Lob SH, Boer JH, Porter PG, *et al.* Promoting Best-Care Practices in Childhood Asthma: Quality Improvement in Community Health Centers. *Pediatrics* 2011;128:20; (Originally Published Online June 13, 2011; DOI: 10.1542/Peds.2010-1962 .

44 Lozano P, Finkelstein JA, Carey VJ *et al.* Arch Pediatr Adolesc Med: A multisite randomized trial of the effects of physician education and organizational change in chronic-asthma care: health outcomes of the Pediatric Asthma Care Patient Outcomes Research Team II Study. 2004; 158:875-83.

45 Lundborg CS , Wahlstrom R, Oke T, Tomson G, Diwan VK. J Clin Epidemiol: Influencing prescribing for urinary tract infection and asthma in primary care in Sweden: a randomized controlled trial of an interactive educational intervention. 1999; 52:801-12.

46 Mahi-Taright S, Belhocine M, Ait-Khaled N. Int J Tuberc Lung Dis: Can we improve the management of chronic obstructive respiratory disease? The example of asthma in adults. 2004; 8:873-81.

47 Mangione-Smith R, Schonlau M, Chan KS *et al.* Ambulatory Pediatrics: Measuring the effectiveness of a collaborative for quality improvement in pediatric asthma care: Does implementing the chronic care model improve processes and outcomes of care? 2005; 5:75-82.

48 Martens JD, Winkens RA, van der Weijden T, de Bruyn D, Severens JL. BMC Health Serv Res: Does a joint development and dissemination of multidisciplinary guidelines improve prescribing behaviour: a pre/post study with concurrent control group and a randomised trial. 2006; 6:145.

49 Martens JD, van der Weijden T, Severens JL *et al.* Int J Med Inform: The effect of computer reminders on GPs' prescribing behaviour: a cluster-randomised trial. 2007; 76 Suppl 3:S403-16.

50 McCowan C, Neville RG, Ricketts IW, Warner FC, Hoskins G, Thomas GE. Medical Informatics and the Internet in Medicine: Lessons from a randomized controlled trial designed to evaluate computer decision support software to improve the management of asthma. 2001; 26:191-201.

51 Mitchell EA , Didsbury PB, Kruithof N *et al.* Acta Paediatr: A randomized controlled trial of an asthma clinical pathway for children in general practice. 2005; 94:226-33.

52 Newton WP, Lefebvre A, Donahue KE, Bacon T, Dobson A. J Contin Educ Health Prof: Infrastructure for large-scale quality-improvement projects: early lessons from North Carolina Improving Performance in Practice. 2010; 30:106-13.

53 O'Laughlen MC, Hollen PJ, Rakes G, Ting S. Pediatric Asthma,

Allergy and Immunology: Improving pediatric asthma by the MSAGR algorithm: A multicolored, simplified asthma guideline reminder. 2008; 21:119-27.

54 Patel PH, Welsh C, Foggs MB. Dis Manag: Improved asthma outcomes using a coordinated care approach in a large medical group. 2004; 7:102-11.

55 Premaratne UN, Sterne JA, Marks GB, Webb JR, Azima H, Burney PG. BMJ: Clustered randomised trial of an intervention to improve the management of asthma: Greenwich asthma study. 1999; 318:1251-5.

56 Ragazzi H, Keller A, Ehrensberger R, Irani AM. J Urban Health: Evaluation of a practice-based intervention to improve the management of pediatric asthma. 2011; 88 Suppl 1:38-48.

57 Rance K, O'Laughlen M, Ting S. J Pediatr Health Care: Improving asthma care for African American children by increasing national asthma guideline adherence. 2011; 25:235-49.

58 Renzi PM, Ghezzo H, Goulet S, Dorval E, Thivierge RL. Can Respir J: Paper stamp checklist tool enhances asthma guidelines knowledge and implementation by primary care physicians. 2006; 13:193-7.

59 Richman MJ, Poltawsky JS. Stud Health Technol Inform: Partnership for excellence in asthma care: evidence based disease management. 2000; 76:107-21.

60 Ruoff G. Family Medicine: Effects of flow sheet implementation on physician performance in the management of asthmatic patients. 2002; 34:514-7.

61 Saini B, Krass I, Armour C. Annals of Pharmacotherapy: Development, implementation, and evaluation of a community pharmacy-based asthma care model. 2004; 38:1954-60.

62 Schneider A, Wensing M, Biessecker K, Quinzler R, Kaufmann-Kolle P, Szecsenyi J. J Eval Clin Pract: Impact of quality circles for improvement of asthma care: results of a randomized controlled trial. 2008; 14:185-90.

63 Shah S, Sawyer SM, Toelle BG et al. Med J Aust: Improving paediatric asthma outcomes in primary health care: a randomised controlled trial. 2011; 195:405-9.

64 Shapiro A, Gracy D, Quinones W, Applebaum J, Sarmiento A. Arch Pediatr Adolesc Med: Putting guidelines into practice: improving documentation of pediatric asthma management using a decision-making tool. 2011; 165:412-8.

65 Shiffman RN, Freudigman M, Brandt CA, Liaw Y, Navedo DD. Pediatrics: A guideline implementation system using handheld computers for office management of asthma: effects on adherence and patient outcomes. 2000; 105:767-73.

66 Smeele IJ, Grol RP, van Schayck CP, van den Bosch WJ, van den Hoogen HJ, Muris JW. Qual Health Care: Can small group education and peer review improve care for patients with asthma/chronic obstructive pulmonary disease? 1999; 8:92-8.

67 Sondergaard J, Andersen M, Vach K, Kragstrup J, Maclure M, Gram LF. Eur J Clin Pharmacol: Detailed postal feedback about prescribing to asthma patients combined with a guideline statement showed no impact: a randomised controlled trial. 2002; 58:127-32.

68 Stergachis A, Gardner JS, Anderson MT, Sullivan SD. Journal of the American Pharmaceutical Association (Washington,D.C.: 1996): Improving pediatric asthma outcomes in the community setting: does pharmaceutical care make a difference? 2002; 42:743-52.

69 Suh DC, Shin SK, Okpara I, Voytovich RM, Zimmerman A. Am J Manag Care: Impact of a targeted asthma intervention program on treatment costs in patients with asthma. 2001; 7:897-906.

70 Sulaiman ND, Barton CA, Liaw ST et al. Fam Pract: Do small group workshops and locally adapted guidelines improve asthma patients' health outcomes? A cluster randomized controlled trial. 2010; 27:246-54.

71 Thyne SM, Marmor AK, Madden N, Herrick G. Paediatric and Perinatal Epidemiology: Comprehensive asthma management for

of Clinical Epidemiology: Improving drug treatment in general practice. 2000; 53:762-72.

75   Weinberger M, Murray MD, Marrero DG *et al.* Journal of the American Medical Association: Effectiveness of pharmacist care for patients with reactive airways disease: A randomized controlled trial. 2002; 288:1594-602.

76   Yawn BP, Bertram S, Wollan P. Journal of Asthma and Allergy: Introduction of asthma APGAR tools improve asthma management in primary care practices. 2008; 1-10.

underserved children. 2007; 21:29-34.

72   To T, Cicutto L, Degani N, McLimont S, Beyene J. Med Care: Can a community evidence-based asthma care program improve clinical outcomes?: a longitudinal study. 2008; 46:1257-66.

73   Veninga CC, Lagerløv P, Wahlström R, *et al.* Evaluating an educational intervention to improve the treatment of asthma in four european countries. American Journal of Respiratory and Critical Care Medicine:1999; 160:1254-62.

74   Veninga CCM , Denig P, Zwaagstra R, Haaijer-Ruskamp FM. Journal

Evidence Table 2. Healthcare provider characteristics

Author, year	Arm	n at Baseline	Type of Healthcare Provider	Practice Setting	Practice Specialty	Service Area	Insurance Type	International study / Insurance
Ables AZ, 2002[1]	Education and Reminders	NR	Nurse, Physician	Community Health Center, Other	Family Medicine	NR	NR	NR
Armour C., 2007[2]	Arm A: Control	25	Pharmacist	NR	NR	Rural, Urban	NR	No
Armour C., 2007[2]	Arm B: Pharmacy Asthma Care Program (PACP)	32	Pharmacist	NR	NR	Rural, Urban	NR	NR
Baker R., 2003[3]	Arm A: Guidelines only	27	General Practitioner	NR	General Practice	NR	NR	Yes
Baker R., 2003[3]	Arm B: Guidelines with audit criteria	27	General Practitioner	NR	General Practice	NR	NR	NR
Baker R., 2003[3]	Arm C: Guidelines with audit criteria and feedback	27	General Practitioner	NR	General Practice	NR	NR	NR
Bell L.M., 2010[4]	Arm A: UP Control	NR	Pediatrician	Academic	Pediatric Medicine	Urban	NR	No
Bell L.M., 2010[4]	Arm B: UP intervention	NR	Pediatrician	Academic	Pediatric Medicine	Urban	NR	NR
Bell L.M., 2010[4]	Arm C: SP Control	NR	Pediatrician	NR	Pediatric Medicine	Suburban	NR	NR
Bell L.M., 2010[4]	Arm D: SP Intervention	NR	Pediatrician	NR	Pediatric Medicine	Suburban	NR	NR
Bender B. G., 2011[5]	Arm A: Education, Coaching and Toolkit	Arm A+B = 372	NR	NR	NR	NR	NR	No
Bender B. G., 2011[5]	Arm B:	Arm A+B = 372	Nurse, Physician, Physician Assistant, Medical assistants,	Other	Primary Care	NR	NR	NR

E-10

Author, year	Arm	n at Baseline	Type of Healthcare provider	Practice Setting	Practice Specialty	Service Area	Insurance Type	International study / Insurance
Blackstien-Hirsch P., 2000[6]	Education	59	practice managers, office staff, Physician	NR	Family Medicine	Suburban	NR	NR
Brown R, 2004[7]	Arm A: Control	11	Pediatrician	NR	Primary Care	NR	NR	No
Brown R, 2004[7]	Arm B: Education	12	Pediatrician	NR	Primary Care	NR	NR	NR
Bryce FP, 1995[8]	Arm A: Control	NR	General Practitioner, Nurse	NR	General Practice	Rural, Urban	Uninsured	No
Bryce FP, 1995[8]	Arm B: Reminders and Tools	NR	General Practitioner	NR	General Practice	Rural, Urban	NR	NR
Cabana M. D., 2006[9]	Arm A:Control	43	Primary Healthcare	NR	Primary Care	NR	Commercial/Private, n: 376 (83) Medicaid/Medicare, n: 48 (11)	No
Cabana M. D., 2006[9]	Arm B: Physician Asthma Care Education (PACE)	51	Primary Healthcare	NR	Primary Care	NR	Commercial/Private, n: 307 (73) Type2: Medicaid/Medicare, n: 71 (17)	NR
Cho S. H., 2010[10]	Decision Support,	377	Allergist, General Practitioner, Physician	NR	NR	NR	NR	NR
Clark NM, 1998[11]	Arm A:	37	Pediatrician, Physician	Private Practice	Pediatric Medicine	NR	NR	No
Clark NM, 1998[11]	Arm B: Education	37	Pediatrician, Physician	Private Practice	Pediatric Medicine	NR	NR	NR
Cloutier M. M., 2002[12]	Decision support	172	Nurse, Nurse Practitioner, Other, Pediatrician, Physician, Physician Assistant Advanced practice nurses, Family practice	NR	Primary Care	Urban	Medicaid/Medicare, n: NR (84)	No
Cloutier M. M., 2005[13]	Decision support	151	Nurse, Nurse Practitioner, Pediatrician, Physician Assistant, Primary	Academic, Community Health Center, Other	Primary Care	Urban	Medicaid/Medicare	NR

Author, year	Arm	n at Baseline	Type of Healthcare provider	Practice Setting	Practice Specialty	Service Area	Insurance Type	International study / Insurance
			Health care pediatric residents, medical students					
Cloutier M.M., 2009[13] [14]	Decision support	NR	Pediatrician	NR	NR	Urban	NR	NR
Cloutier M.M., 2012 [15]	Control	44	Nurse practioner, pediatrician, physician assistant	Other	Pediatric medicine	8 urban and 16 private practices total. Arm A: 12 practices	NR	No.
Cloutier M.M., 2012 [15]	Arm B: Physician-directed interventions	44	Nurse Practitioner, pediatrician, physician assistant	Other	Pediatric medicine	8 urban and 16 private practices total. Arm B: 12 practices.	NR	No.
Coleman C. I., 2003[16]	Arm A: Patient specific information: Prescribers with patients on 'high dose'	NR	Pharmacist Prescriber	NR	NR	NR	NR	No
Coleman C. I., 2003[16]	Arm B: Patient specific information: Prescribers with patients on 'low dose'	NR	Pharmacist Prescriber	NR	NR	NR	NR	NR
Cowie R. L., 2001[17]	Arm A: Basic Education	NR	NR	NR	NR	Urban	NR	Yes
Cowie R. L., 2001[17]	Arm B: Intermediate Education	NR	NR	NR	NR	Urban	NR	NR
Cowie R. L., 2001[17]	Arm C: Intensive Education	NR	NR	NR	NR	Urban	NR	NR
Daniels E.	Arm A:	Arm A+B:	General Practitioner,	Community	NR	Rural, Urban	Uninsured, n: 67200	No

E-12

Author, year	Arm	n at Baseline	Type of Healthcare provider	Practice Setting	Practice Specialty	Service Area	Insurance Type	International study / Insurance
C., 2005[18]	Control	163	Internist, Nurse Practitioner, Pediatrician, Physician, Physician Assistant staff	Health Center			Type2: Medicaid/Medicare, n: 48419	
Daniels E. C., 2005[18]	Arm B: Education	Arm A+B: 163	General Practitioner, Internist, Nurse Practitioner, Other, Pediatrician, Physician, Physician Assistant staff	Community Health Center	NR	Rural, Urban	Uninsured, n: 30713 Type2: Medicaid/Medicare, n: 38059	NR
Davis AM, 2010[19]	Decision Support	NR	Physician Family medicine residents	Community Health Center	Family Medicine	NR	NR	NR
Davis R. S., 2004[20]	Arm A: Guidelines only	Arm A+B: 20	Primary Healthcare	Other	Primary Care	NR	NR	No
Davis R. S., 2004[20]	Arm B: Education and Toolkit	Arm A+B: 20	Primary Healthcare	Other	Primary Care	NR	NR	NR
de Vries T. W., 2010[21]	Arm A: Control	Arm A+B+C: 9	General Practitioner	NR	General Practice	NR	NR	Yes
de Vries T. W., 2010[21]	Arm B: Feedback	Arm A+B+C: 9	Pharmacists, General Practitioner	NR	General Practice	NR	NR	NR
de Vries T. W., 2010[21]	Arm C: 2002	Arm A+B+C: 9	Pharmacists, General Practitioner, Pediatrician	NR	NR	NR	NR	NR
Eccles M., 2002[22]	Arm A: angina	NR	General Practitioner	NR	General Practice	NR	NR	Yes
Eccles M., 2002[22]	Arm B: asthma	NR	General Practitioner	NR	General Practice	NR	NR	NR
Fairall L., 2010[23]	Arm A: Control	Arm A+B: 148	Nurse	NR	Primary Care	Rural	NR	Yes
Fairall L., 2010[23]	Arm B: Intervention	Arm A+B: 148	Nurse	NR	Primary Care	Rural	NR	NR
Feder G, 1995[24]	Arm A: Diabetes Education	NR	General Practitioner	Private Practice	General Practice	Urban	NR	Yes: International study; no insurance info.

Author, year	Arm	n at Baseline	Type of Healthcare provider	Practice Setting	Practice Specialty	Service Area	Insurance Type	International study / Insurance
Feder G, 1995[24]	Arm B: Education, Reminders and Audit	NR	General Practitioner	Private Practice	General Practice	Urban	NR	NR.
Finkelstein J. A., 2005[25] [26]	Arm A: Control	Arm A+B+C: 228	NR	NR		NR	NR	No
Finkelstein J. A., 2005[25] [26]	Arm B: PLE Intervention	Arm A+B+C: 228	NR	NR		NR	NR	NR
Finkelstein J. A., 2005[25] [26]	Arm C: Planned Care Intervention	Arm A+B+C: 228	NR	NR		NR	NR	NR
Foster J. M., 2007[27]	Arm A: Education and Feedback (Delayed)	12	General Practitioner	NR	General Practice	Inner City, Rural, Urban	NR	Yes
Foster J. M., 2007[27]	Arm B: Education and Feedback	11	General Practitioner	NR	General Practice	Inner City, Rural, Urban	NR	NR
Fox P., 2007[28]	Quality Improvement	NR	Nurse, Nurse Practitioner, Physician caregivers, administrative staff	Community Health Center	NR	NR	Commercial/Private (4.7-23.6) Uninsured (10.6-13.2) Medicaid/Medicare (52.1-75.1)	NR
Frankowski B. L., 2006[29]	Multimodal: Education and Feedback	NR	Nurse, Pediatrician, Primary Healthcare	Community Health Center, Other	Primary Care	NR	Medicaid/Medicare, n: 55 (47.4)	NR
Glasgow N. J., 2003[30]	Arm A: Control	12	General Practitioner	NR	General Practice	NR	NR	No
Glasgow N.	Arm	12	General Practitioner	NR	General Practice	NR	NR	NR

E-14

Author, year	Arm	n at Baseline	Type of Healthcare provider	Practice Setting	Practice Specialty	Service Area	Insurance Type	International study / Insurance
J., 2003[30]	B: Intervention							
Gorton T. A., 1995[31]	Arm A: Guidelines only	22	Primary Healthcare	NR	Family Medicine, General Practice, Internal Medicine, Pediatric Medicine, Primary Care	NR	NR	No
Gorton T. A., 1995[31]	Arm B: Education and Detailing	NR	Primary Healthcare	NR	Family Medicine, General Practice, Internal Medicine, Pediatric Medicine, Primary Care	NR	NR	NR
Gorton T. A., 1995[31]	Arm C: Education on Computer	NR	Primary Healthcare	NR	Family Medicine, General Practice, Internal Medicine, Pediatric Medicine, Primary Care	NR	NR	NR
Gorton T. A., 1995[31]	Arm D: Education – multimedia	NR	Primary Healthcare	NR	Primary Care	NR	NR	NR
Hagmolen of ten Have, W., 2008[32]	Arm C: Education and Guidelines and individualized treatment advice	38	General Practitioner	Community Health Center	NR	NR	NR	NR
Hagmolen, W., 2008[32]	Arm A: Guidelines only	34	General Practitioner	Community Health Center	NR	NR	NR	Yes
Hagmolen, W., 2008[32]	Arm B: Education and Guidelines	34	General Practitioner	Community Health Center	NR	NR	NR	NR
Halterman J. S., 2005[33]	Arm A: Control	NR	NR	NR	NR	NR	Medicaid/Medicare, n: 54 (70.1)	No

Author, year	Arm	n at Baseline	Type of Healthcare provider	Practice Setting	Practice Specialty	Service Area	Insurance Type	International study / Insurance
Halterman J. S., 2005[33]	Arm B: Intervention	NR	NR	NR	NR	NR	Medicaid/Medicare, n: 46 (63)	NR
Halterman J.S., 2006[34]	Arm A: Control	NR	Nurse Practitioner, Pediatrician, Physician	Academic	Pediatric Medicine	Inner City	Medicaid/Medicare, n: 89 (78.1)	No
Halterman J.S., 2006[34]	Arm B: Intervention	NR	Nurse Practitioner, Pediatrician, Physician	Academic	Pediatric Medicine	Inner City	Medicaid/Medicare, n: 81 (72.3)	NR
Herborg H., 2001[35,36]	Arm A: Control	64	General Practitioner, Other, Pharmacist, Pharmacy assistant	Other	Other	NR	NR	Yes
Herborg H., 2001[35,36]	Arm B: Therapeutic Outcomes Monitoring (TOM)	75	General Practitioner, Other, Pharmacist, Pharmacy assistant	Other	Other	NR	NR	NR
Holton C., 2011[37]	Arm A: Control	45	General Practitioner	NR	General Practice	NR	NR	Yes
Holton C., 2011[37]	Arm B: Spirometry training	127	General Practitioner	NR	General Practice	NR	NR	NR
Homer CJ, 2005[38]	Arm A: Control	NR	Nurse, Physician Front office staff	Community Health Center, Other, Private Practice	NR	NR, Urban	Medicaid/Medicare (10)	No
Homer CJ, 2005[38]	Arm B: Learning collaborative	NR	Nurse, Other, Physician Front office staff	Community Health Center, Other, Private Practice	NR	NR, Urban	Medicaid/Medicare (10)	NR
Horswell R., 2008[39]	HCSD's DM program	NR	Physician	Community Health Center, Other	NR	NR	Uninsured	NR
Hoskins G., 1997[40]	Arm A: Before intervention	91	General Practitioner	NR	General Practice	NR	NR	No
Hoskins G., 1997[40]	Arm B: Education and Feedback	91	General Practitioner	NR	General Practice	NR	NR	NR
Kattan M., 2006[41]	Arm A: Control	NR	Nurse Practitioner, Physician Assistant, Primary Healthcare	Community Health Center, Other, Private	Family Medicine, General Practice, Other, Pediatric	Urban	Medicaid/Medicare (35) Type2: Managed care	No

Author, year	Arm	n at Baseline	Type of Healthcare provider	Practice Setting	Practice Specialty	Service Area	Insurance Type	International study / Insurance
				Practice	Medicine		(25.5) Type3: Uninsured (17)	
Kattan M., 2006[41]	Arm B: Intervention	435	Nurse Practitioner, Physician Assistant, Primary Healthcare	Community Health Center, Other, Private Practice	NR	Urban	Medicaid/Medicare (28.7) Type2: Managed care(25.3) Type3: Uninsured (21.4)	NR
Lesho E. P., 2005[42]	Decision Support	NR	Primary Healthcare	Other	Primary Care	NR	NR	NR
Liaw S. T., 2008[43]	Arm A: Control	18	General Practitioner	NR	General Practice	Urban	NR	Yes
Liaw S. T., 2008[43]	Arm B: Control (unrelated education)	15	General Practitioner	NR	General Practice	Urban	NR	NR
Liaw S. T., 2008[43]	Arm C: Education and Guidelines	18	General Practitioner	NR	General Practice	Urban	NR	NR
Lob S. H., 2011[44]	Longitudinal Evaluation Group – Patient-level Interview Sample	NR	Physician, Nurse Practitioner	Community Health Center	Pediatric Primary Care	NR	None (7.5) Medi-Cal MC (60.5) Medi-Cal FFS (6.6) Other government programs (19.1) Private (5.5) Other (0.8)	No.
Lob S. H., 2011[44]	Cross-sectional Random Sample – Clinic-level Chart Review, T1	NR	Physician, Nurse Practitioner	Community Health Center	Pediatric Primary Care	NR	None (9.2) Medi-Cal MC (51.7) Medi-Cal FFS (8.0) Other government programs (16.9) Private (13.6) Other (0.6)	NR
Lob S. H., 2011[44]	Cross-sectional Random Sample – Clinic-level Chart Review, T2	NR	Physician, Nurse Practitioner	Community Health Center	Pediatric Primary Care	NR	None (7.7) Medi-Cal MC (61.6) Medi-Cal FFS (6.4) Other government programs (12.1) Private (10.7) Other (1.5)	NR

Author, year	Arm	n at Baseline	Type of Healthcare provider	Practice Setting	Practice Specialty	Service Area	Insurance Type	International study / Insurance
Lob S. H., 2011[44]	Cross-sectional Random Sample – Clinic-level Chart Review, T3	NR	Physician, Nurse Practitioner	Community Health Center	Pediatric Primary Care	NR	None (8.6) Medi-Cal MC (58.4) Medi-Cal FFS (10.5) Other government programs (11.2) Private (9.9) Other (1.3)	NR
Lozano P., 2004[26]	Arm A: Control	NR	Primary Healthcare	Other	Primary Care	NR	NR	NR
Lozano P., 2004[26]	Arm B: Peer leader education	NR	Primary Healthcare	Other	Primary Care	NR	NR	NR
Lozano P., 2004[26]	Arm C: Chronic care model	NR	Primary Healthcare	Other	Primary Care	NR	NR	NR
Lundborg C. S., 1999[45]	Arm A: Control	104	General Practitioner	NR	General Practice	NR	Uninsured	No
Lundborg C. S., 1999[45]	Arm B: Education and Feedback	100	General Practitioner	NR	General Practice	NR	Uninsured	NR
Mahi-Taright S., 2004[46]	Education	50	General Practitioner	Community Health Center	General Practice	Rural	NR	NR
Mangione-Smith R., 2005[47]	Arm A: Control	NR	"Health care providers"	Community Health Center	Primary Care	Rural, Urban	Uninsured (4) Commercial/Private/ PPO-FFS (40) HMO (56)	No
Mangione-Smith R., 2005[47]	Arm B: Learning collaborative	NR	"Health care providers"	Community Health Center	Primary Care	Rural, Urban	Uninsured (9) Commercial/Private/ PPO-FFS (47) HMO (44)	NR
Martens J. D., 2006[48]	Arm A: Control	54	General Practitioner	NR	NR	NR	NR	Yes
Martens J. D., 2006[48]	Arm B: Guidelines and involved in development	53	General Practitioner	NR	NR	NR	NR	NR
Martens J.	Arm C:	26	General Practitioner	NR	NR	NR	NR	NR

Author, year	Arm	n at Baseline	Type of Healthcare provider	Practice Setting	Practice Specialty	Service Area	Insurance Type	International study / Insurance
D., 2006[48]	Guidelines only							
Martens J. D., 2007[49]	Arm A: cholesterol	28	General Practitioner	Academic, NR	General Practice	NR	NR	Yes
Martens J. D., 2007[49]	Arm B: antibiotics, asthma/COP	25	General Practitioner	Academic, NR	General Practice	NR	NR	NR
McCowan C, 2001[50]	Arm A: Control	NR	General Practitioner		General Practice	NR	Uninsured	No
McCowan C, 2001[50]	Arm B: Intervention	NR	General Practitioner		General Practice	NR	NR	NR
Mitchell E. A., 2005[51]	Arm A: Control	Arm A+B: 270	General Practitioner		NR	NR	NR	Yes
Mitchell E. A., 2005[51]	Arm B: Intervention	Arm A+B: 270	General Practitioner		NR	NR	NR	NR
Newton W. P., 2010[52]	Decision Support	NR	Nurse, Physician Practice managers, other staff	Academic, Community Health Center, Private Practice	Family Medicine, Internal Medicine, Pediatric Medicine	NR	NR	NR
O'Laughlen MC, 2008[53]	MSAGR group	6	General Practitioner, Nurse Practitioner Family Medicine	Community Health Center	Family Medicine, General Practice	Rural	NR	NR
Premaratne U. N., 1999[54]	Arm A: Control	NR	Nurse practice nurses	NR	General Practice	NR	NR	No
Premaratne U. N., 1999[54]	Arm B: Education	NR	Nurse practice nurses	NR	General Practice	NR	NR	NR
Ragazzi H., 2011[55]	Practice 1	Arm A, B: 26-28	Nurse, Pediatrician	Private Practice	Pediatric Medicine	Inner City	Medicaid/Medicare (90)	NR
Ragazzi H., 2011[55]	Practice 2	Arm A, B: 26-28	Nurse, Pediatrician	Private Practice	Pediatric Medicine	Inner City	Medicaid/Medicare (90)	NR
Ragazzi H., 2011[55]	Practice 3	NR	Nurse, Pediatrician	Community Health Center	Pediatric Medicine	Inner City	Medicaid/Medicare (90)	NR
Rance K., 2011[56]	Decision Support	4	Nurse Practitioner, Pediatrician	NR	Pediatric Medicine, Primary Care	Urban	NR	NR
Renzi P. M., 2006[57]	Arm A:Group 4 (control)	NR	Primary Healthcare	Private Practice	NR	NR	NR	No

Author, year	Arm	n at Baseline	Type of Healthcare provider	Practice Setting	Practice Specialty	Service Area	Insurance Type	International study / Insurance
Renzi P. M., 2006[57]	Arm B: Group 1 (stamp)	NR	Primary Healthcare	Private Practice	NR	NR	NR	NR
Renzi P. M., 2006[57]	Arm C: Group 2 (stamp + CME)	NR	Primary Healthcare	Private Practice	NR	NR	NR	NR
Richman M. J, 2000[58]	Feedback	29	Pediatrician	NR	Pediatric Medicine, Primary Care	Urban	Medicaid/Medicare,	No
Ruoff G., 2002[59]	Arm A: Before the Flow Sheet	17	Family physicians	Community Health Center	Family Medicine	NR	NR	No
Ruoff G., 2002[59]	Arm B: After implementation of the Flow Sheet	17	Family physicians	Community Health Center	Family Medicine	NR	NR	NR
Saini B, 2004[60]	Arm A: Control 1	13	General Practitioner, Pharmacist	NR	NR	NR	NR	No
Saini B, 2004[60]	Arm B: Control 2	12	Pharmacist	NR		NR	NR	NR
Saini B, 2004[60]	Arm C: Education	NR	Pharmacist	NR	NR	NR	Uninsured	NR
Schneider A., 2008[61]	Arm A: traditional quality circle	Arm A+B+C: 96	General Practitioner	NR	General Practice	NR	NR	Yes
Schneider A., 2008[61]	Arm B: benchmark quality circle	Arm A+B+C: 96	General Practitioner	NR	General Practice	NR	NR	NR
Schneider A., 2008[61]	Arm C: combined arms	Arm A+B+C: 96	General Practitioner	NR	General Practice	NR	NR	NR
Shah S., 2011[62]	Arm A: Control	Arm A+B: 150	General Practitioner	NR	General Practice	Urban	NR	Yes
Shah S., 2011[62]	Arm B: Practitioner Asthma Communication and Education (PACE)	Arm A+B: 150	General Practitioner	NR	General Practice	Urban	NR	NR

Author, year	Arm	n at Baseline	Type of Healthcare provider	Practice Setting	Practice Specialty	Service Area	Insurance Type	International study / Insurance
Shapiro A., 2011[63]	SBHC	SBHC + NYCHP: 25	Nurse, Physician	Community Health Center	Primary Care	Inner City	Medicaid/Medicare (67), Uninsured (17)	NR
Shapiro A., 2011[63]	NYCHP	SBHC + NYCHP: 25	Nurse, Physician	Community Health Center	Primary Care	Inner City	Medicaid/Medicare (76) Type2: Uninsured (24)	NR
Shiffman R. N., 2000[64]	Arm A: Sole physician arm, pre-post, patient arm, pre	11	Pediatrician	NR	Pediatric Medicine, Primary Care	Inner City, Rural, Suburban, Urban	NR	No
Sondergaard J., 2002[65]	Arm A: control	141	General Practitioner	NR	General Practice	NR	NR	Yes
Sondergaard J., 2002[65]	Arm B: Individual patient count data feedback	77	General Practitioner	NR	General Practice	NR	NR	NR
Sondergaard J., 2002[65]	Arm C: Aggregate data feedback	74	General Practitioner	NR	General Practice	NR	NR	NR
Stergachis A, 2002[66]	Arm A: Control	NR	Pharmacist	Community Health Center, Other, Private Practice	Other	Rural, Urban	managed care, n: 113 (74) Commercial/Private, n: 23 (115) Medicaid/Medicare, n: 4 (3)	No
Stergachis A, 2002[66]	Arm B: Education	35	Pharmacist	Community Health Center, Other, Private Practice	Other	Rural, Urban	managed care, n: 97 (76) Commercial/Private, n: 25(20) Medicaid/Medicare, n: 2 (2)	NR
Suh D. C., 2001[67]	Feedback	NR	NR	NR	NR	NR	NR	NR
Sulaiman N. D., 2010[68]	Arm A: Control (unrelated education)	18	General Practitioner	NR	General Practice	Urban	NR	Yes
Sulaiman N. D., 2010[68]	Arm B: Education	18	General Practitioner	NR	General Practice	Urban	NR	NR

E-21

Author, year	Arm	n at Baseline	Type of Healthcare provider	Practice Setting	Practice Specialty	Service Area	Insurance Type	International study / Insurance
	and guidelines							
Sulaiman N. D., 2010[68]	Arm C: Guidelines	15	General Practitioner	NR	General Practice	Urban	NR	NR
Thyne S.M., 2007[69]	Arm A: Time 1, 2002-2003	NR	Pediatric medical providers," "urgent care clinicians"	Academic, Other	NR	Urban	NR	No
Thyne S.M., 2007[69]	Arm B:	NR	Pediatric medical providers	Community Health Center	Pediatric Medicine	Urban	NR	NR
Thyne S.M., 2007[69]	Arm B: Time 2, 2003-2004	NR	Pediatric medical Providers," "urgent care clinicians"	Academic, Other	NR	Urban	NR	NR
Thyne S.M., 2007[69]	Arm C: Time 3, 2004-2005	NR	Pediatric medical Providers," "urgent care clinicians"	Academic, Other	NR	Urban	NR	NR
To T. 2008[70]	PCAPP Intervention	NR	Primary Healthcare	Community Health Center, Other	NR	Inner City, Rural, Urban	NR	NR
Veninga CCM, 1999[71]	Arm A: Netherlands	181	General Practitioner	NR	General Practice	NR	NR	Yes
Veninga CCM, 1999[71]	Arm B: Sweden	204	General Practitioner	NR	General Practice	NR	NR	NR
Veninga CCM, 1999[71]	Arm C: Norway	199	General Practitioner	NR	General Practice	NR	NR	NR
Veninga CCM, 1999[71]	Arm D: Slovakia	81	Allergist, Pulmonologist	NR	Other	NR	NR	NR
Veninga CCM, 2000[72]	Arm A: UTI	91	General Practitioner	NR	General Practice	NR	NR	Yes
Veninga CCM, 2000[72]	Arm B: Education and Feedback	90	General Practitioner	NR	General Practice	NR	NR	NR
Weinberger M, 2002[73]	Arm A: Control	NR	Pharmacist	Private Practice	NR	NR	NR	No
Weinberger M, 2002[73]	Arm B: Peak Flow Meter Monitoring Control Group	NR	Pharmacist	Private Practice	NR	NR	Uninsured	NR
Weinberger	Arm C:	NR	Pharmacist	NR	NR	NR	NR	NR

Author, year	Arm	n at Baseline	Type of Healthcare provider	Practice Setting	Practice Specialty	Service Area	Insurance Type	International study / Insurance
M, 2002[73]	Pharmaceutical Care Program Group							
Weinberger M, 2002[73]	Arm D:	NR	NR	Private Practice	NR	NR	NR	NR
Yawn BP, 2008[74]	Education and Feedback	211	Nurse Practitioner, Physician, Physician Assistant	Community Health Center, Private Practice	Family Medicine, Other	Rural, Suburban	NR	NR

FFS = fee for service; HMO = Health Maintenance Organization; MC = Managed Care; NR = Not Reported; NYCHP = New York Children's Hospital Project; PPO = Preferred Provider Organization; UTI = Urinary Tract Infection

References

1 Ables AZ, Godenick MT, Lipsitz SR. Family Medicine: Improving family practice residents' compliance with asthma practice guidelines. 2002; 34:23-8.

2 Armour C, Bosnic-Anticevich S, Brillant M et al. Thorax: Pharmacy Asthma Care Program (PACP) improves outcomes for patients in the community. 2007; 62:496-502.

3 Baker R, Fraser RC, Stone M, Lambert P, Stevenson K, Shiels C. Br J Gen Pract: Randomised controlled trial of the impact of guidelines, prioritized review criteria and feedback on implementation of recommendations for angina and asthma. 2003; 53:284-91.

4 Bell LM, Grundmeier R, Localio R et al. Pediatrics: Electronic health record-based decision support to improve asthma care: a cluster-randomized trial. 2010; 125:e770-7.

5 Bender BG, Dickinson P, Rankin A, Wamboldt FS, Zittleman L, Westfall JM. J Am Board Fam Med: The Colorado Asthma Toolkit Program: a practice coaching intervention from the High Plains Research Network. 2011; 24:240-8.

6 Blackstien-Hirsch P, Anderson G, Cicutto L, McIvor A, Norton P. Journal of Asthma: Implementing continuing education strategies for family physicians to enhance asthma patients' quality of life. 2000; 37:247-57.

7 Brown R, Bratton SL, Cabana MD, Kaciroti N, Clark NM. Chest: Physician asthma education program improves outcomes for children of low-income families. 2004; 126:369-74.

8 Bryce FP, Neville RG, Crombie IK, Clark RA, McKenzie P. British Medical Journal: Controlled trial of an audit facilitator in diagnosis and treatment of childhood asthma in general practice. 1995; 310:838-42.

9 Cabana MD, Slish KK, Evans D et al. Pediatrics: Impact of physician asthma care education on patient outcomes. 2006; 117:2149-57.

E-23

10 Cho SH, Jeong JW, Park HW *et al.* J Asthma: Effectiveness of a computer-assisted asthma management program on physician adherence to guidelines. 2010; 47:630-6.

11 Clark N, Gong M, Schork, M, *et al.* Impact of education for physicians on patient outcomes. Pediatrics 1998; 101(5):831-6.

12 Cloutier MM , Wakefield DB, Carlisle PS, Bailit HL, Hall CB. Arch Pediatr Adolesc Med: The effect of Easy Breathing on asthma management and knowledge. 2002; 156:1045-51.

13 Cloutier MM , Hall CB, Wakefield DB, Bailit H. J Pediatr: Use of asthma guidelines by primary care providers to reduce hospitalizations and emergency department visits in poor, minority, urban children. 2005; 146:591-7.

14 Cloutier MM , Grosse SD, Wakefield DB, Nurmagambetov TA, Brown CM. American Journal of Managed Care: The economic impact of an urban asthma management program. 2009; 15:345-51.

15 Vital signs: asthma prevalence, disease characteristics, and self-management education: United States, 2001--2009. MMWR Morb Mortal Wkly Rep 2011; 60(17):547-52.

16 Coleman CI, Reddy P, Laster-Bradley NM, Dorval S, Munagala B, White CM. Ann Pharmacother: Effect of practitioner education on adherence to asthma treatment guidelines. 2003; 37:956-61.

17 Cowie RL, Underwood MF, Mack S. Can Respir J: The impact of asthma management guideline dissemination on the control of asthma in the community. 2001; 8 Suppl A:41A-5A.

18 Daniels EC, Bacon J, Denisio S *et al.* J Asthma: Translation squared: improving asthma care for high-disparity populations through a safety net practice-based research network. 2005; 42:499-505.

19 Davis AM, Cannon M, Ables AZ, Bendyk H. Family Medicine: Using the electronic medical record to improve asthma severity documentation and treatment among family medicine residents. 2010; 42:334-7.

20 Davis RS, Bukstein DA, Luskin AT, Kailin JA, Goodenow G. Ann Allergy Asthma Immunol: Changing physician prescribing patterns through problem-based learning; an interactive, teleconference case-based education program and review of problem-based learning. 2004; 93:237-42.

21 de Vries TW , van den Berg PB, Duiverman EJ, de Jong-van den Berg LT. Arch Dis Child: Effect of a minimal pharmacy intervention on improvement of adherence to asthma guidelines. 2010; 95:302-4.

22 Eccles M, McColl E, Steen N *et al.* BMJ: Effect of computerised evidence based guidelines on management of asthma and angina in adults in primary care: cluster randomised controlled trial. 2002; 325:941.

23 Fairall L, Bachmann MO, Zwarenstein M *et al.* Trop Med Int Health: Cost-effectiveness of educational outreach to primary care nurses to increase tuberculosis case detection and improve respiratory care: economic evaluation alongside a randomised trial. 2010; 15:277-86.

24 Feder G, Griffiths C, Highton C, Eldridge S, Spence M, Southgate L. British Medical Journal: Do clinical guidelines introduced with practice based education improve care of asthmatic and diabetic patients? A randomised controlled trial in general practices in east London. 1995; 311:1473-8.

25 Finkelstein JA, Lozano P, Fuhlbrigge AL *et al.* Health Serv Res: Practice-level effects of interventions to improve asthma care in primary care settings: the Pediatric Asthma Care Patient Outcomes Research Team. 2005; 40:1737-57.

26 Lozano P, Finkelstein JA, Carey VJ *et al.* Arch Pediatr Adolesc Med: A multisite randomized trial of the effects of physician education and organizational change in chronic-asthma care: health outcomes of the Pediatric Asthma Care Patient Outcomes Research Team II Study. 2004; 158:875-83.

27 Foster JM, Hoskins G, Smith B, Lee AJ, Price D, Pinnock H. BMC Fam Pract: Practice development plans to improve the primary care management of acute asthma: randomised controlled trial. 2007;

8:23.

28 Fox P, Porter PG, Lob SH, Boer JH, Rocha DA, Adelson JW. Pediatrics: Improving asthma-related health outcomes among low-income, multiethnic, school-aged children: Results of a demonstration project that combined continuous quality improvement and community health worker strategies. 2007; 120:e902-e911.

29 Frankowski BL, Keating K, Rexroad A et al. J Sch Health: Community collaboration: concurrent physician and school nurse education and cooperation increases the use of asthma action plans. 2006; 76:303-6.

30 Glasgow NJ, Ponsonby AL, Yates R, Beilby J, Dugdale P. BMJ: Proactive asthma care in childhood: general practice based randomised controlled trial. 2003; 327:659.

31 Gorton TA, Cranford CO, Golden WE, Walls RC, Pawelak JE. Arch Fam Med: Primary care physicians' response to dissemination of practice guidelines. 1995; 4:135-42.

32 Hagmolen of ten Have W, van den Berg NJ, van der Palen J, van Aalderen WM, Bindels PJ. Prim Care Respir J: Implementation of an asthma guideline for the management of childhood asthma in general practice: a randomised controlled trial. 2008; 17:90-6.

33 Halterman JS, McConnochie KM, Conn KM et al. Archives of Pediatrics and Adolescent Medicine: A randomized trial of primary care provider prompting to enhance preventive asthma therapy. 2005; 159:422-7.

34 Halterman JS, Fisher S, Conn KM et al. Archives of Pediatrics & Adolescent Medicine: Improved preventive care for asthma: a randomized trial of clinician prompting in pediatric offices. 2006; 160:1018-25.

35 Herborg H, Soendergaard B, Jorgensen T, et al. J Am Pharm Assoc (Wash): Improving drug therapy for patients with asthma-part 2: Use of antiasthma medications. 2001; 41:551-9.

36 Herborg H, Soendergaard B, Froekjaer B, et al. Improving drug therapy for patients with asthma–part 1: Patient outcomes. J Am Pharm Assoc (Wash) 2001; (4):539-50.

37 Holton C, Crockett A, Nelson M, et al. International Journal for Quality in Health Care: Does spirometry training in general practice improve quality and outcomes of asthma care? 2011; 23:545-53.

38 Homer CJ, Forbes P, Horvitz L, Peterson LE, Wypij D, Heinrich P. Archives of Pediatrics and Adolescent Medicine: Impact of a quality improvement program on care and outcomes for children with asthma. 2005; 159:464-9.

39 Horswell R, Butler MK, Kaiser M et al. Dis Manag: Disease management programs for the underserved. 2008; 11:145-52.

40 Hoskins G, Neville RG, Smith B, Clark RA. Health Bull (Edinb): Does participation in distance learning and audit improve the care of patients with acute asthma attacks? The General Practitioners in Asthma Group. 1997; 55:150-5.

41 Kattan M, Crain EF, Steinbach S et al. Pediatrics: A randomized clinical trial of clinician feedback to improve quality of care for inner-city children with asthma. 2006; 117:e1095-103.

42 Lesho EP, Myers CP, Ott M, Winslow C, Brown JE. Mil Med: Do clinical practice guidelines improve processes or outcomes in primary care? 2005; 170:243-6.

43 Liaw ST, Sulaiman ND, Barton CA et al. BMC Fam Pract: An interactive workshop plus locally adapted guidelines can improve general practitioners asthma management and knowledge: a cluster randomised trial in the Australian setting. 2008; 9:22.

44 Lob SH, Boer JH, Porter PG, et al. Promoting Best-Care Practices in Childhood Asthma: Quality Improvement in Community Health Centers. Pediatrics 2011;128:20; Originally Published Online June 13, 2011; DOI: 10.1542/Peds.2010-1962 .

45 Lundborg CS , Wahlstrom R, Oke T, Tomson G, Diwan VK. J Clin

Epidemiol: Influencing prescribing for urinary tract infection and asthma in primary care in Sweden: a randomized controlled trial of an interactive educational intervention. 1999; 52:801-12.

46 Mahi-Taright S, Belhocine M, Ait-Khaled N. Int J Tuberc Lung Dis: Can we improve the management of chronic obstructive respiratory disease? The example of asthma in adults. 2004; 8:873-81.

47 Mangione-Smith R, Schonlau M, Chan KS et al. Ambulatory Pediatrics: Measuring the effectiveness of a collaborative for quality improvement in pediatric asthma care: Does implementing the chronic care model improve processes and outcomes of care? 2005; 5:75-82.

48 Martens JD, Winkens RA, van der Weijden T, de Bruyn D, Severens JL. BMC Health Serv Res: Does a joint development and dissemination of multidisciplinary guidelines improve prescribing behaviour: a pre/post study with concurrent control group and a randomised trial. 2006; 6:145.

49 Martens JD, van der Weijden T, Severens JL et al. Int J Med Inform: The effect of computer reminders on GPs' prescribing behaviour: a cluster-randomised trial. 2007; 76 Suppl 3:S403-16.

50 McCowan C, Neville RG, Ricketts IW, Warner FC, Hoskins G, Thomas GE. Medical Informatics and the Internet in Medicine: Lessons from a randomized controlled trial designed to evaluate computer decision support software to improve the management of asthma. 2001; 26:191-201.

51 Mitchell EA, Didsbury PB, Kruithof N et al. Acta Paediatr: A randomized controlled trial of an asthma clinical pathway for children in general practice. 2005; 94:226-33.

52 Newton WP, Lefebvre A, Donahue KE, Bacon T, Dobson A. J Contin Educ Health Prof: Infrastructure for large-scale quality-improvement projects: early lessons from North Carolina Improving Performance in Practice. 2010; 30:106-13.

53 O'Laughlen MC, Hollen PJ, Rakes G, Ting S. Pediatric Asthma,

Allergy and Immunology: Improving pediatric asthma by the MSAGR algorithm: A multicolored, simplified, asthma guideline reminder. 2008; 21:119-27.

54 Premaratne UN, Sterne JA, Marks GB, Webb JR, Azima H, Burney PG. BMJ: Clustered randomised trial of an intervention to improve the management of asthma: Greenwich asthma study. 1999; 318:1251-5.

55 Ragazzi H, Keller A, Ehrensberger R, Irani AM. J Urban Health: Evaluation of a practice-based intervention to improve the management of pediatric asthma. 2011; 88 Suppl 1:38-48.

56 Rance K, O'Laughlen M, Ting S. J Pediatr Health Care: Improving asthma care for African American children by increasing national asthma guideline adherence. 2011; 25:235-49.

57 Renzi PM, Ghezzo H, Goulet S, Dorval E, Thivierge RL. Can Respir J: Paper stamp checklist tool enhances asthma guidelines knowledge and implementation by primary care physicians. 2006; 13:193-7.

58 Richman MJ, Poltawsky JS. Stud Health Technol Inform: Partnership for excellence in asthma care: evidence-based disease management. 2000; 76:107-21.

59 Ruoff G. Family Medicine: Effects of flow sheet implementation on physician performance in the management of asthmatic patients. 2002; 34:514-7.

60 Saini B, Krass I, Armour C. Annals of Pharmacotherapy: Development, implementation, and evaluation of a community pharmacy-based asthma care model. 2004; 38:1954-60.

61 Schneider A, Wensing M, Biessecker K, Quinzler R, Kaufmann-Kolle P, Szecsenyi J. J Eval Clin Pract: Impact of quality circles for improvement of asthma care: results of a randomized controlled trial. 2008; 14:185-90.

62 Shah S, Sawyer SM, Toelle BG et al. Med J Aust: Improving paediatric asthma outcomes in primary health care: a randomised

controlled trial. 2011; 195:405-9.

63 Shapiro A, Gracy D, Quinones W, Applebaum J, Sarmiento A. Arch Pediatr Adolesc Med: Putting guidelines into practice: improving documentation of pediatric asthma management using a decision-making tool. 2011; 165:412-8.

64 Shiffman RN, Freudigman M, Brandt CA, Liaw Y, Navedo DD. Pediatrics: A guideline implementation system using handheld computers for office management of asthma: effects on adherence and patient outcomes. 2000; 105:767-73.

65 Sondergaard J, Andersen M, Vach K, Kragstrup J, Maclure M, Gram LF. Eur J Clin Pharmacol: Detailed postal feedback about prescribing to asthma patients combined with a guideline statement showed no impact: a randomised controlled trial. 2002; 58:127-32.

66 Stergachis A, Gardner JS, Anderson MT, Sullivan SD. Journal of the American Pharmaceutical Association (Washington,D.C. : 1996): Improving pediatric asthma outcomes in the community setting: does pharmaceutical care make a difference? 2002; 42:743-52.

67 Suh DC, Shin SK, Okpara I, Voytovich RM, Zimmerman A. Am J Manag Care: Impact of a targeted asthma intervention program on treatment costs in patients with asthma. 2001; 7:897-906.

68 Sulaiman ND, Barton CA, Liaw ST et al. Fam Pract: Do small group workshops and locally adapted guidelines improve asthma patients'

health outcomes? A cluster randomized controlled trial. 2010; 27:246-54.

69 Thyne SM, Marmor AK, Madden N, Herrick G. Paediatric and Perinatal Epidemiology: Comprehensive asthma management for underserved children. 2007 21:29-34.

70 To T, Cicutto L, Degani N, McLimont S, Beyene J. Med Care: Can a community evidence-based asthma care program improve clinical outcomes?: a longitudinal study. 2008; 46:1257-66.

71 Veninga CC, Lagerløv P, Wahlström R,et al. Evaluating an educational intervention to improve the treatment of asthma in four european countries. American Journal of Respiratory and Critical Care Medicine:1999; 160: 1254-62.

72 Veninga CCM , Denig P, Zwaagstra R, Haaijer-Ruskamp FM. Journal of Clinical Epidemiology: Improving drug treatment in general practice. 2000; 53:762-72.

73 Weinberger M, Murray MD, Marrero DG et al. Journal of the American Medical Association: Effectiveness of pharmacist care for patients with reactive airways disease: A randomized controlled trial. 2002; 288:1594-602.

74 Yawn BP, Bertram S, Wollan P. Journal of Asthma and Allergy: Introduction of asthma APGAR tools improve asthma management in primary care practices. 2008; 1-10.

Evidence Table 3. Patient characteristics

Author, Year	Arm (n)	Age in years	Women n (%)	Race	Asthma Severity, n(%) (Degree of control if reported)	# of Acute Asthma visits/given timeframe
Ables AZ, 2002[1]	Education and reminders(126)	Mean: 26	n: 85(67.5)	White-n: 46 White(36.5), Black-n: 77 Black(61.1), Latino-n: 2, Latino(1.6), A/P-n: 1,A/P(0.8)	Intermittent (25) Mild (0) Moderate (0) Severe (25)	NR
Armour C., 2007[2]	Arm A: Control (186)	Mean: 51	(60.8)	NR	Mild, n: 3 (1.6) Moderate n: 50 (27.2) Severe, n: 131 (71.2)	NR
Armour C., 2007[2]	Arm B: Pharmacy Asthma Care Program [PACP](165)	Mean: 49	(69.7)	NR	Mild, n: 5 (3) Moderate, n: 15 (9.1) Severe, n: 145 (87.9)	NR
Baker R., 2003[3]	Arm A: Guidelines only(483)	Mean: 50	n: 249(51.6)	NR	NR	NR
Baker R., 2003[3]	Arm B: Guidelines with audit criteria(510)	Mean: 49	n: 294(57.7)	NR	NR	NR
Baker R., 2003[3]	Arm C: Guidelines with audit criteria and feedback (489)	Mean: 45	n: 288(58.9)	NR	NR	NR
Bell L.M., 2010[4]	Arm A: UP Control(5192)	NR	NR	White(1) Black(96), Latino(1),A/P(NR),Ot her(1)	NR	NR
Bell L.M., 2010[4]	Arm B: UP intervention(5040)	NR	NR	White(13) Black(80), Latino(3),A/P(NR),Ot her(8)	NR	NR
Bell L.M., 2010[4]	Arm C: SP Control(3843)	NR	NR	White(80) Black(5), Latino(5),A/P(NR),Ot her(15)	NR	NR
Bell L.M., 2010[4]	Arm D: up Control (5375)	NR	NR	White(40) Black(50), Latino(3),A/P(999),Ot her(10)	NR	NR
Brown R, 2004[5]	Arm A: Control(122)	NR	n: 37(30.3)	White-n: 91 White(74.6), Black-n: 13 Black(10.7), Latino-n: 13, Latino(10.7), Other-n: 5,Other(4.1)	Moderate, Severe, n: 112 (91.8)	NR
Brown R, 2004[5]	Arm B: Education(157)	NR	n: 42(26.7)	White-n: 113 White(72), Black-n:	Moderate, Severe, n: 134 (85.4)	NR

Author, Year	Arm (n)	Age in years	Women n (%)	Race	Asthma Severity, n(%) (Degree of control if reported)	# of Acute Asthma visits/given timeframe
				27 Black(17.2), Latino-n: 12, Latino(7.6), Other-n: 5,Other(3.2)		
Bryce FP, 1995[6]	Arm A: Control Group(1563)	NR	NR	NR	NR	NR
Bryce FP, 1995[6]	Arm B: Reminders and tools(1585)	NR	NR	NR	NR	NR
Cabana M. D., 2006[7]	Arm A: Control(452)	Mean: 7	n: 168	NR	Persistent asthma, n: 172 (38)	Hospital admissions per year: 0.12 +/- 0.47 (Mean +/- Std. Dev.); ED asthma visits per year: 0.66 +/- 1.8; emergent doctor visits per year: 1.7 +/- 2.5
Cabana M. D., 2006[7]	Arm B: Physician Asthma Care Education [PACE](418)	Mean: 7	n: 148	NR	Persistent asthma, n: 153 (36)	Hospital admissions per year: 0.14 +/- 0.0.54 (Mean +/- Std. Dev.); ED asthma visits per year: 0.85 +/- 2.0 ; emergent doctor visits per year: 1.8 +/-3.3
Cho S. H., 2010[8]	Decision Support (2042)	Mean: 51,	n: 1096(53.7)	NR	Mild, n: 519 ⁻25.4) Moderate, n 1234 (60.4) Severe, n: 239 (14.2)	NR
Clark NM, 1998[9]	Arm B: Education(637)	Range: 1-12	(30)	White(NR) Black(15), Latino(15)	NR	NR
Cloutier M. M., 2002[10]	Pre-intervention (860)	NR	NR	NR	NR	NR
Cloutier M. M., 2002[10]	Post-intervention (860)	NR	NR	NR	NR	NR
Cloutier M. M., 2005[11]	Decision support (3748)	NR	n: 1638(44)	White-n: 50 White(1), Black-n: 825 Black(22), Latino-n: 2436, Latino(65), Other-n: 437,Other(12)	NR	NR
Cloutier M.M., 2009[12]	Decision support (3298)	NR	NR	White(5) Black(22), Latino(65),Other (7)	Mild (29) Moderate (▼) Severe (2)	NR

Study	Arm	Age	n (%)	Race/Ethnicity		
Cloutier M.M., 2012[13]	Arm A: Control ()	NR	NR	NR	NR	NR
Cloutier M.M., 2012[13]	Arm B: Patient-directed interventions	NR	NR	NR	NR	NR
Coleman C. I., 2003[14]	Arm A: Patient specific information: Prescribers with patients on 'high dose' (510)	Mean: 46	n: 393(77)	White-n: 172 White(34), Black-n: 103 Black(20), Latino-n: 220, Latino(43), A/P-n: 14,A/P(3), Other-n: 1,Other(0.1)	NR	NR
Coleman C. I., 2003[14]	Arm B: Patient specific information: Prescribers with patients on 'low dose' (135)	Mean: 46	n: 79(59)	White-n: 48 White(36), Black-n: 36 Black(27), Latino-n: 49, Latino(36), A/P-n: 2,A/P(1), Other-n: 0,Other(0)	NR	NR
Cowie R. L., 2001[15]	Arm A: Basic Education(NR)	Mean: 39,	NR	NR	NR	NR
Cowie R. L., 2001[15]	Arm B: Intermediate Education(NR)	Mean: 45,	NR	NR	NR	NR
Cowie R. L., 2001[15]	Arm C: Intensive Education(NR)	Mean: 46,	NR	NR	NR	NR
Daniels E. C., 2005[16]	Arm A: Control (136079)	NR	NR	Black(57.9), Latino(10.1)	NR	NR
Daniels E. C., 2005[16]	Arm B: Education (90555)	NR	NR	Black(26.9), Latino(2.3)	NR	NR
Davis AM, 2010[17]	Decision Support(180)	Mean: 32	n: 125(69.4)	White-n: 48 White(26.7), Black-n: 129 Black(71.7), Latino-n: 3, Latino(1.7), A/P-n: 0,A/P(0)	NR	NR
de Vries T. W., 2010[18]	Arm A: Control (3527)	NR	NR	NR	NR	NR
de Vries T. W., 2010[18]	Arm B: Feedback(1447)	NR	NR	NR	NR	NR
de Vries T. W., 2010[18]	Arm C: 2002(3612)	NR	NR	NR	NR	NR
Eccles M., 2002[19]	Arm A: angina (4851)	NR	NR	NR	NR	NR
Eccles M., 2002[19]	Arm B: asthma (4960)	NR	NR	NR	NR	NR

Author, Year	Arm (n)	Age in years	Women n (%)	Race	Asthma Severity, n(%) (Degree of control if reported)	# of Acute Asthma visits/given timeframe
Fairall L., 2010[20]	Arm A: Control	Mean: 44,	n: 660(66.1)	NR	NR	NR
Fairall L., 2010[20]	Arm B: Intervention(1000)	Mean: 45	n: 643(64.3)	NR	NR	NR
Feder G, 1995[21]	Arm A: Diabetes education	NR	NR	NR	NR	NR
Feder G, 1995[21]	Arm B: Education and reminders audit	NR	NR	NR	NR	NR
Finkelstein J. A., 2005[22]	Arm B: PLE Intervention(2003)	NR	NR	NR	NR	NR
Finkelstein J. A., 2005[22]	Arm C: Planned Care Intervention (1635)	NR	NR	NR	NR	NR
Foster J. M., 2007[23]	Arm A: Education and Feedback (delayed)(133)	Mean: 40,	(68)	NR	NR	NR
Foster J. M., 2007[23]	Arm B: Education and Feedback(54)	Mean: 38,	(56)	NR	NR	NR
Fox P., 2007[24]	Chart review sample (280)	Mean: 11, Median: 10	(38.6)	White(13.6) Black(16.4), Latino(66.1),Other (3.9)	Mild Intermittent (47.1) Mild persistent (27.9) Moderate (24)	NR
Frankowski B. L., 2006[25]	Multimodal: Education and Feedback(150)	NR	NR	NR	NR	NR
Glasgow N. J., 2003[26]	Arm A: Control (73)	NR	(45)	NR	NR	NR
Glasgow N. J., 2003[26]	Arm B: Intervention (101)	NR	(35)	NR	NR	NR
Gorton T. A., 1995[27]	Arm A: Guidelines only	NR	NR	NR	NR	NR
Gorton T. A., 1995[27]	Arm B: Education and Detailing	NR	NR	NR	NR	NR
Gorton T. A., 1995[27]	Arm C: Education on computer	NR	NR	NR	NR	NR
Gorton T. A., 1995[27]	Arm D:Education – multimedia	NR	NR	NR	NR	NR
Gorton T. A., 1995[27]	Arm C:	NR	NR	NR	NR	NR
Hagmolen, W.,, 2008[28]	Arm A: Guidelines only(98)	Mean: 11	n: 41	NR	NR	NR
Hagmolen, W.,,	Arm B: Education and	Mean: 11	n: 58	NR	NR	NR

Author, Year	Arm (n)	Age in years	Women n (%)	Race	Asthma Severity, n(%) (Degree of control if reported)	# of Acute Asthma visits/given timeframe
2008[28]	Guidelines(133)					
Hagmolen, W., 2008[28]	Arm C: Education and Guidelines and individualized treatment advice(131)	Mean: 11	n: 62	NR	NR	NR
Halterman J. S., 2005[29]	Arm A: Control (77)	NR	n: 31(40.3)	White-n: 7 White(9.1), Black-n: 48 Black(62.3), Latino(22.1), A/P-NR, A/P(NR), Other-n: 22, Other(28.6)	No. of visit: 4(+) symptom days per week over 4 weeks: 21 (27.3%) 4(+) symptom nights per week over past 4 wks: 13 (27.3%)	3(+) acute visits in the past yr: 23 (30.3%) 1(+) hospitalization in past yr: 5 (6.5%).
Halterman J. S., 2005[29]	Arm B: Intervention (73)	NR	n: 32(43.8)	White-n: 10 White(13.7), Black-n: 41 Black(56.2), Latino-n: 20, Latino(27.4), A/P-NR, A/P(NR), Other-n: 22, Other(30.1)	No. of visit: 4(+) symptom days per week over 4 weeks: 18 (25.4%) 4(+) symptom nights per week over past 4 wks: 11 (15.1%)	3(+) acute visits in the past yr: 24 (32.9%) 1(+) hospitalization in past yr: 3 (4.1%).
Halterman J.S., 2006[30]	Arm A: Control(124)	NR	n: 38(33)	White-n: 13 White(11.4), Black-n: 74 Black(64.9), Latino-n: 37, Latino(32.5), A/P-NR, A/P(NR), Other-n: 27, Other(23.7)	Mild, n: 19 (16.7) Moderate, n: 47 (41.2) Severe, n: 48 (42.1)	NR
Halterman J.S., 2006[30]	Arm B: Intervention(122)	NR	n: 57(51)	White-n: 9 White(8), Black-n: 71 Black(63.4), Latino-n: 30, Latino(26.8), A/P-NR, A/P(NR), Other-n: 32, Other(26.8)	Mild, n: 29 (25.9) Moderate, n: 45 (40.2) Severe, n: 38 (33.9)	NR
Herborg H., 2001[31][32]	Arm B: Therapeutic Outcomes Monitoring [TOM](NR)	Mean: 45,	NR	NR	NR	NR
Herborg, H., 2001[31][32]	Arm A: Control(NR)	Mean: 39,	NR	NR	NR	NR
Holton C., 2011[33]	Arm A: Control (157)	Mean: 55,	n: 106 (67.5)	NR	Mild, n: 106 (67.5) Controlled, n: 123 (78.4) Not well-Controlled: 26	NR

Author, Year	Arm (n)	Age in years	Women n (%)	Race	Asthma Severity, n(%) (Degree of control if reported)	# of Acute Asthma visits/given timeframe
		(16.5)			Poorly controlled n: 8 (5.1)	
Holton C., 2011[33]	Arm B: Spirometry training (240)	Mean: 58,	n: 162(67.5)	NR	Mild n: 164 68.3) Controlled, n: 165 (68.7) Not well-Controlled, n: 58 (24.2) Poorly controlled n: 17 (7.1)	NR
Homer CJ, 2005[34]	Arm A: Control(337)	Median: 9, Range: 2.6-16.7	n: 134(40)	White(43) Black(27),Other(30)	NR	NR
Homer CJ, 2005[34]	Arm B: Learning collaborative (294)	Median: 8, Range: 2.5-16.4	n: 107(36)	White(50) Black(28), Other(22)	NR	NR
Horswell R., 2008[35]	HCSD's DM program(2199)	NR	NR	NR	NR	NR
Hoskins G., 1997[36]	Arm A: Before intervention (782)	NR	NR	NR	NR	NR
Hoskins G., 1997[36]	Arm B: Education and Feedback(669)	NR	NR	NR	NR	NR
Kattan M., 2006[37]	Arm A: Control(466)	Mean: 8	(37.1)	White(6.4) Black(38.8), Latino(39.9),A/P(1.3), Other(9.7)	NR	Mean ED visits: 3.0; unscheduled clinic visits: 5.5; hospitalizations: 0.8.
Kattan M., 2006[37]	Arm B: Intervention(471)	Mean: 8	(39.5)	White(7.4) Black(40.3), Latino(40.3),A/P(1.1), Other(8.5)	NR	Mean ED visits: 3.0; unscheduled clinic visits: 5.6; hospitalizations: 1.1
Lesho E. P., 2005[38]	Decision Support (330)	NR	NR	NR	NR	553/pre-intervention; 193/post intervention
Lob S. H., 2011[39]	Longitudinal Evaluation Group – Patient-level Interview (761)	Mean: 7.4, Median: 6.9, Range: 0-18	(41.3)	Black (6.7) Hispanic (85.3) White (3.9) Other (4.1)	Intermittent: 22.6 Mild Persistent: 49.2 Mod Persistent: 25.8 Severe Persistent: 2.3	NR
Lob S. H., 2011[39]	Cross-sectional Random Sample - Clinic-level Chart Review, T1 (680)	Mean:7.8, Median: 7.0, Range: 0-18	(40.4)	Black (10.9) Hispanic (76.9) White (5.9) Other (6.3)	Intermittent:43.9 Mild Persistent: 36.0 Mod Persistent: 19.9 Severe Persistent: 0.3	NR

Study	Intervention/Arm	Age		Race/Ethnicity	Severity	Other
Lob S. H., 2011[39]	Cross-sectional Random Sample - Clinic-level Chart Review, T2 (680)	Mean: 8.0, Median: 7.5), Range: 0-18	(42.1)	Black (10.9) Hispanic (76.9) White (5.9) Other (6.3)	Intermittent: 42.3 Mild Persistent:34.1 Mod Persistent: 22.0 Severe Persistent: 1.7	NR
Lob S. H., 2011[39]	Cross-sectional Random Sample - Clinic-level Chart Review, T3 (680)	Mean: 8.1, Median: 7.7 Range: 0-18	(40.6)	Black (10.9) Hispanic (76.9) White (5.9) Other (6.3)	Intermittent: 36.3 Mild Persistent: 44.5 Mod Persistent: 18.0 Severe Persistent 1.2	NR
Lozano P., 2004[40]	Arm A: Control(199)	Mean: 10	n: 139	White-n: 70, Black-n: 13, Latino-n: 6, Other-n: 11	NR	NR
Lozano P., 2004[40]	Arm B: Chronic care model(226)	Mean: 9	n: 169	White-n: 58, Black-n: 22, Latino-n: 6, Other-n: 14	NR	NR
Lozano P., 2004[40]	Planned care intervention (213)	Mean: 9	n: 151	White-n: 69, Black-n: 18, Latino-n: 4, Other-n: 9	NR	22/past year
Lundborg C. S., 1999[41]	Arm A: Control arm(1333)	NR	NR	NR	NR	NR
Lundborg C. S., 1999[41]	Arm B: Education and Feedback(1121)	NR	NR	NR	NR	NR
Mahi-Taright S., 2004[42]	Education(49)	NR	NR	NR	NR	24/past year
Mangione-Smith R., 2005[43]	Arm A: Control(126)	Mean: 10,	(34)	White(43) Black(23), Latino(22),A/P(NR),Other(12)	Scale: NAEPP, Persistent: Intermittent (50) Mild (24) Moderate, Severe (26)	NR
Mangione-Smith R., 2005[43]	Arm B: Learning collaborative(385)	Mean: 9,	(43)	White(19) Black(30), Latino(29), Other(22)	Scale: NAEPP, Persistent: Intermittent (64) Mild (20) Moderate, Severe (16)	NR
Martens J. D., 2007[44]	Arm A: (24160)	NR	NR	NR	NR	NR
Martens J. D., 2007[44]	Arm B: (35748)	NR	NR	NR	NR	NR
McCowan C, 2001[45]	Arm A: Control (330)	Mean: 37,	n: 176(53)	NR	NR	NR
McCowan C, 2001[45]	Arm B: Decision support (147)	Mean: 33,	n: 75 (51)	NR	NR	NR
Mitchell E. A., 2005[46]	Arm B: Intervention (NR)	NR	NR	NR	NR	NR

Author, Year	Arm (n)	Age in years	Women n (%)	Race	Asthma Severity, n(%) (Degree of control if reported)	# of Acute Asthma visits/given timeframe
O'Laughlen MC, 2008[47]	Arm B: MSAGR group(24)	Mean: 9, NR, Range: 5-12	n: 8(33)	White-n: 21 White(88), Black-n: 2 Black(8), Latino-NR, Latino(NR), A/P-NR,A/P(NR), Other-n: 1,Other(4)	Mild, n: 22 (92) Moderate, r: 2 (8)	NR
Patel P . H., 2004[48]	Organizational Change (451)	NR	NR	NR	NR	NR
Premaratne U. N., 1999[49]	Arm A: Control(14410)	NR	NR	NR	NR	NR
Premaratne U. N., 1999[49]	Arm B: Education (9900)	NR	NR	NR	NR	NR
Ragazzi H., 2011[50]	Arm B: Practice 1(17)	NR	NR	NR	NR	NR
Ragazzi H., 2011[50]	Arm C: Practice 2(26)	NR	NR	NR	NR	NR
Rance K., 2011[51]	Arm B: (41)	Range: 5-17 years	n: 19	NR	Mild, n: 5 (12) Moderate, π 29 (70) Severe, n: 7 (17)	NR
Richman M. J, 2000[52]	Feedback(228)	NR	NR	NR	NR	NR
Ruoff G., 2002[53]	Arm A: Before the Flow Sheet(122)	NR	NR	NR	NR	NR
Ruoff G., 2002[53]	Arm B: After implementation of the Flow Sheet(122)	NR	NR	NR	NR	NR
Saini B, 2004[54]	Arm A: Control 1(22)	Mean: 52,	NR (73)	NR	NR	hospitalizations past year = 0.1 +/- 0.6
Saini B, 2004[54]	Arm B: Control 2(28)	Mean: 42,	NR (79)	NR	NR	hospitalizations past year = 1.3 +/- 4.1
Saini B, 2004[54]	Arm C: Education (52)	Mean: 43,	NR(61)	NR	NR	hospitalizations past year = 0.18 +/- 0.6
Schneider A., 2008[55]	Arm A: traditional quality circle(NR)	NR	NR	NR	NR	NR
Schneider A., 2008[55]	Arm B: benchmark quality circle(NR)	NR	NR	NR	NR	NR
Schneider A.,	Arm C: combined	Mean: 57	n: 158(61.7)	NR	Gina asthma severity	NR

Author, Year	Arm (n)	Age in years	Women n (%)	Race	Asthma Severity, n(%) (Degree of control if reported)	# of Acute Asthma visits/given timeframe
2008[55]	arms(256)				2005, Persistent Intermittent, n: 59 (23.3) Mild, n: 63 (24.6) Moderate, n: 92 (35.9)	
Shah S., 2011[56]	Arm A: Control (107)	Mean: 3	NR	NR	NR	NR
Shah S., 2011[56]	Arm B: Practitioner Asthma Communication and Education (PACE) (110)	Mean: 2	NR	NR	NR	NR
Shapiro A., 2011[57]	Arm B: (200)	NR, Range: <2-18	n: 84(42)	NR	NR	Pre-toolbox: 61(30.3%); Post 1: 39(19.5%)
Shapiro A., 2011[57]	Arm C: (197)	NR, Range: <2-18	n: 81(41.1)	NR	NR	Pre-toolbox: 66(33.5%); Post 1: 59(23.7%)
Shiffman R. N., 2000[58]	Arm A: Sole physician arm, pre-post; patient arm, pre(91)	Mean: 10, NR, Range: 5-17.4	NR	NR	As defined by AAP practice guideline, 1994: Mild, n: 71 (78) Moderate, n: 20 (22)	NR
Shiffman R. N., 2000[58]	Arm B: patient arm, post(74)	Mean: 11, NR, Range: 5-17.8	NR	NR	Scale: as defined by AAP practice guideline, 1994: Mild, n: 44 (59) Moderate, n: 27 (36) Severe, n: 3 (4)	NR
Smeele I. J., 1999[59]	Arm A: No intervention(223)	Mean: 49	(59)	NR	NR	NR
Smeele I. J., 1999[59]	Arm B: Education(210)	Mean: 52	(62)	NR	NR	NR
Stergachis A, 2002[60]	Arm A: Control(177)	Mean: 12	n: 58(33)	NR	NR	NR
Stergachis A, 2002[60]	Arm B: Education(153)	Mean: 12	n: 60(39)	NR	NR	NR
Suh D. C., 2001[61]	Arm A: (566)	Mean: 26,	n: 330(58.3)	NR	NR	NR
Suh D. C., 2001[61]	Arm B: Feedback(1050)	Mean: 30,	n: 617(58.8)	NR	NR	NR
Sulaiman N. D., 2010[62]	Arm A: Control [unrelated education] (121)	Range: 2-14 years	n: 40(40.8)	NR	Mild n: 42 (43.3) Moderate, Severe, n: 55 (56.7)	NR

Author, Year	Arm (n)	Age in years	Women n (%)	Race	Asthma Severity, n(%) (Degree of control if reported)	# of Acute Asthma visits/given timeframe
Sulaiman N. D., 2010[62]	Arm B: Education and guidelines(156)	Range: 2-14 years	n: 45(35.7)	NR	Mild, n: 70 (55.6) Moderate, Severe, n: 56 (44.4)	NR
Sulaiman N. D., 2010[62]	Arm C: Guidelines only(134)	Range: 2-14 years	n: 38(36.2)	NR	Mild, n: 62 (56.4) Moderate, Severe, n: 48 (43.6)	NR
Thyne S.M., 2007[63]	Arm A: Time 1, 2002-2003(NR)	NR	NR	NR	NR	NR
Thyne S.M., 2007[63]	Arm A: Time 1, 2002-2003(NR)	NR	NR	NR	NR	NR
Thyne S.M., 2007[63]	Arm B: Time 2, 2003-2004(NR)	NR	NR	NR	NR	NR
Thyne S.M., 2007[63]	Arm B: Time 2, 2003-2004(NR)	NR	NR	NR	NR	NR
Thyne S.M., 2007[63]	Arm C: Time 3, 2004-2005(NR)	NR	NR	NR	NR	NR
Thyne S.M., 2007[63]	Arm C: Time 3, 2004-2005(NR)	NR	NR	NR	NR	NR
To T., 2008[64]	Arm B: Intervention(1408)	Mean: 26	n: 869(61.72)	NR	NR	NR
Veninga CCM, 1999[65]	Arm A: Netherlands	NR	NR	NR	NR	NR
Veninga CCM, 1999[65]	Arm B: Intervention (NR)	NR	NR	NR	NR	NR
Veninga CCM, 1999[65]	Arm C: Norway	NR	NR	NR	NR	NR
Veninga CCM, 1999[65]	Arm D: Slovakia	NR	NR	NR	NR	NR
Veninga CCM, 2000[66]	Arm A: UTI(NR)	NR	NR	NR	NR	NR
Veninga CCM, 2000[66]	Arm B: Education and Feedback(NR)	NR	NR	NR	NR	NR
Weinberger M, 2002[67]	Arm A: Control(165)	Mean: 45,	n: 139(84.2)	White-n: 145 White(87.9)	NR	NR
Weinberger M, 2002[67]	Arm B: Peak Flow Meter Monitoring Control Group(233)	Mean: 47,	n: 190(81.6)	White-n: 189 White(81.1)	NR	NR
Weinberger M, 2002[67]	Arm C: Education, Feedback, Pay-for-	Mean: 45,	n: 210(80.2)	White-n: 197 White(75.2)	NR	NR

Author, Year	Arm (n)	Age in years	Women n (%)	Race	Asthma Severity, n(%) (Degree of control if reported)	# of Acute Asthma visits/given timeframe
Yawn BP, 2008[68]	performance(262) Arm B: Education and Feedback(840)	NR	NR	NR	NR	NR

AAP = Asthma Action Plan; A/P = Asian/Pacific Islander; HCSD = Health Care Services Division; NAEPP = National Asthma Education and Prevention Program; NR = Not Reported; PACP = Pharmacy Asthma Care Program; PACE = Physician Asthma Care Program; PACE = Physician Asthma Care Education; PLE = Peer Leader Education; TOM = Therapeutic Outcomes Monitoring; SP= Suburban Practice; UP = Urban Practice; UTI = Urinary Tract Infection

References

1 Ables AZ, Godenick MT, Lipsitz SR. Family Medicine: Improving family practice residents' compliance with asthma practice guidelines. 2002; 34:23-8.

2 Armour C, Bosnic-Anticevich S, Brillant M et al. Thorax: Pharmacy Asthma Care Program (PACP) improves outcomes for patients in the community. 2007; 62:496-502.

3 Baker R, Fraser RC, Stone M, Lambert P, Stevenson K, Shiels C. Br J Gen Pract: Randomised controlled trial of the impact of guidelines, prioritized review criteria and feedback on implementation of recommendations for angina and asthma. 2003; 53:284-91.

4 Bell LM, Grundmeier R, Localio R et al. Pediatrics: Electronic health record-based decision support to improve asthma care: a cluster-randomized trial. 2010; 125:e770-7.

5 Brown R, Bratton SL, Cabana MD Kaciroti N, Clark NM. Chest: Physician asthma education program improves outcomes for children of low-income families. 2004; 126:369-74.

6 Bryce FP, Neville RG, Crombie IK, Clark RA, McKenzie P. British Medical Journal: Controlled trial of an audit facilitator in diagnosis and treatment of childhood asthma in general practice. 1995; 310:838-42.

7 Cabana MD, Slish KK, Evans D et al. Pediatrics: Impact of physician asthma care education on patient outcomes. 2006; 117:2149-57.

8 Cho SH, Jeong JW, Park HW et al. J Asthma: Effectiveness of a computer-assisted asthma management program on physician adherence to guidelines. 2010; 47:680-6.

9 Clark N, Gong M, Schork, M, et al. Impact of education for physicians on patient outcomes. Pediatrics 1998; 101(5):831-6.

10 Cloutier MM , Wakefield DB, Carlisle PS, Bailit HL, Hall CB. Arch Pediatr Adolesc Med: The effect of Easy Breathing on asthma management and knowledge. 2002; 156:1045-51.

11 Cloutier MM , Hall CB, Wakefield DB, Bailit H. J Pediatr: Use of

increase tuberculosis case detection and improve respiratory care: economic evaluation alongside a randomised trial. 2010; 15:277-86.

21 Feder G, Griffiths C, Highton C, Eldridge S, Spence M, Southgate L. British Medical Journal: Do clinical guidelines introduced with practice based education improve care of asthmatic and diabetic patients? A randomised controlled trial in general practices in east London. 1995; 311:1473-8.

22 Finkelstein JA, Lozano P, Fuhlbrigge AL et al. Health Serv Res: Practice-level effects of interventions to improve asthma care in primary care settings: the Pediatric Asthma Care Patient Outcomes Research Team. 2005; 40:1737-57.

23 Foster JM, Hoskins G, Smith B, Lee AJ, Price D, Pinnock H. BMC Fam Pract: Practice development plans to improve the primary care management of acute asthma: randomised controlled trial. 2007; 8:23.

24 Fox P, Porter PG, Lob SH, Boer JH, Rocha DA, Adelson JW. Pediatrics: Improving asthma-related health outcomes among low-income, multiethnic, school-aged children: Results of a demonstration project that combined continuous quality improvement and community health worker strategies. 2007; 120:e902-e911.

25 Frankowski BL, Keating K, Rexroad A et al. J Sch Health: Community collaboration: concurrent physician and school nurse education and cooperation increases the use of asthma action plans. 2006; 76:303-6.

26 Glasgow NJ, Ponsonby AL, Yates R, Beilby J, Dugdale P. BMJ: Proactive asthma care in childhood: general practice based randomised controlled trial. 2003; 327:659.

27 Gorton TA, Cranford CO, Golden WE, Walls RC, Pawelak JE. Arch Fam Med: Primary care physicians' response to dissemination of practice guidelines. 1995; 4:135-42.

28 Hagmolen of ten Have W, van den Berg NJ, van der Palen J, van

asthma guidelines by primary care providers to reduce hospitalizations and emergency department visits in poor, minority, urban children. 2005; 146:591-7.

12 Cloutier MM, Grosse SD, Wakefield DB, Nurmagambetov TA, Brown CM. American Journal of Managed Care: The economic impact of an urban asthma management program. 2009; 15:345-51.

13 Cloutier MM, Tennen H, Wakefield DB, Brazil K, Hall CB. Improving clinician self-efficacy does not increase asthma guideline use by primary care clinicians. Acad. Pediatr. 2012; 12(4):312-8.

14 Coleman CI, Reddy P, Laster-Bradley NM, Dorval S, Munagala B, White CM. Ann Pharmacother: Effect of practitioner education on adherence to asthma treatment guidelines. 2003; 37:956-61.

15 Cowie RL, Underwood MF, Mack S. Can Respir J: The impact of asthma management guideline dissemination on the control of asthma in the community. 2001; 8 Suppl A:41A-5A.

16 Daniels EC, Bacon J, Denisio S et al. J Asthma: Translation squared: improving asthma care for high-disparity populations through a safety net practice-based research network. 2005; 42:499-505.

17 Davis AM, Cannon M, Ables AZ, Bendyk H. Family Medicine: Using the electronic medical record to improve asthma severity documentation and treatment among family medicine residents. 2010; 42:334-7.

18 de Vries TW, van den Berg PB, Duiverman EJ, de Jong-van den Berg LT. Arch Dis Child: Effect of a minimal pharmacy intervention on improvement of adherence to asthma guidelines. 2010; 95:302-4.

19 Eccles M, McColl E, Steen N et al. BMJ: Effect of computerised evidence based guidelines on management of asthma and angina in adults in primary care: cluster randomised controlled trial. 2002; 325:941.

20 Fairall L, Bachmann MO, Zwarenstein M et al. Trop Med Int Health: Cost-effectiveness of educational outreach to primary care nurses to

28. Aalderen WM, Bindels PJ. Prim Care Respir J: Implementation of an asthma guideline for the management of childhood asthma in general practice: a randomised controlled trial. 2008; 17:90-6.

29. Halterman JS, McConnochie KM, Conn KM et al. Archives of Pediatrics and Adolescent Medicine: A randomized trial of primary care provider prompting to enhance preventive asthma therapy. 2005; 159:422-7.

30. Halterman JS, Fisher S, Conn KM et al. Archives of Pediatrics & Adolescent Medicine: Improved preventive care for asthma: a randomized trial of clinician prompting in pediatric offices. 2006; 160:1018-25.

31. Herborg H, Soendergaard B, Jorgensen T et al. J Am Pharm Assoc (Wash): Improving drug therapy for patients with asthma--part 2: Use of antiasthma medications. 2001; 41:551-9.

32. Herborg H. SBFBeal. Improving drug therapy for patients with asthma--part 1: Patient outcomes. J Am Pharm Assoc (Wash) 2001; (4):539-50.

33. Holton C, Crockett A, Nelson M et al. International Journal for Quality in Health Care: Does spirometry training in general practice improve quality and outcomes of asthma care? 2011; 23:545-53.

34. Homer CJ, Forbes P, Horvitz L, Peterson LE, Wypij D, Heinrich P. Archives of Pediatrics and Adolescent Medicine: Impact of a quality improvement program on care and outcomes for children with asthma. 2005; 159:464-9.

35. Horswell R, Butler MK, Kaiser M et al. Dis Manag: Disease management programs for the underserved. 2008; 11:145-52.

36. Hoskins G, Neville RG, Smith B, Clark RA. Health Bull (Edinb): Does participation in distance learning and audit improve the care of patients with acute asthma attacks? The General Practitioners in Asthma Group. 1997; 55:150-5.

37. Kattan M, Crain EF, Steinbach S et al. Pediatrics: A randomized clinical trial of clinician feedback to improve quality of care for inner-city children with asthma. 2006; 117:e1095-103.

38. Lesho EP, Myers CP, Ott M, Winslow C, Brown JE. Mil Med: Do clinical practice guidelines improve processes or outcomes in primary care? 2005; 170:243-6.

39. Lob SH, Boer JH, Porter PG, et al. Promoting Best-Care Practices in Childhood Asthma: Quality Improvement in Community Health Centers. Pediatrics 2011;128;20; Originally Published Online June 13, 2011; DOI: 10.1542/Peds.2010-1962 .

40. Lozano P, Finkelstein JA, Carey VJ et al. Arch Pediatr Adolesc Med: A multisite randomized trial of the effects of physician education and organizational change in chronic-asthma care: health outcomes of the Pediatric Asthma Care Patient Outcomes Research Team II Study. 2004; 158:875-83.

41. Lundborg CS, Wahlstrom R, Oke T, Tomson G, Diwan VK. J Clin Epidemiol: Influencing prescribing for urinary tract infection and asthma in primary care in Sweden: a randomized controlled trial of an interactive educational intervention. 1999; 52:801-12.

42. Mahi-Taright S, Belhocine M, Ait-Khaled N. Int J Tuberc Lung Dis: Can we improve the management of chronic obstructive respiratory disease? The example of asthma in adults. 2004; 8:873-81.

43. Mangione-Smith R, Schonlau M, Chan KS et al. Ambulatory Pediatrics: Measuring the effectiveness of a collaborative for quality improvement in pediatric asthma care: Does implementing the chronic care model improve processes and outcomes of care? 2005; 5:75-82.

44. Martens JD, van der Weijden T, Severens JL et al. Int J Med Inform: The effect of computer reminders on GPs' prescribing behaviour: a cluster-randomised trial. 2007; 76 Suppl 3:S403-16.

45. McCowan C, Neville RG, Ricketts IW, Warner FC, Hoskins G, Thomas GE. Medical Informatics and the Internet in Medicine: Lessons from a randomized controlled trial designed to evaluate

computer decision support software to improve the management of asthma. 2001; 26:191-201.

46 Mitchell EA , Didsbury PB, Kruithof N *et al.* Acta Paediatr: A randomized controlled trial of an asthma clinical pathway for children in general practice. 2005; 94:226-33.

47 O'Laughlen MC, Hollen PJ, Rakes G, Ting S. Pediatric Asthma, Allergy and Immunology: Improving pediatric asthma by the MSAGR algorithm: A multicolored, simplified, asthma guideline reminder. 2008; 21:119-27.

48 Patel PH, Welsh C, Foggs MB. Dis Manag: Improved asthma outcomes using a coordinated care approach in a large medical group. 2004; 7:102-11.

49 Premaratne UN, Sterne JA, Marks GB, Webb JR, Azima H, Burney PG. BMJ: Clustered randomised trial of an intervention to improve the management of asthma: Greenwich asthma study. 1999; 318:1251-5.

50 Ragazzi H, Keller A, Ehrensberger R, Irani AM. J Urban Health: Evaluation of a practice-based intervention to improve the management of pediatric asthma. 2011; 88 Suppl 1:38-48.

51 Rance K, O'Laughlen M, Ting S. J Pediatr Health Care: Improving asthma care for African American children by increasing national asthma guideline adherence. 2011; 25:235-49.

52 Richman MJ, Poltawsky JS. Stud Health Technol Inform: Partnership for excellence in asthma care: evidence-based disease management. 2000; 76:107-21.

53 Ruoff G. Family Medicine: Effects of flow sheet implementation on physician performance in the management of asthmatic patients. 2002; 34:514-7.

54 Saini B, Krass I, Armour C. Annals of Pharmacotherapy: Development, implementation, and evaluation of a community pharmacy-based asthma care model. 2004; 38:1954-60.

55 Schneider A , Wensing M, Biessecker K, Quinzler R, Kaufmann-Kolle P, Szecsenyi J. J Eval Clin Pract: Impact of quality circles for improvement of asthma care: results of a randomized controlled trial. 2008; 14:185-90.

56 Shah S, Sawyer SM, Toelle BG *et al.* Med J Aust: Improving paediatric asthma outcomes in primary health care: a randomised controlled trial. 2011; 195:405-9.

57 Shapiro A, Gracy D, Quinones W, Applebaum J, Sarmiento A. Arch Pediatr Adolesc Med: Putting guidelines into practice: improving documentation of pediatric asthma management using a decision-making tool. 2011; 165:412-8.

58 Shiffman RN , Freudigman M, Brandt CA, Liaw Y, Navedo DD. Pediatrics: A guideline implementation system using handheld computers for office management of asthma: effects on adherence and patient outcomes. 2000; 105:767-73.

59 Smeele IJ, Grol RP, van Schayck CP, van den Bosch WJ, van den Hoogen HJ, Muris JW. Qual Health Care: Can small group education and peer review improve care for patients with asthma/chronic obstructive pulmonary disease? 1999; 8:92-8.

60 Stergachis A, Gardner JS, Anderson MT, Sullivan SD. Journal of the American Pharmaceutical Association (Washington,D.C. : 1996): Improving pediatric asthma outcomes in the community setting: does pharmaceutical care make a difference? 2002; 42:743-52.

61 Suh DC, Shin SK, Okpara I, Voytovich RM, Zimmerman A. Am J Manag Care: Impact of a targeted asthma intervention program on treatment costs in patients with asthma. 2001; 7:897-906.

62 Sulaiman ND , Barton CA, Liaw ST *et al.* Fam Pract: Do small group workshops and locally adapted guidelines improve asthma patients' health outcomes? A cluster randomized controlled trial. 2010; 27:246-54.

63 Thyne SM, Marmor AK, Madden N, Herrick G. Paediatric and Perinatal Epidemiology: Comprehensive asthma management for

Journal of Clinical Epidemiology: Improving drug treatment in general practice. 2000; 53:762-72.

67 Weinberger M, Murray MD, Marrero DG *et al.* Journal of the American Medical Association: Effectiveness of pharmacist care for patients with reactive airways disease: A randomized controlled trial. 2002; 288:1594-602.

68 Yawn BP, Bertram S, Wollan P. Journal of Asthma and Allergy: Introduction of asthma APGAR tools improve asthma management in primary care practices. 2008; 1-10.

underserved children. 2007; 21:29-34.

64 To T, Cicutto L, Degani N, McLimont S, Beyene J. Med Care: Can a community evidence-based asthma care program improve clinical outcomes?: a longitudinal study. 2008; 46:1257-66.

65 Veninga CC, Lagerløv P, Wahlström R, *et al.* Evaluating an educational intervention to improve the treatment of asthma in four european countries. American Journal of Respiratory and Critical Care Medicine:1999; 160:1254-62.

66 Veninga CCM, Denig P, Zwaagstra R, Haaijer-Ruskamp FM.

Evidence Table 4. Intervention characteristics

Author, Year	Arm Name	Type of Intervention	Type of delivery	Duration of Intervention	Frequency of Intervention
Ables AZ, 2002[1]	Education and Reminders	Education, Reminders	In person ,Conducted by: Peer , Group , Paper, EMR: No	4 months	NR
Armour C., 2007[2]	Arm A: Control	Other trained on risk assessment, spirometry and the control protocol during a 1 day workshop	Mode :In person ,Conducted by: External Person , Group, EMR: No,	1 day	NR
Armour C., 2007[2]	Arm B: Pharmacy Asthma Care Program (PACP)	Other they were given an asthma education manual & were trained on risk assessment, pathophysiology of asthma, asthma medications, the NAC 6 step asthma management plan, patient education, goal setting, adherence assessment, spirometry & the PACP protocol	In person, Conducted by: External Person, , Group, EMR: No	2 days	NR
Baker R., 2003[3]	Arm A:Guidelines only	Other: distribution of guidelines alone	Paper, EMR: No	NR	single event
Baker R., 2003[3]	Arm B: Guidelines with audit criteria	Other distribution of guideline recommendations in prioritized review criteria format (according to strength of evidence and impact on outcome)	Paper, EMR: No	NR	single event
Baker R., 2003[3]	Arm C: Guidelines with audit criteria and feedback	Feedback, Other distribution of review criteria supplemented with feedback	Conducted by: External Person , Group, Paper, EMR: No, "feedback on actual practice performance was prepared from the results of the first data collection and presented as text, tables, and charts comparing details of individual practice performance with other participating practices."	NR	single event
Bell L.M., 2010[4]	Arm A: UP Control	Education	In person ,Conducted by: Peer, Group, EMR: No	NR	NR
Bell L.M., 2010[4]	Arm B: UP intervention	Decision Support, Education, Reminders	Electronic, EMR: No	NR	NR
Bell L.M., 2010[4]	Arm C: SP Control	Education	In Person ,Conducted by: Peer , Group, EMR: No	NR	NR

Author, Year	Arm Name	Type of Intervention	Type of delivery	Duration of Intervention	Frequency of Intervention
Bell L. M., 2010[4]	Arm D: SP Control	Decision Support, Education, Reminders	Electronic, EMR: No	NR	NR
Bender B. G., 2011[5]	Education, Coaching, Toolkit	Education, Other Guidelines	In person , Conducted by: External Person, Group, EMR: No	NR	2 clinician town hall meetings, 4 patient focus group meetings then 1 full day coaching session then 2 4-hour review visits at the clinics
Blackstien-Hirsch P., 2000[6]	Education	Education, Other, Physician Detailing medical grand rounds, newsletters, workshop	In person , Conducted by: External Person , Group, EMR: No	NR	NR
Brown R, 2004[7]	Arm A:Control	Standard practice	EMR: No		
Brown R, 2004[7]	Arm B: Education	Education, Other Guideline	In person , Conducted by: External Person, Group, EMR: No	NR	2 2-3hour sessions held over 2-3 weeks
Bryce FP, 1995[8]	Arm A:Control	NR	EMR: No	NR	NR
Bryce FP, 1995[8]	Arm B: Reminders and Tools	Education, Feedback, Other Peak flow meters supplies, portable nebulizers for use	Electronic ,Conducted by: External Person , Individual, EMR: No	12 months	NR
Cabana M. D., 2006[9]	Arm A:Control	Standard practice	EMR: No	NR	NR
Cabana M. D., 2006[9]	Arm B: Physician Asthma Care Education (PACE)	Education	In person , Conducted by: External Person , Group, EMR: No	2.5 hours	2
Cho S. H., 2010[10]	Decision Support	Decision Support, Education	In person , Conducted by: External Person , Group, Electronic, EMR: No	3 months	3 follow-up visits with 4-week intervals
Clark NM, 1998[11]	Arm B: Education	Education, Other Interactive seminar to guide physicians to examine ways to develop a partnership with their patients. Used lectures, videos, case studies, etc.	In person , Conducted by: External Person , Group, EMR: No	3 weeks	2 meetings
Cloutier M. M., 2002[12]	Decision support	Decision Support, Education	In person , Conducted by: External Person , NR , Paper, EMR: No, Easy Breathing: A detailed survey regarding symptoms, triggers, personal and family history is given to ALL patients; clinicians have an	4 hours	Duration above is of education, frequency is once

E-44

Author, Year	Arm Name	Type of Intervention	Type of delivery	Duration of Intervention	Frequency of Intervention
			instrument to assess severity for those diagnosed with asthma; template for creating asthma treatment plan		
Cloutier M. M., 2005[13]	Decision support	Decision Support, Education	In person , Conducted by: External Person , Group , Electronic, EMR: No	NR	NR
Cloutier M.M., 2009[14]	Decision support	Decision Support, Education	In person , Conducted by: External Person , Paper, EMR: No	1 year	2-hr per week (edu)
Cloutier M.M., 2012[15]	Arm A: Control	Audit, Education, Feedback, Organizational Change, Both arms received ongoing support from Easy Breathing staff.	In person, Conducted by: External person, Group, EMR: No. Control: Education, some practice-level detailing.	36 months	Bi-weekly
Cloutier M.M., 2012[15]	Arm B: Physician-directed intervention	Audit, Education, Feedback, Organizational Change, Audit, Physician Detailing. Multiple interventions	In person, Conducted by: External person, Group, EMR: No. Clinicians in Arm B (active arm) were offered multiple interventions to increase self-efficacy. Toolbox: VCR, tapes, instruction sheets for each inhaler, peak flow meters and graphs, brochures, luncheon seminars (topics: office management of asthma, spirometry, spacers, peak flow meters). Eight monthly 30-minute teleconferences were offered at 3 different times ndoor airway quality, allergic rhinitis, and adolescent adherence to therapy. Miniature fellowships consisting of a 1/2 day of shadowing an asthma specialist were also offered. Three national experts participated in grand rounds and dinner symposia that were open to all physicians, but intervention clinicians received personal invitations. Individual provider feedback on performance including number of children enrolled in Easy Breathing, number of treatment plans submitted, and percent of treatment plans that	36 months	NR

Author, Year	Arm Name	Type of Intervention	Type of delivery	Duration of Intervention	Frequency of Intervention
			adhered to the national asthma guidelines were distributed quarterly.		
Cloutier M.M. 2012 [15]	Arm B: Physician-directed intervention	NR	NR	NR	NR
Coleman C. I., 2003 [16]	Arm A: Patient specific information: Prescribers with patients on 'high dose'	NR	EMR: No	NR	NR
Coleman C. I., 2003 [16]	Arm B: Patient specific information: Prescribers with patients on 'low dose'	Feedback	Electronic , Conducted by: External Person , Individual, EMR: No	1 month	1
Cowie R. L., 2001 [17]	Arm A: Basic Education	Education, Other Patient education by nurse educator, with report to the PCP; dissemination of guidelines to physicians; public education forums	In person , Conducted by: External Person , Group, EMR: No, The clinician education was "several conventional medical education programs directed at physicians in the area"	1year	for patient education, this occurred every 6 weeks for one year (the duration above); The education for health professionals occurred "several" times.
Cowie R. L., 2001 [17]	Arm B: Intermediate Education	Education, Other Everything in A plus "development of an asthma clinic" in the table, but what is described sounds like staff training in "patient assessment, education, & counseling"	In person, Conducted by: External Person, EMR: No, The type Yes. B is describing the additional education component, the staff training. It is unclear if this is individual or group.	NR	NR
Cowie R. L., 2001 [17]	Arm C: Intensive Education	Education, Other Everything in B plus "intensive asthma education of the public and health professionals, and publicity campaign"	In Person, Conducted by: External Person, Group, EMR: No, This was "multipronged", but had an intensive full day asthma course that is described in Yesc.	NR	NR
Daniels E. C., 2005 [18]	Arm A: Control	Other, Standard practice "Copies of the national asthma guidelines and one asthma resource kit" p. 500)	EMR: No	NR	NR
Daniels E. C., 2005 [18]	Arm B: Education	Education, Other "asthma flow sheet in "Microsoft Word format" (p. 501), "documentation tools"	In person , Conducted by: External Person , Group, EMR: No	0.5 day	2
Davis AM, 2010 [19]	Decision Support	Other Guidelines	In person , Conducted by: Peer , Group, EMR: No	NR	once

Author, Year	Arm Name	Type of Intervention	Type of delivery	Duration of Intervention	Frequency of Intervention
Davis R. S., 2004[20]	Arm A: Guidelines only	Standard practice	EMR: No	NR	NR
Davis R. S., 2004[20]	Arm B: Education and Toolkit	Education, Other Guidelines	Electronic ,Conducted by: External Person , Group, EMR: No	NR	NR
de Vries T. W., 2010[21]	Arm A: Control	Standard practice	EMR: No	NR	NR,
de Vries T. W., 2010[21]	Arm B: Feedback	Education	In person ,Conducted by: External Person , Individual, EMR: No	NR	NR
de Vries T. W., 2010[21]	Arm C:2002	NR	EMR: No	NR	NR
Eccles M., 2002[22]	Arm A: angina	Decision support, Education, Other Distribution of the guideline	In person, Conducted by: External Person , Group , Electronic, EMR:- Yes, "The system offered suggestions for management (including prescribing) informed by the content of the patient's record"; "the guideline was, however, a separate path w/l the clinical system, & it was not possible. To access all other parts...from guideline"	12months	Guideline: once Education: one time training on use of system
Eccles M., 2002[22]	Arm B: asthma	Decision Support, Education, Other Distribution of the guideline	In person, Conducted by: External Person, Group, Electronic, EMR:- Yes, "The system offered suggestions for management (including prescribing) informed by the content of the patient's record"; "the guideline was, however, a separate path w/i the clinical system, & it was not possible to access all other parts...from ..guideline"	12 months	Guideline: once Education: one time training on use of system
Fairall L., 2010[23]	Arm A: Control	Standard practice	EMR: No	3months	NR
Fairall L., 2010[23]	Arm B: Intervention	Decision Support, Education, Other Nurse practitioners were permitted to prescribe inhaled corticosteroids for asthma (previously, could only renew existing physician-initiated Rx's).	In person ,Conducted by: External Person , Group, EMR: No	3 months	3-4 educational outreach workshops (1-3 hours each)
Feder G, 1995[24]	Arm A: Diabetes Education	Other similar approach to active arm, but all content was	EMR: No	NR	NR

E-47

Author, Year	Arm Name	Type of Intervention	Type of delivery	Duration of Intervention	Frequency of Intervention
		about diabetes			
Feder G, 1995[24]	Arm B: Education, Reminders and Audit	Audit, Education, Reminders	In person , Conducted by: External Person , Group , Paper, EMR: No	6 months	3 sessions
Finkelstein J. A., 2005[25]	Arm A: Control	Standard practice received copies of NAEPP guidelines	EMR: No	NR	NR
Finkelstein J. A., 2005[25]	Arm B: PLE Intervention	Education, Feedback, Reminders	In person , Conducted by: Peer , Group, EMR: No	3 hour	2
Finkelstein J. A., 2005[25]	Arm C:Planned Care Intervention	Education Same as in Arm B, with the addition of an asthma nurse educator who worked with families (symptoms assessment, provide self-management support).	In Person , Conducted by: Peer , Group, EMR: No	3 hour	2
Foster J. M., 2007[26]	Arm A: Education and Feedback (delayed)	Audit, Feedback, Other Formulation of a practice development plan	Mode :In person , Conducted by: External Person , Group, EMR: No	NR	Once
Foster J. M., 2007[26]	Arm B: Education and Feedback	Audit, Education, Feedback, Other Formulation of a development plan	Electronic, Conducted by: External Person , Group, EMR: No	NR	Once
Fox P 2007[27]	Quality improvement	Continuous quality improvement (CQI) and the addition of a community health worker, with central technical assistance (TA).	In person. Conducted by: Peer , Group. EMR: No.	NR	Monthly CQI team meetings at each site and monthly meetings of all CQI teams with TA
Frankowski B. L., 2006[28]	Multimodal: Education and Feedback	Education, Feedback, Organizational Change, Other Guidelines	In person , Conducted by: External Person , Group, EMR: No	NR	NR
Glasgow N. J., 2003[29]	Arm B: Intervention	Decision Support The 3+ visit plan	Paper, EMR: No	12 months	NR
Gorton T. A., 1995[30]	Arm A:Control comparison site	Standard practice	EMR: No	NR	NR
Gorton T. A., 1995[30]	Arm B: Education and Detailing	Education, Physician Detailing 45 page guideline, decline summary, Detailing calls by peer physician, CME conference, audiocassette	In person , Conducted by: Peer , Individual, EMR: No	4 months	two telephone calls
Gorton T. A., 1995[30]	Arm B: Education on computer	Education, Other45 page guideline, four "hypertext" computer modules, Computer conference	In Person , Conducted by: External Person , Group, EMR: No	4months	3 different times
Gorton T. A.,	Arm B: Education	45 -Page guideline, Four	Electronic , Conducted by: External	4months	one a week for 4

Author, Year	Arm Name	Type of Intervention	Type of delivery	Duration of Intervention	Frequency of Intervention
1995[30]	multimedia	fascimile messages, Four posters, CME conference, Audiocassette, Videocassette	Person , Group, EMR: No		weeks: Four Fascimile messages One a month for 4-months: four posters
Hagmolen, W., 2008[31]	Arm A: Guidelines only	Other distribution of a guideline	EMR: No	NR	guideline: once,
Hagmolen, W., 2008[31]	Arm B: Education and Guidelines	Education, Other distribution of a guideline	In person ,Conducted by: NR , Group, EMR: No	NR	guideline: once education: once
Hagmolen, W., 2008[31]	Arm C: Education and Guidelines and individualized treatment advice	Education, Other distribution of a guideline	In Person ,Conducted by: External Person , Individual, EMR: No	NR	guideline: once education: once individual treatment advice: varied, median 5 range 1-13
Halterman J. S., 2005[32]	Arm A: Control	Standard practice	EMR: No	NR	NR
Halterman J. S., 2005[32]	Arm B: Intervention	Decision Support	Paper, EMR: No	NR	NR
Halterman J.S., 2006[33]	Arm A: Control	Standard practice	EMR: No	NR	NR,
Halterman J.S., 2006[33]	Arm B: Intervention	Decision Support Intervention elaborated: "single-page prompt including the child's symptoms and guideline recommendations given to the clinician at the time of visit"	Paper, EMR: No	NR	1
Herborg H., 2001[34] & 35	Arm A:Control	Standard practice	EMR: No	1year	none,
Herborg H., 2001[34] & 35	Arm B: Therapeutic Outcomes Monitoring (TOM)	Clinical Pharmacy Service, Other "TOM" training for pharmacists= Therapeutic outcomes monitoring	EMR: No, The pharmacy service was in person visits where they identify problems with drug therapy, outline goals, and develop an individual intervention and monitoring plan	1 year	once per month (pharmacists interacting with patients),
Holton C., 2011[36]	Arm A:Control	NR	EMR: No	NR	NR
Holton C., 2011[36]	Arm B: Spirometry training	Education	In person, Conducted by: External Person, Group, EMR: No	2 hours	once
Homer CJ,	Arm A:Control	Standard practice	EMR: No	NR	NR

Author, Year	Arm Name	Type of Intervention	Type of delivery	Duration of Intervention	Frequency of Intervention
2005[37]					
Homer CJ, 2005[37]	Arm B: Learning collaborative	Learning collaborative based on Breakthrough Series methodology	In person, Conducted by: Peer, Group, EMR: No	10 months	3 one-day learning sessions; coaching and support through bi-weekly conference calls and periodic performance feedback
Horswell R., 2008[38]	HCSD's DM program	Decision Support, Feedback, Reminders	Electronic, EMR:-Yes, CLIQ (Clinical Inquiry) incorporates a "prevention page" and "Yes6 real-time data interfaces from clinical and administrative feeder systems"	3 years	continuous
Hoskins G., 1997[39]	Arm A: Before intervention	NR	EMR: No	NR	NR
Hoskins G., 1997[39]	Arm B: Education and Feedback	Audit, Education, Feedback	Conducted by: External Person , Individual, EMR: No	12 months	NR
Kattan M., 2006[40]	Arm A:Control	Standard practice	EMR: No	1 year	once every 2 months
Kattan M., 2006[40]	Arm B: Intervention	Decision Support, Feedback	Paper, EMR: No	1 year	once every 2 months
Lesho E. P., 2005[41]	Decision Support	Decision Support, Education, Other Guidelines	In person , Conducted by: NR , Group , Paper, EMR: No	NR	NR
Liaw S. T., 2008[42]	Arm A:Control	Standard practice	EMR: No	NR	NR
Liaw S. T., 2008[42]	Arm B:Control (unrelated education)	Education, Other education on unrelated topic	EMR: No	NR	NR
Liaw S. T., 2008[42]	Arm C: Education and Guidelines	Education	In person, Conducted by: External Person, Group, EMR: No	3 hours	twice
Lob S. H., 2011[43]	Longitudinal Evaluation Group – Patient-level Interview Survey	Organizational Change, Quality Improvement (Continuous Quality Improvement [CQI]), Decision Support, Flow Sheet	In person, Conducted by: External Team, Group, EMR: No.	NR	Teleconferences engaging clinician champions (once per month) and all-site participants (bimonthly). Feedback: progress reports given 1-2 times per month. Annual program-wide meetings/site visits.
Lob S. H., 2011[43]	Cross-sectional Random Sample – Clini-level Review	Organizational Change, Quality Improvement (Continuous Quality Improvement [CQI]),	In person, Conducted by: External Team, Group, EMR: No.	NR	Teleconferences engaging clinician champions (once per

Author, Year	Arm Name	Type of Intervention	Type of delivery	Duration of Intervention	Frequency of Intervention
	Samples (T1-T3)	Decision Support, Flow Sheet			month) and all-site participants (bimonthly). Feedback: progress reports given 1-2 times per month. Annual program-wide meetings/site visits.
Lozano P., 2004[44]	Arm A:Control	Standard practice	EMR: No		NR
Lozano P., 2004[44]	Arm B: Peer leader education	Education, Other, Physician Detailing, Reminders Guidelines	Electronic, Conducted by: External Person, Group, Paper, EMR: No	NR	NR
Lozano P., 2004[44]	Arm C: Chronic care model	Education, Organizational Change, Physician Detailing, Reminders Guidelines	In Person, Conducted by: External Person, Individual, Paper, EMR: No	10 hours	4-5 PAC visits over 2 years
Lundborg C. S., 1999[45]	Arm A:Control	Education, Feedback	In person, Conducted by: External Person, Group, EMR: No	NR	2 sessions
Lundborg C. S., 1999[45]	Arm B: Education and Feedback	Education, Feedback	In person, Conducted by: External Person, Group, EMR: No	NR	2 sessions
Mahi-Taright S., 2004[46]	Education	Education	In person, Conducted by: External Person, Group, EMR: No	2.5 days	once
Mangione-Smith R.,, 2005[47]	Arm A:Control	Standard practice	EMR: No	NR	NR
Mangione-Smith R.,, 2005[47]	Arm B: Learning collaborative	Breakthrough Collaborative Series Quality Improvement	In person, Conducted by: External Person, Group, EMR: No	12.5 months	3 two-day learning sessions, followed by action periods of 2-6 months (PDSA cycles).
Martens J. D., 2006[48]	Arm A: Control	Standard practice	EMR: No	NR	NR
Martens J. D., 2006[48]	Arm B: Guidelines and involved in development	Other making of guideline and final guideline dissemination	Paper, EMR: No	NR	NR
Martens J. D., 2006[48]	Arm C: Guidelines only	Other making of guideline and final guideline dissemination	Paper, EMR: No	NR	NR
Martens J. D., 2007[49]	Arm B	Reminders	Electronic, EMR:-Yes	1 year	Based on frequency of prescriptions
Martens, J.D., 2007[49]	Arm A	Reminders	Electronic, EMR:-Yes, When a GP prescribed a drug, the GP was prompted to enter diagnosis related information and codes, which, in	1 year	Based on frequency of prescriptions

Author, Year	Arm Name	Type of Intervention	Type of delivery	Duration of Intervention	Frequency of Intervention
			addition to stored information, was used by the computer to generate reminders		
McCowan C, 2001[50]	Arm A: Control	Standard practice	EMR: No	6months	NR
McCowan C, 2001[50]	Arm B: Intervention	Decision Support	Electronic, EMR: No	6 months	NR
Mitchell E. A., 2005[51]	Arm A:Control	Standard practice	EMR: No	9months	NR
Mitchell E. A., 2005[51]	Arm B: Intervention	Decision Support, Education	In person , Group, EMR: No	2 hours	1
Newton W. P., 2010[52]	Decision Support	Organizational Change	EMR: No	2 years	NR
O'Laughlen MC, 2008[53]	MSAGR group B	Decision Support, Education, Reminders	In person , Individual , Paper, EMR: No	2 months	1
Patel P. H., 2004[54]	Organizational Change	Education, Organizational Change, Other Guidelines	In person ,Conducted by: Peer , Group , Paper, EMR: No	NR	NR
Premaratne U. N., 1999[55]	Arm A:Control	NR	EMR: No	NR	NR
Premaratne U. N., 1999[55]	Arm B: Education	Education	In person ,Conducted by: External Person, Group, EMR: No	NR	NR
Ragazzi H., 2011[56]	Practice 1	Decision Support, Education, Organizational Change	In person ,Conducted by: Peer , Group, Electronic, EMR: No	1 hour	6-8 sessions during the 1st 4 months
Ragazzi H., 2011[56]	Practice 2	Decision Support, Education, Organizational Change	In Person ,Conducted by: Peer , Group, Electronic, EMR: No	1hour	6-8 sessions during the 1st 4 months
Ragazzi H., 2011[56]	Practice 3	Decision Support, Education, Organizational Change	In Person ,Conducted by: Peer , Group, Electronic, EMR: No	1hour	6-8 sessions during the 1st 4 months
Rance K., 2011[57]	Decision Support	Education Reminders	In person ,Conducted by: External Person , Group , Electronic, EMR:-Yes	6 weeks	1 workshop
Renzi P. M., 2006[58]	Arm A:Group 4 (Control)	Other, Standard practice copy of Canadian Clinical Practice Guidelines	EMR: No	NR	NR
Renzi P. M., 2006[58]	Arm B:Group 1	Education, Other, Reminders written instructions for stamp; verbal encouragement to use stamp; asked to have 6 patients to sign informed consent to have charts reviewed	In person, EMR: No	30 minutes	once at 6 months, once 12 months after enrollment
Renzi P. M.,	Arm C: Group 2	Education , Other, Reminders	In Person, EMR: No	30min	NR

Author, Year	Arm Name	Type of Intervention	Type of delivery	Duration of Intervention	Frequency of Intervention
2006[58]		written instructions for stamp; verbal encouragement to use stamp			
Renzi P. M., 2006[58]	Arm D	Other, Reminders written instructions sent by mail	mail, EMR: No	NR	NR
Richman M. J., 2000[59]	Feedback	Audit, Education, Feedback, Other, Reminders Distribution of practice recommendations	In person. Conducted by: External Person, Group Paper, EMR: No, reminder stickers attached to charts	6 months	NR
Ruoff G., 2002[60]	Arm A: Before the Flow Sheet	NR	EMR: No	NR	NR
Ruoff G., 2002[60]	After implementation of the Flow Sheet	Flow sheet	Paper, EMR: No	6 months	one time
Saini B, 2004[61]	Arm A: Control 1	NR	EMR: No	NR	NR
Saini B, 2004[61]	Arm B: Control 2	NR	EMR: No	NR	
Saini B, 2004[61]	Arm C: Education	Education, Other, Standard practice Service--Provide specialized care to patients, i.e. asthma education, device monitoring, set goals with patient	In Person , Conducted by: External Person , Individual, EMR: No	6months	NR
Schneider A., 2008[62]	Arm A: traditional quality circle	Audit, Feedback, Other moderated discussion of feedback results	In person , Conducted by: External Person , Group, EMR: No	NR	NR
Schneider A., 2008[62]	Arm B: benchmark quality circle	Audit, Feedback, Other moderated discussion of feedback results with identification of best performers	In person , Conducted by:	NR	NR External Person Group, EMR:0
Shah S., 2011[63]	Arm B: Practitioner Asthma Communication and Education (PACE)	Education	In person , Conducted by: Peer , Group, EMR: No	6 hours	2 3-hour workshops held 1 week apart
Shapiro A., 2011[64]	Arm A:Control	Decision Support, Reminders	Paper, EMR: No	NR	NR
Shapiro A., 2011[64]	Arm B:Intervention	Reminders	Electronic, EMR: No	NR	NR
Shiffman R. N., 2000[65]	Arm A: Sole physician arm, pre-post; patient arm, pre	Other Control time period, pre-intervention	EMR: No	NR	NR,

Author, Year	Arm Name	Type of Intervention	Type of delivery	Duration of Intervention	Frequency of Intervention
Shiffman R. N., 2000[65]	Arm B: Patient arm, post	Decision Support	Electronic, EMR: No, Custom software on a Newton Message Pad, which provided: structured documentation recommendations based on the guideline assistance with calculation of PEFR and medication doses printed encounter summaries and prescriptions	NR	NR
Smeele I. J., 1999[66]	Arm A: Control	No intervention	In person, Conducted by: Peer, Group, EMR: No	12 months	once
Smeele I. J., 1999[66]	Arm B: Education	Education and peer review program	In person, Conducted by: Peer, Group, EMR: No	12 months	once
Sondergaard J., 2002[67]	Arm A:Control	Feedback	Conducted by: External Person, Individual, EMR: No, not described, except that feedback was given on an unrelated subject	6months	3 times (every 3 months)
Sondergaard J., 2002[67]	Arm B: Individual patient count data feedback	Audit, Feedback	Conducted by: External Person, Individual, EMR: No, The individual feedback group received information about their patients use of ICS relative to their Beta agonist use.	6 months	3 times (every 3 months)
Sondergaard J., 2002[67]	Arm C: Aggregate data feedback	Audit, Feedback	Conducted by: External Person, Individual, EMR: No, The aggregate group received feedback on the number of ICS packages and inhaled beta agonist packages dispensed in one year per YesNoNo patients, with comparison data from other practices.	6months	3 times (every 3 months)
Stergachis A, 2002[68]	Arm A:Control	Standard practice	EMR: No	NR	NR
Stergachis A, 2002[68]	Arm B: Education	Other Guidelines	EMR: No	8 hours	once
Suh D. C., 2001[69]	Arm A: Pre-intervention	Standard practice	EMR: No	NR	NR
Suh D. C., 2001[69]	Arm B: Post-intervention	Audit, Feedback, Other educational mailings to patients, Providers received	Conducted by: External Person, Individual, EMR: No, patients were identified who either overused quick	1 year	every 3 months for mailings to patients and one time mailing to

E-54

Author, Year	Arm Name	Type of Intervention	Type of delivery	Duration of Intervention	Frequency of Intervention
		asthma management fact sheet and patient profiles	relief meds (one or more short acting inhaler per month, or 8 or more/year) or patients who seemed to be non-compliant with long term controller meds. A management fact sheet was sent with the patient		physicians
Sulaiman N. D., 2010[70]	Arm A:Control (unrelated education)	Education	In person ,Conducted by: Peer , Group, EMR: No	6hours	Twice
Sulaiman N. D., 2010[70]	Arm B: Education and Guidelines	Education, Other Guidelines	In person ,Conducted by: Peer , Group, Paper, EMR: No	6 hours	Twice
Sulaiman N. D., 2010[70]	Arm C: Guidelines only	Other Guidelines	Paper, EMR: No	6hours	Twice
Thyne S.M., 2007[71]	Arm A:Control	NR	EMR: No	NR	NR
Thyne S.M., 2007[71]	Arm B: Time 1, 2002-2003	Decision support, Education, Feedback, Other Posting and distribution of guidelines, posting of local medical plan formularies	In person, EMR: No, Intervention includes: Yes. quarterly presentations; 2. an "ongoing education campaign" 3 as noted in "other" above; 4. An asthma discharge planning form for urgent care that guides clinicians to classify and rx asthma; 5. asthma clinic staff feedback	NR	Education: quarterly
Thyne S.M., 2007[71]	Arm C	Education, Feedback, Organizational Change	In person, Conducted by: Peer, Group, EMR: No, Medical provider education campaign designed to improve compliance with the national guidelines for asthma management.	3 years	Quarterly
To T., 2008[72]	PCAPP Intervention	Decision Support, Education decision support = flow-chart	Paper, EMR: No	3 hours	once
Veninga CCM, 1999[73]	Arm A: Netherlands	Audit, Education, Feedback	In person ,Conducted by: Peer , Group, EMR: No	5months	2 group meetings, average 7.8 weeks (+/-3.0 weeks) between meetings
Veninga CCM, 1999[73]	Arm B:Sweden	Audit, Education, Feedback	In person ,Conducted by: Peer , Group, EMR: No	6 months	2 group meetings, average 10.3 weeks (+/- 7.2 weeks) between meetings, Mode: In

E-55

Author, Year	Arm Name	Type of Intervention	Type of delivery	Duration of Intervention	Frequency of Intervention
					person Conducted by: Peer Group, EMR:0
Veninga CCM, 1999[73]	Arm C:Norway	Audit, Education, Feedback	In Person, Conducted by: Peer , Group, EMR: No	4months	2 group meetings, average 1.3 weeks (+/- 1.3 weeks) between meetings
Veninga CCM, 1999[73]	Arm D: Slovakia	Audit, Education, Feedback	In Person, Conducted by: Peer , Group, EMR: No	3months	single group meeting
Veninga CCM, 2000[74]	Arm A: UTI	Audit, Education, Feedback	In person,Conducted by: Peer , Group, EMR: No, "self-learning auditing program for peer groups". Control group discussed UTI issues	NR	Twice
Veninga CCM, 2000[74]	Arm B: Education and Feedback	Audit, Education, Feedback	In person,Conducted by: Peer, Group, EMR: No, "self-learning auditing program for peer groups". Conducted in already established peer groups. Moderated by regular group members, after training by researchers. Discussed case vignettes in the first meeting, and individualized feedback. on prescribing in 2n	NR	Twice
Weinberger M, 2002[75]	Arm A: Usual Care Control Group	4 hour training session on different topics than Pharmaceutical care	EMR: No	NR	NR
Weinberger M, 2002[75]	Arm B: Peak Flow Meter Monitoring Control Group	Other received Peak flow meter, instructions, monthly calls to elicit PEFRs but not PEFR data provided to pharmacists. Did received 4 hour training but topics different than pharmaceutical care	In person ,Conducted by: External Person , Individual, EMR: No	NR	NR
Weinberger M, 2002[75]	Arm C: Education, Feedback, pay-for-performance	Decision Support, Education, Pay-for-Performance/Quality Incentive	Conducted by: External Person , Individual, EMR: No	12	Mode: Electronic
Yawn BP, 2008[76]	Education and Feedback	Audit, Decision Support, Education Documentation tool	In person ,Conducted by: External Person , Individual, EMR: No	6 hours	NR

CME = Continued Medical Education; CQI = Continuous Quality Improvement; EMR = Electronic Medical Records; GP = General Practitioner; ICS = Inhaled Corticosteroids; PCAPP = Primary Care Asthma Pilot Project;MSAGR = Multicolored, Simplified, Asthma Guideline Reminder; NAC = National Asthma Campaign; NAEPP = National Asthma

Education and Prevention Program; NR = Not Reported; PACE = Practitioner Asthma Communication and Education; PACP = Pharmacy Asthma Care Program; PDSA = Plan-Do-Study-Act; PEFR = Peak Exploratory Flow Rate; PLE = Peer Leader Education; TA = Technical Assistance; TOM = Therapeutic Outcomes Monitoring; UTI = Urinary Tract Infection;

References

1 Ables AZ, Godenick MT, Lipsitz SR. Family Medicine: Improving family practice residents' compliance with asthma practice guidelines. 2002; 34:23-8.

2 Armour C, Bosnic-Anticevich S, Brillant M *et al.* Thorax: Pharmacy Asthma Care Program (PACP) improves outcomes for patients in the community. 2007; 62:496-502.

3 Baker R, Fraser RC, Stone M, Lambert P, Stevenson K, Shiels C. Br J Gen Pract: Randomised controlled trial of the impact of guidelines, prioritized review criteria and feedback on implementation of recommendations for angina and asthma. 2003; 53:284-91.

4 Bell LM, Grundmeier R, Localio R *et al.* Pediatrics: Electronic health record-based decision support to improve asthma care: a cluster-randomized trial. 2010; 125:e770-7.

5 Bender BG, Dickinson P, Rankin A, Wamboldt FS, Zittleman L, Westfall JM. J Am Board Fam Med: The Colorado Asthma Toolkit Program: a practice coaching intervention from the High Plains Research Network. 2011; 24 :240-8.

6 Blackstien-Hirsch P, Anderson G, Cicutto L, McIvor A, Norton P. Journal of Asthma: Implementing continuing education strategies for family physicians to enhance asthma patients' quality of life. 2000; 37:247-57.

7 Brown R, Bratton SL, Cabana MD, Kaciroti N, Clark NM. Chest: Physician asthma education program improves outcomes for children of low-income families. 2004; 126:369-74.

8 Bryce FP, Neville RG, Crombie IK, Clark RA, McKenzie P. British Medical Journal: Controlled trial of an audit facilitator in diagnosis and treatment of childhood asthma in general practice. 1995; 310:838-42.

9 Cabana MD, Slish KK, Evans D *et al.* Pediatrics: Impact of physician asthma care education on patient outcomes. 2006; 117:2149-57.

10 Cho SH, Jeong JW, Park HW *et al.* J Asthma: Effectiveness of a computer-assisted asthma management program on physician adherence to guidelines. 2010; 47:680-6.

11 Clark N, Gong M, Schork M, *et al.* Impact of education for physicians on patient outcomes. Pediatrics 1998; 101(5):831-6.

12 Cloutier MM , Wakefield DB, Carlisle PS, Bailit HL, Hall CB. Arch Pediatr Adolesc Med: The effect of Easy Breathing on asthma management and knowledge. 2002; 156:1045-51.

13 Cloutier MM , Hall CB, Wakefield DB, Bailit H. J Pediatr: Use of asthma guidelines by primary care providers to reduce hospitalizations and emergency department visits in poor, minority, urban children. 2005; 146:591-7.

14 Cloutier MM , Grosse SD, Wakefield DB, Nurmagambetov TA, Brown CM. American Journal of Managed Care: The economic impact of an urban asthma management program. 2009; 15:345-51.

15 Cloutier MM , Tennen H, Wakefield DB, Brazil K, Hall CB. Improving clinician self-efficacy does not increase asthma guideline

use by primary care clinicians. Acad. Pediatr. 2012; 12(4):312-8.

16 Coleman CI, Reddy P, Laster-Bradley NM, Dorval S, Munagala B, White CM. Ann Pharmacother: Effect of practitioner education on adherence to asthma treatment guidelines. 2003; 37:956-61.

17 Cowie RL, Underwood MF, Mack S. Can Respir J: The impact of asthma management guideline dissemination on the control of asthma in the community. 2001; 8 Suppl A:41A-5A.

18 Daniels EC, Bacon J, Denisio S et al. J Asthma: Translation squared: improving asthma care for high-disparity populations through a safety net practice-based research network. 2005; 42:499-505.

19 Davis AM, Cannon M, Ables AZ, Bendyk H. Family Medicine: Using the electronic medical record to improve asthma severity documentation and treatment among family medicine residents. 2010; 42:334-7.

20 Davis RS, Bukstein DA, Luskin AT, Kailin JA, Goodenow G. Ann Allergy Asthma Immunol: Changing physician prescribing patterns through problem-based learning: an interactive, teleconference case-based education program and review of problem-based learning. 2004; 93:237-42.

21 de Vries TW , van den Berg PB, Duiverman EJ, de Jong-van den Berg LT. Arch Dis Child: Effect of a minimal pharmacy intervention on improvement of adherence to asthma guidelines. 2010; 95:302-4.

22 Eccles M, McColl E, Steen N et al. BMJ: Effect of computerised evidence based guidelines on management of asthma and angina in adults in primary care: cluster randomised controlled trial. 2002; 325:941.

23 Fairall L, Bachmann MO, Zwarenstein M et al. Trop Med Int Health: Cost-effectiveness of educational outreach to primary care nurses to increase tuberculosis case detection and improve respiratory care: economic evaluation alongside a randomised trial. 2010; 15:277-86.

24 Feder G, Griffiths C, Highton C, Eldridge S, Spence M, Southgate L.

British Medical Journal: Do clinical guidelines introduced with practice based education improve care of asthmatic and diabetic patients? A randomised controlled trial in general practices in east London. 1995; 311:1473-8.

25 Finkelstein JA, Lozano P, Fuhlbrigge AL et al. Health Serv Res: Practice-level effects of interventions to improve asthma care in primary care settings: the Pediatric Asthma Care Patient Outcomes Research Team. 2005; 40:1737-57.

26 Foster JM, Hoskins G, Smith B, Lee AJ, Price D, Pinnock H. BMC Fam Pract: Practice development plans to improve the primary care management of acute asthma: randomised controlled trial. 2007; 8:23.

27 Fox P, Porter PG, Lob SH, Boer JH, Rocha DA, Adelson JW. Pediatrics: Improving asthma-related health outcomes among low-income, multiethnic, school-aged children: Results of a demonstration project that combined continuous quality improvement and community health worker strategies. 2007; 120:e902-e911.

28 Frankowski BL, Keating K, Rexroad A et al. J Sch Health: Community collaboration: concurrent physician and school nurse education and cooperation increases the use of asthma action plans. 2006; 76:303-6.

29 Glasgow NJ, Ponsonby AL, Yates R, Beilby J, Dugdale P. BMJ: Proactive asthma care in childhood: general practice based randomised controlled trial. 2003; 327:659.

30 Gorton TA, Cranford CO, Golden WE, Walls RC, Pawelak JE. Arch Fam Med: Primary care physicians' response to dissemination of practice guidelines. 1995; 4:135-42.

31 Hagmolen of ten Have W, van den Berg NJ, van der Palen J, van Aalderen WM, Bindels PJ. Prim Care Respir J: Implementation of an asthma guideline for the management of childhood asthma in general practice: a randomised controlled trial. 2008; 17:90-6.

32 Halterman JS, McConnochie KM, Conn KM et al. Archives of Pediatrics and Adolescent Medicine: A randomized trial of care provider prompting to enhance preventive asthma therapy. 2005; 159:422-7.

33 Halterman JS, Fisher S, Conn KM et al. Archives of Pediatrics & Adolescent Medicine: Improved preventive care for asthma: a randomized trial of clinician prompting in pediatric offices. 2006; 160:1018-25.

34 Herborg H, Soendergaard B, Jorgensen T, et al. J Am Pharm Assoc (Wash): Improving drug therapy for patients with asthma-part 2: Use of antiasthma medications. 2001; 41:551-9.

35 Herborg H, Soendergaard B, Froekjaer B, et al. Improving drug therapy for patients with asthma--part 1: Patient outcomes. J Am Pharm Assoc (Wash) 2001; (4):539-50.

36 Holton C, Crockett A, Nelson M, et al. International Journal for Quality in Health Care: Does spirometry training in general practice improve quality and outcomes of asthma care? 2011; 23:545-53.

37 Homer CJ, Forbes P, Horvitz L, Peterson LE, Wypij D, Heinrich P. Archives of Pediatrics and Adolescent Medicine: Impact of a quality improvement program on care and outcomes for children with asthma. 2005; 159:464-9.

38 Horswell R, Butler MK, Kaiser M, et al. Dis Manag: Disease management programs for the underserved. 2008; 11:145-52.

39 Hoskins G, Neville RG, Smith B, Clark RA. Health Bull (Edinb): Does participation in distance learning and audit improve the care of patients with acute asthma attacks? The General Practitioners in Asthma Group. 1997; 55:150-5.

40 Kattan M, Crain EF, Steinbach S et al. Pediatrics: A randomized clinical trial of clinician feedback to improve quality of care for inner-city children with asthma. 2006; 117:e1095-103.

41 Lesho EP, Myers CP, Ott M, Winslow C, Brown JE. Mil Med: Do clinical practice guidelines improve processes or outcomes in primary care? 2005; 170:243-6.

42 Liaw ST, Sulaiman ND, Barton CA et al. BMC Fam Pract: An interactive workshop plus locally adapted guidelines can improve general practitioners asthma management and knowledge: a cluster randomised trial in the Australian setting. 2008; 9:22.

43 Lob SH, Boer JH, Porter PG, et al. Promoting Best-Care Practices in Childhood Asthma: Quality Improvement in Community Health Centers. Pediatrics 2011;128:20; Originally Published Online June 13, 2011; DOI: 10.1542/Peds.2010-1962 .

44 Lozano P, Finkelstein JA, Carey VJ et al. Arch Pediatr Adolesc Med: A multisite randomized trial of the effects of physician education and organizational change in chronic-asthma care: health outcomes of the Pediatric Asthma Care Patient Outcomes Research Team II Study. 2004; 158:875-83.

45 Lundborg CS, Wahlstrom R, Oke T, Tomson G, Diwan VK. J Clin Epidemiol: Influencing prescribing for urinary tract infection and asthma in primary care in Sweden: a randomized controlled trial of an interactive educational intervention. 1999; 52:801-12.

46 Mahi-Taright S, Belhocine M, Ait-Khaled N. Int J Tuberc Lung Dis: Can we improve the management of chronic obstructive respiratory disease? The example of asthma in adults. 2004; 8:873-81.

47 Mangione-Smith R, Schonlau M, Chan KS et al. Ambulatory Pediatrics: Measuring the effectiveness of a collaborative for quality improvement in pediatric asthma care: Does implementing the chronic care model improve processes and outcomes of care? 2005; 5:75-82.

48 Martens JD, Winkens RA, van der Weijden T, de Bruyn D, Severens JL. BMC Health Serv Res: Does a joint development and dissemination of multidisciplinary guidelines improve prescribing behaviour: a pre/post study with concurrent control group and a randomised trial. 2006; 6:145.

49   Martens JD, van der Weijden T, Severens JL et al. Int J Med Inform: The effect of computer reminders on GPs' prescribing behaviour: a cluster-randomised trial. 2007; 76 Suppl 3:S403-16.

50   McCowan C, Neville RG, Ricketts IW, Warner FC, Hoskins G, Thomas GE. Medical Informatics and the Internet in Medicine: Lessons from a randomized controlled trial designed to evaluate computer decision support software to improve the management of asthma. 2001; 26:191-201.

51   Mitchell EA, Didsbury PB, Kruithof N et al. Acta Paediatr: A randomized controlled trial of an asthma clinical pathway for children in general practice. 2005; 94:226-33.

52   Newton WP, Lefebvre A, Donahue KE, Bacon T, Dobson A. J Contin Educ Health Prof: Infrastructure for large-scale quality-improvement projects: early lessons from North Carolina Improving Performance in Practice. 2010; 30:106-13.

53   O'Laughlen MC, Hollen PJ, Rakes G, Ting S. Pediatric Asthma, Allergy and Immunology: Improving pediatric asthma by the MSAGR algorithm: A multicolored, simplified, asthma guideline reminder. 2008; 21:119-27.

54   Patel PH, Welsh C, Foggs MB. Dis Manag: Improved asthma outcomes using a coordinated care approach in a large medical group. 2004; 7:102-11.

55   Premaratne UN, Sterne JA, Marks GB, Webb JR, Azima H, Burney PG. BMJ: Clustered randomised trial of an intervention to improve the management of asthma: Greenwich asthma study. 1999; 318:1251-5.

56   Ragazzi H, Keller A, Ehrensberger R, Irani AM. J Urban Health: Evaluation of a practice-based intervention to improve the management of pediatric asthma. 2011; 88 Suppl 1:38-48.

57   Rance K, O'Laughlen M, Ting S. J Pediatr Health Care: Improving asthma care for African American children by increasing national asthma guideline adherence. 2011; 25:235-49.

58   Renzi PM, Ghezzo H, Goulet S, Dorval E, Thivierge RL. Can Respir J: Paper stamp checklist tool enhances asthma guidelines knowledge and implementation by primary care physicians. 2006; 13:193-7.

59   Richman MJ, Poltawsky JS. Stud Health Technol Inform: Partnership for excellence in asthma care: evidence-based disease management. 2000; 76:107-21.

60   Ruoff G. Family Medicine: Effects of flow sheet implementation on physician performance in the management of asthmatic patients. 2002; 34:514-7.

61   Saini B, Krass I, Armour C. Annals of Pharmacotherapy: Development, implementation, and evaluation of a community pharmacy-based asthma care model. 2004; 38:1954-60.

62   Schneider A, Wensing M, Biessecker K, Quinzler R, Kaufmann-Kolle P, Szecsenyi J. J Eval Clin Pract: Impact of quality circles for improvement of asthma care: results of a randomized controlled trial. 2008; 14:185-90.

63   Shah S, Sawyer SM, Toelle BG et al. Med J Aust: Improving paediatric asthma outcomes in primary health care: a randomised controlled trial. 2011; 195:405-9.

64   Shapiro A, Gracy D, Quinones W, Applebaum J, Sarmiento A. Arch Pediatr Adolesc Med: Putting guidelines into practice: improving documentation of pediatric asthma management using a decision-making tool. 2011; 165:412-8.

65   Shiffman RN, Freudigman M, Brandt CA, Liaw Y, Navedo DD. Pediatrics: A guideline implementation system using handheld computers for office management of asthma: effects on adherence and patient outcomes. 2000; 105:767-73.

66   Smeele IJ, Grol RP, van Schayck CP, van den Bosch WJ, van den Hoogen HJ, Muris JW. Qual Health Care: Can small group education and peer review improve care for patients with asthma/chronic obstructive pulmonary disease? 1999; 8:92-8.

67 Sondergaard J, Andersen M, Vach K, Kragstrup J, Maclure M, Gram LF. Eur J Clin Pharmacol: Detailed postal feedback about prescribing to asthma patients combined with a guideline statement showed no impact: a randomised controlled trial. 2002; 58:127-32.

68 Stergachis A, Gardner JS, Anderson MT, Sullivan SD. Journal of the American Pharmaceutical Association (Washington,D.C. : 1996): Improving pediatric asthma outcomes in the community setting: does pharmaceutical care make a difference? 2002; 42:743-52.

69 Suh DC, Shin SK, Okpara I, Voytovich RM, Zimmerman A. Am J Manag Care: Impact of a targeted asthma intervention program on treatment costs in patients with asthma. 2001; 7:897-906.

70 Sulaiman ND, Barton CA, Liaw ST et al. Fam Pract: Do small group workshops and locally adapted guidelines improve asthma patients' health outcomes? A cluster randomized controlled trial. 2010; 27:246-54.

71 Thyne SM, Marmor AK, Madden N, Herrick G. Paediatric and Perinatal Epidemiology: Comprehensive asthma management for underserved children. 2007; 21:29-34.

72 To T, Cicutto L, Degani N, McLimont S, Beyene J. Med Care: Can a community evidence-based asthma care program improve clinical outcomes?: a longitudinal study. 2008; 46:1257-66.

73 Veninga CC, Lagerløv P, Wahlström R, et al. Evaluating an educational intervention to improve the treatment of asthma in four european countries. American Journal of Respiratory and Critical Care Medicine:1999; 160:1254-62.

74 Veninga CCM, Denig P, Zwaagstra R, Haaijer-Ruskamp FM. Journal of Clinical Epidemiology: Improving drug treatment in general practice. 2000; 53:762-72.

75 Weinberger M, Murray MD, Marrero DG, et al. Journal of the American Medical Association: Effectiveness of pharmacist care for patients with reactive airways disease: A randomized controlled trial. 2002; 288:1594-602.

76 Yawn BP, Bertram S, Wollan P. Journal of Asthma and Allergy: Introduction of asthma APGAR tools improve asthma management in primary care practices. 2008; 1-10.

Evidence Table 5. Clinical Outcomes Baseline and End of Treatment

Author, Year	Arm	Clinical Outcome	Definition of Scale	Range of Scale	Were outcomes measured over a period of at least 12 months?	Is there enough information to determine seasonality?	Measurement at Baseline N n (%) mean SD	Measurement at end of treatment N n (%) mean SD	Measurement at last follow-up N n (%) mean SD	Were outcomes adjusted?
Richman, 2000[16]	Feedback	Missed days of school	Percent reporting 0 school absence due to asthma in past 6 months	0-100	No	No	N: 228 n with outcomes: 114 (49)	N: 317 n with outcomes: 158 (38)	NR	No.
Baker, 2002 [37]	Arm A- Guidelines only	Rescue use of short- acting B2 agonists	In patients using beta 2 agonists, compliance has been checked	NR	NR	NR	N: 347 n with outcomes: 285 n with events: 285 (82.1)	N: 396 n with outcomes: 324 n with events: 324 (81.8)	NR	No.
Baker, 2002 [37]	Arm B- Guidelines with audit criteria	Rescue use of short- acting B2 agonists	In patients using beta 2 agonists, compliance has been checked	NR	NR	NR	N: 386 n with outcomes: 335 n with events: 335 (86.8)	N: 403 n with outcomes: 328 n with events: 328 (81.4)	NR	No.
Baker, 2002 [37]	Arm C- Guidelines with audit criteria and feedback	Rescue use of short- acting B2 agonists	In patients using beta 2 agonists, compliance has been checked	NR	NR	NR	N: 349 n with outcomes: 300 n with events: 300 (86)	N: 405 n with outcomes: 345 n with events: 345 (85.2)	NR	No.
Baker, 2003 [37]	Arm A- Guidelines only	Patient perceptions	patients are satisfied that everything possible was done	NR	NR	NR	N: 420 n with outcomes: 357 (85)	NR	N: 478 n with outcomes: 410 (85.8)	No

Author, Year	Arm	Clinical Outcome	Definition of Scale	Range of Scale	Were outcomes measured over a period of at least 12 months?	Is there enough information to determine seasonality?	Measurement at Baseline N n (%) mean SD	Measurement at end of treatment N n (%) mean SD	Measurement at last follow-up N n (%) mean SD	Were outcomes adjusted?
			to treat asthma							
Baker,2003 [37]	Arm B- Guidelines with audit criteria	Patient perceptions	patients are satisfied that everything possible was done to treat asthma	NR	NR	NR	N: 446 n with outcomes: 364 (81.6)	NR	N: 466 n with outcomes: 379 (81.3)	No
Baker,2003 [37]	Arm C- Guidelines with audit criteria and feedback	Patient perceptions	patients are satisfied that everything possible was done to treat asthma	NR	NR	NR	N: 395 n with outcomes: 338 (85.6)	NR	N: 463 n with outcomes: 390 (84.2)	No
Baker,2003 [37]	Arm A- Guidelines only	Patient perceptions	patients are satisfied with explanations given by the doctor about asthma	NR	NR	NR	N: 417 n with outcomes: 327 (78.4)	NR	N: 471 n with outcomes: 377 (80)	No
Baker,2003 [37]	Arm B- Guidelines with audit criteria	Patient perceptions	patients are satisfied with explanations given by the doctor about asthma	NR	NR	NR	N: 444 n with outcomes: 337 (75.9)	NR	N: 462 n with outcomes: 354 (76.6)	No
Baker,2003 [37]	Arm C- Guidelin	Patient perceptions	patients are satisfied	NR	NR	NR	N: 394 n with outcomes:	NR	N: 457 n with	No

Author, Year	Arm	Clinical Outcome	Definition of Scale	Range of Scale	Were outcomes measured over a period of at least 12 months?	Is there enough information to determine seasonality?	Measurement at Baseline N n (%) mean SD	Measurement at end of treatment N n (%) mean SD	Measurement at last follow-up N n (%) mean SD	Were outcomes adjusted?
	es with audit criteria and feedbac k		with explanation s given by the doctor about asthma				321 (81.5)		outcomes: 366 (80.1)	
Baker,2003 [37]	Arm A-Guidelin es only	Symptom Score	mean symptom score	NR	NR	NR	N: 406 Mean: 36.2 SD: 23.9	NR	N: 453 Mean: 34.1 SD: 22.7	No
Baker,2003 [37]	Arm B-Guidelin es with audit criteria	Symptom Score	mean symptom score	NR	NR	NR	N: 424 Mean:34 SD:22	NR	N: 440 Mean:33.1 SD:21.8	No
Baker,2003 [37]	Arm C-Guidelin es with audit criteria and feedbac k	Symptom Score	mean symptom score	NR	NR	NR	N: 378 Mean:30.4 SD:20.5	NR	N: 443 Mean: 33.8 SD:22.3	No
Bell,2009 [32]	Arm A-UP control	Lung function tests	Spirometry performed	NR	NR	Yes. The education period was from October 13 2006, to April 15, 2007, and the intervention 2 (follow up) period was from October 16, 2007, to April 15, 2008.	N: 647 n with outcomes: 101,(16)	N: 690 n with outcomes: 150,(22)	NR	No.
Bell,2009 [32]	Arm B-	Lung	Spirometry	NR	NR	Yes. The	N: 586	N: 604	NR	No.

Author, Year	Arm	Clinical Outcome	Definition of Scale	Range of Scale	Were outcomes measured over a period of at least 12 months?	Is there enough information to determine seasonality?	Measurement at Baseline N n (%) mean SD	Measurement at end of treatment N n (%) mean SD	Measurement at last follow-up N n (%) mean SD	Were outcomes adjusted?
	UP intervention	function tests	performed			education period was from October 13, 2006, to April 15, 2007, and the intervention 2 (follow up) period was from October 16, 2007, to April 15, 2008.	n with outcomes: 87 (15)	n with outcomes: 147 (24)		
Bell, 2009[32]	Arm C-Suburban Practice Control	Lung function tests	Spirometry performed	NR	NR	Yes. The education period was from October 13, 2006, to April 15, 2007, and the intervention 2 (follow up) period was from October 16, 2007, to April 15, 2008.	N: 129 n with outcomes: 10 (8)	N: 155 n with outcomes: 2 (1)	NR	No.
Bell, 2009[32]	Arm D-Suburban Practice intervention	Lung function tests	Spirometry performed	NR	NR	Yes. The education period was from October 13, 2006, to April 15, 2007, and the intervention 2 (follow up) period was from October	N: 387 n with outcomes: 30 (8)	N: 464 n with outcomes: 67 (14)	NR	No.

Author, Year	Arm	Clinical Outcome	Definition of Scale	Range of Scale	Were outcomes measured over a period of at least 12 months?	Is there enough information to determine seasonality?	Measurement at Baseline N n (%) mean SD	Measurement at end of treatment N n (%) mean SD	Measurement at last follow-up N n (%) mean SD	Were outcomes adjusted?
						16, 2007, to April 15, 2008.				
Brown, 2004[21]	<$20,000 annual household income	Emergency department visits	Yearly rates of emergency department visits	NR	Yes	No	NR	NR	N: 19 Mean:1.441	Yes. Medications, asthma severity, parental education
Brown, 2004[21]	Medicaid Insurance	Emergency department visits	Yearly rate of emergency department visit	NR	Yes	No	NR	NR	N: 47 Mean:0.709	Yes. Medications, asthma severity, parental education
Brown, 2004[21]	Non-Medicaid Insurance	Emergency department visits	Yearly rate of emergency department visits	NR	NR	NR	NR	NR	N: 115 Mean:0.225	Yes. Medications, asthma severity, parental education
Brown, 2004[21]	≥$20,000 annual household income	Emergency department visits	Yearly rate of emergency department visits	NR	Yes	No	NR	NR	N: 115 Mean:0.232	Yes. Medications, asthma severity, parental education
Brown, 2004[21]	<$20,000 annual household income	Emergency department visits	Yearly rates of emergency department visits	NR	Yes	No	NR	NR	N: 17 Mean:0.208	Yes. Medications, asthma severity, parental

Author, Year	Arm	Clinical Outcome	Definition of Scale	Range of Scale	Were outcomes measured over a period of at least 12 months?	Is there enough information to determine seasonality?	Measurement at Baseline N n (%) mean SD	Measurement at end of treatment N n (%) mean SD	Measurement at last follow-up N n (%) mean SD	Were outcomes adjusted?
										education
Brown, 2004[21]	Medicaid Insurance	Emergency department visits	Yearly rate of emergency department visit	NR	Yes	No	NR	NR	N: 65 Mean:0.264	Yes. Medications, asthma severity, parental education
Brown, 2004[21]	Non-Medicaid Insurance	Emergency department visits	Yearly rate of emergency department visits	NR	NR	NR	NR	NR	N: 92, Mean:0.27	Yes. Medications, asthma severity, parental education
Brown, 2004[21]	≥$20,000 annual household income	Emergency department visits	Yearly rate of emergency department visits	NR	Yes	No	NR	NR	N: 140, Mean:0.262	Yes. Medications, asthma severity, parental education
Brown, 2004[21]	<$20,000 annual household income	hospitalizations	Yearly rate of hospitalizations	NR	Yes	No	NR	NR	N: 19, Mean:0.029	Yes. Medications, asthma severity, parental education
Brown, 2004[21]	Medicaid Insurance	hospitalizations	Yearly rate of hospitalizations	NR	NR	NR	NR	NR	N: 47, Mean:0.052	Yes. Medications, asthma severity, parental education

Author, Year	Arm	Clinical Outcome	Definition of Scale	Range of Scale	Were outcomes measured over a period of at least 12 months?	Is there enough information to determine seasonality?	Measurement at Baseline N n (%) mean SD	Measurement at end of treatment N n (%) mean SD	Measurement at last follow-up N n (%) mean SD	Were outcomes adjusted?
Brown,2004[21]	≥$20,000 annual household income	hospitalizations	Yearly rate of hospitalizations	NR	NR	NR	NR	NR	N: 103, Mean:0.037	Yes. Medications, asthma severity, parental education
Brown,2004[21]	Non-Medicaid Insurance	hospitalizations	Yearly rate of hospitalizations	NR	NR	NR	NR	NR	N: 75, Mean:0.034	Yes. Medications, asthma severity, parental education
Brown,2004[21]	<$20,000 annual household income	hospitalizations	Yearly rate of hospitalizations	NR	Yes	No	NR	NR	N: 19, Mean:0.029	Yes. Medications, asthma severity, parental education
Brown,2004[21]	Medicaid Insurance	hospitalizations	Yearly rate of hospitalizations	NR	NR	NR	NR	NR	N: 47, Mean:0.052	Yes. Medications, asthma severity, parental education
Brown,2004[21]	≥20,000 annual household income	hospitalizations	Yearly rate of hospitalizations	NR	NR	NR	NR	NR	N: 103, Mean:0.037	Yes. Medications, asthma severity, parental education
Brown,200	Non-	hospitalizatio	Yearly rate	NR	NR	NR	NR	NR	N: 75,	Yes.

Author, Year	Arm	Clinical Outcome	Definition of Scale	Range of Scale	Were outcomes measured over a period of at least 12 months?	Is there enough information to determine seasonality?	Measurement at Baseline N n(%) mean SD	Measurement at end of treatment N n(%) mean SD	Measurement at last follow-up N n(%) mean SD	Were outcomes adjusted?
4[21]	Medicaid Insurance	ns	of hospitalizations						Mean:0.034	Medications, asthma severity, parental education
Brown,2004[21]	<$20,000 annual household income	hospitalizations	Yearly rate of hospitalizations	NR	Yes	No	NR	NR	N: 17, Mean:0	Yes. Medications, asthma severity, parental education
Brown,2004[21]	Medicaid Insurance	hospitalizations	Yearly rate of hospitalizations	NR	NR	NR	NR	NR	N: 65, Mean:0.012	Yes. Medications, asthma severity, parental education
Brown,2004[21]	≥20,000 annual household income	hospitalizations	Yearly rate of hospitalizations	NR	NR	NR	NR	NR	N: 140, Mean:0.013	Yes. Medications, asthma severity, parental education
Brown,2004[21]	Non-Medicaid Insurance	hospitalizations	Yearly rate of hospitalizations	NR	NR	NR	NR	NR	N: 92, Mean:0.013	Yes. Medications, asthma severity, parental education
Brown,2004[21]	Non-Medicai	hospitalizations	Yearly rate of	NR	NR	NR	NR	NR	N: 92, Mean:0.013	Yes. Medicatio

Author, Year	Arm	Clinical Outcome	Definition of Scale	Range of Scale	Were outcomes measured over a period of at least 12 months?	Is there enough information to determine seasonality?	Measurement at Baseline N n (%) mean SD	Measurement at end of treatment N n (%) mean SD	Measurement at last follow-up N n (%) mean SD	Were outcomes adjusted?
	d Insurance		hospitalizations							ns, asthma severity, parental education
Bryce, 1995 [26]	Arm A-Control	Emergency department visits	No of patients attending Accident and emergency departments	NR	NR	NR	N: 1563 n with events: 6	NR	N: 1563 n with events: 6	No.
Bryce, 1995 [26]	Arm B-Education	Emergency department visits	No of patients attending: Accident and emergency departments	NR	NR	NR	N: 1585 n with events: 12	NR	N: 1585 n with events: 5	No.
Bryce, 1995 [26]	Arm A-Control	hospitalizations	No of patients admitted	NR	NR	NR	N: 1563 n with events: 13	NR	N: 1563 , n with events: 28	No.
Bryce, 1995 [26]	Arm B-Education	hospitalizations	No of patients admitted	NR	NR	NR	N: 1585 n with events: 22	NR	N: 1585 , n with events: 25	No.
Clark, 1998 [20]	Arm A-	Emergency department visits	NR	NR	NR	NR	NR	Mean:0.67	NR	Yes. Baseline scores and group assignment.
Clark, 1998 [20]	Arm B-Education	Emergency department visits	NR	NR	NR	NR	NR	Mean:0.65	NR	Yes. Baseline scores

Author, Year	Arm	Clinical Outcome	Definition of Scale	Range of Scale	Were outcomes measured over a period of at least 12 months?	Is there enough information to determine seasonality?	Measurement at Baseline N n (%) mean SD	Measurement at end of treatment N n (%) mean SD	Measurement at last follow-up N n (%) mean SD	Were outcomes adjusted?
										and group assignment.
Clark, 1998[2]	Arm A-	hospitalizations	NR	NR	NR	NR	NR	Mean:0.076	NR	Yes. Baseline scores and group assignment.
Clark, 1998[2]	Arm B-Education	hospitalizations	NR	NR	NR	NR	NR	Mean:0.081	NR	Yes. Baseline scores and group assignment.
Cloutier,2002[40]	Arm A-Decision support: mild, intermittent	Rescue use of short-acting B2 agonists	No. of bronchodilator prescriptions per child per year	NR	Yes	NR	N: NR Mean:1.28	NR	N: NR Mean:1.64 SD:NR	No
Cloutier,2002[40]	Arm B-Decision support: mild, persistent	Rescue use of short-acting B2 agonists	No. of bronchodilator prescriptions per child per year	NR	Yes	NR	N: NR Mean:2.329	NR	N: NR Mean:2.56	No
Cloutier,2002[40]	Arm C-Decision support: moderate, persiste	Rescue use of short-acting B2 agonists	No. of bronchodilator prescriptions per child per year	NR	Yes	NR	N: NR Mean:4.06	NR	N: NR Mean:4.52	No

Author, Year	Arm	Clinical Outcome	Definition of Scale	Range of Scale	Were outcomes measured over a period of at least 12 months?	Is there enough information to determine seasonality?	Measurement at Baseline N n (%) mean SD	Measurement at end of treatment N n (%) mean SD	Measurement at last follow-up N n (%) mean SD	Were outcomes adjusted?
	nt									
Cloutier, 2002[40]	Arm D-Decision support: severe, persistent	Rescue use of short-acting B2 agonists	No. of bronchodilator prescriptions per child per year	NR	Yes	NR	N: NR Mean:11.33	NR	N: NR Mean:10.15	No
Cloutier, 2009[18]	Decision support	Emergency department visits	NR	NR	NR	NR	6.0 per 100 children	NR	6.1 per 100 children	Yes. Controlled for asthma severity, sex, linic, chronological time, and race/ethnicity.
Cloutier, 2009[18]	Decision support	Emergency department visits	NR	NR	NR	NR	15.4 per 100 children	NR	10.6 per 100 children	Yes. Controlled for asthma severity, sex, linic, chronological time, and race/ethnicity.
Cloutier, 2009[18i]	Decision support	hospitalizations	NR	NR	Yes	NR	7.9 per 100 children	NR	3.4 per 100 children	Yes. Controlled for asthma severity, sex, linic, chronological time, and

Author, Year	Arm	Clinical Outcome	Definition of Scale	Range of Scale	Were outcomes measured over a period of at least 12 months?	Is there enough information to determine seasonality?	Measurement at Baseline N n(%) mean SD	Measurement at end of treatment N n(%) mean SD	Measurement at last follow-up N n(%) mean SD	Were outcomes adjusted?
										race/ethni city.
Cloutier,2009[18i]	Decision support	hospitalizations	NR	NR	NR	NR	0.9 per 100 children	NR	1.2 per 100 children	Yes. Controlled for asthma severity, sex, linic, chronologi cal time, and race/ethni city.
Coleman,2003[12]	Arm A-Comparison group	Emergency department visits	NR	NR	No	No	N: 510 n with outcomes: 510 n with events: 510 Mean: 0.012 SD: 0.11	NR	N: 510 n with outcomes: 510 Mean: 0.008 SD: 0.11	No
Coleman,2003[12]	Arm B-Feedback	Emergency department visits	NR	NR	No	No	N: 135 n with outcomes: 135 Mean:0.02 SD:0.15	NR	N: 135 n with outcomes: 135 Mean: 0 SD: 0	No
Coleman,2003[12]	Arm A-Comparison group	hospitalizations	NR	NR	NR	NR	N: 510 n with outcomes: 510 Mean:0.1 SD:0.44	NR	N: 510 n with outcomes: 510 Mean:0.08 SD:0.4	No
Coleman,2003[12]	Arm B-Feedback	hospitalizations	NR	NR	NR	NR	N: 135 n with outcomes: 135 Mean:0.07 SD:0.35	NR	N: 135 n with outcomes: 135 Mean: 0.04 SD: 0.19	No
Cowie,2001[15]	Arm A-Basic	Emergency department	ED visit in last 12	Yes/No	Yes	NR	NR	N: NR n with outcomes:	NR	No.

Author, Year	Arm	Clinical Outcome	Definition of Scale	Range of Scale	Were outcomes measured over a period of at least 12 months?	Is there enough information to determine seasonality?	Measurement at Baseline N n (%) mean SD	Measurement at end of treatment N n (%) mean SD	Measurement at last follow-up N n (%) mean SD	Were outcomes adjusted?
	educatio n	visits	months					174 n with events: (22)		
Cowie,2001 [15]	Arm B-Interme diate educatio n	Emergency department visits	ED visit in last 12 months	Yes/No	Yes	NR	NR	N: NR n with events, (45)	NR	No.
Cowie,2001 [15]	Arm C-Intensiv e educatio n	Emergency department visits	ED visin in last 12 months	Yes/No	Yes	NR	NR	N: NR n with outcomes: 98 n with events: (36)	NR	No.
Cowie,2001 [15]	Arm A-Basic educatio n	hospitalizatio ns	admitted for asthma in 12 months	Yes/no	Yes	12 months	N: NR	N: NR n with outcomes: 174 n with events: (7.5)	NR	No.
Cowie,2001 [15]	Arm B-Interme diate educatio n	hospitalizatio ns	admitted for asthma in 12 months	Yes/no	NR	NR	NR	N: NR n with outcomes: 55 n with events: (14.5)	NR	No.
Cowie,2001 [15]	Arm C-Intensiv e educatio n	hospitalizatio ns	admitted for asthma in 12 months	Yes/no	NR	NR	NR	N: NR n with outcomes: 98 n with events: (18)	NR	No.
Cowie,2001 [15]	Arm A-Basic educatio n	Rescue use of short-acting B2 agonists	Use of beta2-agonist more than once/day	Yes/no	Yes	NR	NR	N: NR n with outcomes: 174 n with events: NR (34)	NR	No.
Cowie,2001 [15]	Arm B-Interme	Rescue use of short-	Use of beta2-	Yes/no	Yes	NR	NR	N: NR n with outcomes:	NR	No.

Author, Year	Arm	Clinical Outcome	Definition of Scale	Range of Scale	Were outcomes measured over a period of at least 12 months?	Is there enough information to determine seasonality?	Measurement at Baseline N n(%) mean SD	Measurement at end of treatment N n(%) mean SD	Measurement at last follow-up N n(%) mean SD	Were outcomes adjusted?
	diate educatio n	acting B2 agonists	agonist more than once/day					55 n with events: (49)		
Cowie,2001 [15]	Arm C-Intensive educatio n	Rescue use of short-acting B2 agonists	Use of beta2-agonist more than once/day	Yes/no	Yes	NR	NR	N: NR n with outcomes: 98 n with events: (29)	NR	No.
Cowie,2001 [15]	Arm A-Basic educatio n	Symptom Days	Waking at night	Yes/No	Yes	NR	NR	N: NR n with events:(52)	NR	No.
Cowie,2001 [15]	Arm B-Interme diate educatio n	Symptom Days	Waking at night	Yes/No	Yes	NR	NR	N: NR n with outcomes: 55 n with events: 99 (49)	NR	No.
Cowie,2001 [15]	Arm C-Intensiv e educatio n	Symptom Days	Waking at night	Yes/No	Yes	NR	NR	N: NR n with outcomes: 98 n with events: (42)	NR	No.
Finkelstein, 2005 [28i]	Arm A-Control (standard practice)	hospitalizatio ns	Mean	NR	Yes	NR	N: 1531 Mean:0.1 SD:0.06	NR	NR	No
Finkelstein, 2005 [28]	Arm B-PLE Interven tion	hospitalizatio ns	Mean	NR	Yes	NR	N: 2003 Mean:0.13 SD:0.15	NR	NR	No
Finkelstein, 2005 [28]	Arm C-Planned Care	hospitalizatio ns	Mean	NR	Yes	NR	N: 1635 Mean:0.07 SD:0.04	NR	NR	No

Author, Year	Arm	Clinical Outcome	Definition of Scale	Range of Scale	Were outcomes measured over a period of at least 12 months?	Is there enough information to determine seasonality?	Measurement at Baseline N n (%) mean SD	Measurement at end of treatment N n (%) mean SD	Measurement at last follow-up N n (%) mean SD	Were outcomes adjusted?
	Intervention									
Glascow,2003[11]	Arm A-Control	Emergency department visits	Attended emergency department 1-3 times in past 12 months	NR	NR	NR	N: 67 n with outcomes: 15 (22)	NR	N: 71 n with outcomes: 8 (11)	No
Glascow,2003[11]	Arm B-Decision support	Emergency department visits	Attended emergency department 1-3 times in past 12 months	NR	NR	NR	N: 95 n with outcomes: 14 (15)	NR	N: 95 n with outcomes: 4 (4)	No
Glascow,2003[11]	Arm A-Control	Missed days of school	Did not miss any school days with wheezing or asthma in past 12 months†	NR	NR	NR	N: 71 n with outcomes: 23 (32)	NR	N: 71 , n with outcomes: 32,(45)	No
Glascow,2003[11]	Arm B-Decision support	Missed days of school	Did not miss any school days with wheezing or asthma in past 12 months†	NR	NR	NR	N: 101 n with outcomes: 30 (30)	NR	N: 95 , n with outcomes: 49 (26)	No
Gorton,1995[42]	Arm A-appropriateness of self reported use of	Rescue use of short-acting B2 agonists	NR	NR	NR	No Intervention for 4 months	NR	NR	n with outcomes: 17 , Mean:0,SD:0.71	No.

Author, Year	Arm	Clinical Outcome	Definition of Scale	Range of Scale	Were outcomes measured over a period of at least 12 months?	Is there enough information to determine seasonality?	Measurement at Baseline N n (%) mean SD	Measurement at end of treatment N n (%) mean SD	Measurement at last follow-up N n (%) mean SD	Were outcomes adjusted?
	oral agonist prescrip tions for mild asthma									
Gorton,199 5[42]	Arm B-Appropri ateness of self reported use of oral agonist prescrip tions	Rescue use of short-acting B2 agonists	NR	NR	NR	No intervention for 4 months	NR	NR	n with outcomes: 11 Mean:0.05 SD:0.28	No.
Gorton,199 5[42]	Arm C-Appropri ateness of self reported use of oral agonist prescrip tions	Rescue use of short-acting B2 agonists	NR	NR	NR	No Intervention for 4 months	NR	NR	n with outcomes: 17 Mean:0.05 SD:1.33	No.
Gorton,199 5[42]	Arm D-Appropri ateness of self reported use of oral agonist prescrip tions	Rescue use of short-acting B2 agonists	NR	NR	NR	No Intervention for 4 months	NR	NR	n with outcomes: 18 Mean:0.07 0.97	No.

Author, Year	Arm	Clinical Outcome	Definition of Scale	Range of Scale	Were outcomes measured over a period of at least 12 months?	Is there enough information to determine seasonality?	Measurement at Baseline N n (%) mean SD	Measurement at end of treatment N n (%) mean SD	Measurement at last follow-up N n (%) mean SD	Were outcomes adjusted?
Hagmolen, 2008[31]	Arm A- Guidelines only	Lung function tests	FEV1% predicted	0-100	Yes	NR	N: 98 n with outcomes: 98 Mean:96.2, SD:10	NR	N: 98 n with outcomes: 98, Mean:96.7, SE 1.0	Yes. 12 months adjusted for baseline
Hagmolen, 2008[31]	Arm B- Education and guidelines	Lung function tests	FEV1% predicted	0-100	Yes	NR	N: 133 , n with outcomes: 133 , Mean:95. 6,SD:11	NR	N: 133, n with outcomes: 133, Mean:95.6, SE 0.9	Yes. Follow up mean adjusted for baseline
Hagmolen, 2008[31]	Arm C- Guidelines, education, and individualized treatment advice	Lung function tests	FEV1% predicted	0-100	Yes	NR	N: 131, n with outcomes: 131, Mean:96 SD:12	NR	N: 131, n with outcomes: 131, Mean:96 SE 0.9	Yes. 12 months adjusted for baseline
Hagmolen, 2008[31]	Arm A- Guidelines only	Lung function tests	PEF variability	NR	Yes	NR	N: 98 n with outcomes: 98 Mean: 8.8 SD:5	NR	N: 98 n with outcomes: 98, Mean:7.5 SE 0.5	Yes. Follow up mean adjusted for baseline
Hagmolen, 2008[31]	Arm B- Education and guidelines	Lung function tests	PEF variability	NR	Yes	NR	N: 133 n with outcomes: 133 Mean:9.4 SD:5.4	NR	N: 133 n with outcomes: 133, Mean:7.2 SE 0.4	Yes. Follow up mean adjusted for baseline
Hagmolen, 2008[31]	Arm C- Guidelines,	Lung function tests	PEF variability	NR	Yes	NR	N: 131 , n with outcomes: 131, Mean:8.5	NR	N: 131 n with outcomes: 131	Yes. Follow up mean

E-78

Author, Year	Arm	Clinical Outcome	Definition of Scale	Range of Scale	Were outcomes measured over a period of at least 12 months?	Is there enough information to determine seasonality?	Measurement at Baseline N n (%) mean SD	Measurement at end of treatment N n (%) mean SD	Measurement at last follow-up N n (%) mean SD	Were outcomes adjusted?
	education, and individualized treatment advice						SD:5.2		Mean:7.2 SE 0.4	adjusted for baseline
Hagmolen, 2008[31]	Arm A- Guidelines only	Symptom Days	symptom free days	0-14	Yes	NR	N: 98 n with outcomes: 98 median (range): 8.4 (0-14)	NR	N: 98 n with outcomes: 98 Mean:8.6 SE 0.5	Yes. Follow up mean adjusted for baseline
Hagmolen, 2008[31]	Arm B- Education and guidelines	Symptom Days	symptom free days	0-14	Yes	NR	N: 133 n with outcomes: 133 median (range): 6.0 (0-14)	NR	N: 133 n with outcomes: 133 Mean:8.5 SE 0.5	Yes. Follow up mean adjusted for baseline
Hagmolen, 2008[31]	Arm C- Guidelines, education, and individualized treatment advice	Symptom Days	symptom free days	0-14	Yes	NR	N: 131 n with outcomes: 131 median (range): 8.0 (0-14)	NR	N: 131 n with outcomes: 131 Mean:9.1 SE 0.5	Yes. Follow up mean adjusted for baseline
Hagmolen, 2008[31]	Arm A- Guidelines only	Symptom Score	Total symptom score (see mean differences for details)	0-18	Yes	NR	N: 98 n with outcomes: 98 median (range): 0.8 (0-9)	NR	N: 98 n with outcomes: 98 Mean:0.9 SD:NR 0.2	Yes. Follow up mean is "adjusted for baseline"
Hagmolen,	Arm B-	Symptom	Total	0-18	Yes	NR	N: 133	NR	N: 133	Yes.

Author, Year	Arm	Clinical Outcome	Definition of Scale	Range of Scale	Were outcomes measured over a period of at least 12 months?	Is there enough information to determine seasonality?	Measurement at Baseline N n (%) mean SD	Measurement at end of treatment N n (%) mean SD	Measurement at last follow-up N n (%) mean SD	Were outcomes adjusted?
2008[31]	Education and guidelines	Score	symptom score (see mean differences for details)				n with outcomes: 133 median (range): 1.0 (0-8)		n with outcomes: 133 Mean:1.2 SE 0.2	Follow up mean adjusted for baseline
Hagmolen, 2008[31]	Arm C-Guidelines, education, and individualized treatment advice	Symptom Score	Total symptom score (see mean differences for details)	0-18	Yes	NR	N: 131 n with outcomes: 131 median (range): 0.8 (0-10)	NR	N: 131 n with outcomes: 131 Mean:1 SE 0.2	Yes. Follow up mean adjusted for baseline
Hagmolen, 2008[31]	Arm A-Guidelines only	Symptom Score	Nocturnal symptom score	0-9	Yes	NR	N: 98 n with outcomes: 98 median (range): 0.2 (0-5)	NR	N: 98 n with outcomes: 98 Mean:0.3 SE 0.1	Yes. Follow up mean adjusted for baseline
Hagmolen, 2008[31]	Arm B-Education and guidelines	Symptom Score	Nocturnal symptom score	0-9	Yes	NR	N: 133 n with outcomes: 133 median (range): 0.3 (0-3)	NR	N: 133 n with outcomes: 133 Mean:0.5 SE 0.1	Yes. Follow up mean adjusted for baseline
Hagmolen, 2008[31]	Arm C-Guidelines, education, and individualized treatment	Symptom Score	Nocturnal symptom score	0-9	Yes	NR	N: 131 n with outcomes: 131 median (range): 0.2 (0-5)	NR	N: 131 n with outcomes: 131 Mean:0.4 SE 0.1	-1follow up mean adjusted for "baseline"

Author, Year	Arm	Clinical Outcome	Definition of Scale	Range of Scale	Were outcomes measured over a period of at least 12 months?	Is there enough information to determine seasonality?	Measurement at Baseline N n (%) mean SD	Measurement at end of treatment N n (%) mean SD	Measurement at last follow-up N n (%) mean SD	Were outcomes adjusted?
Halterman, 2005[19]	advice Arm A-Control (standard practice)	Emergency department visits	NR	NR	No	No	N: 77	NR	N: 77 n with outcomes: 14 n with events: (19.4)	No.
Halterman, 2005[19]	Arm B-Decision support	Emergency department visits	NR	NR	No	No	N: 73	NR	N: 73 n with outcomes: 8 n with events: (11.8)	No.
Halterman, 2005[19]	Arm A-Control (standard practice)	hospitalizations	NR	NR	NR	NR	N: 77	NR	N: 77 n with outcomes: 3 n with events: (4.2)	No.
Halterman, 2005[19]	Arm B-Decision support	hospitalizations	NR	NR	NR	NR	N: 73	NR	N: 73 n with outcomes: 1 n with events: (1.5)	No.
Herborg, 2001[14]	Arm A-Control (standard practice)	Emergency department visits	number of events per patient	NR	Yes	NR	N: 236	N: 204 Mean:0.021	NR	No.
Herborg, 2001[14]	Arm B-TOM	Emergency department visits	number of events per patient	NR	Yes	NR	N: 264	N: 209 Mean:0.19	NR	No.
Herborg, 2001[14]	Arm A-Control (standard	hospitalizations	mean hospital admissions per patient	NR	Yes	NR	N: 236 Mean:NR	N: 204 Mean:0.058	NR	No.

Author, Year	Arm	Clinical Outcome	Definition of Scale	Range of Scale	Were outcomes measured over a period of at least 12 months?	Is there enough information to determine seasonality?	Measurement at Baseline N n (%) mean SD	Measurement at end of treatment N n (%) mean SD	Measurement at last follow-up N n (%) mean SD	Were outcomes adjusted?
	practice)									
Herborg,2001[14]	Arm B-TOM	hospitalizations	mean hospital admissions per patient	NR	Yes	NR	N: 264	N: 209 Mean:0.019	NR	No.
Herborg,2001[14]	Arm A-Control (standard practice)	Symptom Days	days patients "felt too ill from asthma to work or carry out planned activities"	NR	Yes	NR	N: 236	NR	N: 204 Mean:6.57	No.
Herborg,2001[14]	Arm B-TOM	Symptom Days	days patients "felt too ill from asthma to work or carry out planned activities"	NR	Yes	NR	N: 264	NR	N: 209 Mean:3.81	No.
Herborg,2001[14]	Arm A-Control (standard practice)	Symptom Score	3 item asthma morbidity index	mild (1), moderate(2),	Yes	NR	N: 236 n with outcomes: 201 Mean: 2.1 SEM 0.056	NR	N: 204 n with outcomes: 201 Mean:1.88 SEM 0.060	Yes. Differences among pharmacies and physicians -but unclear how adjusted.
Herborg,2001[14]	Arm B-TOM	Symptom Score	3 item asthma	mild (1), moderate(	Yes	NR	N: 264 n with outcomes:	NR	N: 209 n with	Yes. Difference

Author, Year	Arm	Clinical Outcome	Definition of Scale	Range of Scale	Were outcomes measured over a period of at least 12 months?	Is there enough information to determine seasonality?	Measurement at Baseline N n (%) mean SD	Measurement at end of treatment N n (%) mean SD	Measurement at last follow-up N n (%) mean SD	Were outcomes adjusted?
	intervention		morbidity index	2),			208 Mean:1.99 SEM 0.057		outcomes: 208 Mean:1.52 0.047	s among pharmacies and physicians -but unclear how adjusted.
Herborg,2001[14]	Arm A-Control (standard practice)	urgent doctor visits	physician on call visits, mean number per patient	NR	Yes	NR	N: 236	N: 204 Mean:0.158	NR	No.
Herborg,2001[14]	Arm B-TOM	urgent doctor visits	physician on call visits, mean number per patient	NR	Yes	NR	N: 264	N: 209 Mean:0.067	NR	No.
Herborg,2001[14ii]	Arm A-Control (standard practice)	Quality of Life	Nottingham Health Profile- overall quality of life	0-100	Yes	NR	N: 236 n with outcomes: 204 Mean:11.39 SEM 1.08	N: 204 n with outcomes: 204 Mean:10.32 SEM 1.13	NR	No.
Herborg,2001[14ii]	Arm B-TOM	Quality of Life	Nottingham Health Profile- overall quality of life	0-100	Yes	NR	N: 264 n with outcomes: 209 Mean:8.76 SEM 0.84	N:209 n with outcomes: 209 Mean:4.97 SEM 0.65	NR	No.
Herborg,2001[14ii]	Arm A-Control (standard practice)	Quality of Life	Living with Asthma Questionnaire-QOL specific for	1-3	Yes	NR	N: 236 n with outcomes: 204 Mean:1.68 SEM 0.027	N: 204 n with outcomes: 204 Mean:1.6 SEM 0.031	NR	No.

Author, Year	Arm	Clinical Outcome	Definition of Scale	Range of Scale	Were outcomes measured over a period of at least 12 months?	Is there enough information to determine seasonality?	Measurement at Baseline N n (%) mean SD	Measurement at end of treatment N n (%) mean SD	Measurement at last follow-up N n (%) mean SD	Were outcomes adjusted?
			living with asthma)							
Herborg,2001[14 ii]	Arm B-TOM	Quality of Life	Living with Asthma Questionna ire-QOL specific for living with asthma	1-3	Yes	NR	N: 264 n with outcomes: 209 Mean:1.58 SEM 0.026	N: 209 n with outcomes: 209 Mean:1.41 SEM 0.026	NR	No.
Homer,2005[22]	Arm A-Control (standard practice)	Emergency department visits	NR	NR	NR	NR	N: 337(36)	N: 254(22)	NR	No.
Homer,2005[22]	Arm B-Learning collaborative	Emergency department visits	NR	NR	NR	NR	N: 294(36)	N: 236(17)	NR	No.
Homer,2005[22]	Arm A-Control (standard practice)	Hospitalizations	NR	NR	NR	NR	N: 337 N with events: (9)	N: 254 n with events: (4)	NR	No
Homer,2005[22]	Arm B-Learning collaborative	Hospitalizations	NR	NR	NR	NR	N: 294 n with events: (9)	N: 236 n with events: (2)	NR	No
Horswell,2008[4]	HCSD's DM program	Emergency department visits	# ER visits for respiratory diagnoses per 1,000	NR	NR	NR	191	NR	N: 2199 187	No

Author, Year	Arm	Clinical Outcome	Definition of Scale	Range of Scale	Were outcomes measured over a period of at least 12 months?	Is there enough information to determine seasonality?	Measurement at Baseline N n (%) mean SD	Measurement at end of treatment N n (%) mean SD	Measurement at last follow-up N n (%) mean SD	Were outcomes adjusted?
			patients over past 3 months							
Horswell,2008[4]	HCSD's DM program	hospitalizations	# of hospital admissions for respiratory diagnoses per 1,000 patients over past 3 months	NR	NR	NR	18	NR	N: 2199 11	No
Hoskins,1997[41]	Nebulized broncho dilators	Rescue use of short-acting B2 agonists	NR	NR	Yes	No	N: 782 n with outcomes: 782 n with events: 272 (35)	N: 569 n with outcomes: 669 n with events: 268 (40)	NR	No.
Kattan,2007[6]	Arm A- Control (standard practice)	Emergency department visits	mean # visits per year	NR	No	No	N: 466 Mean:3	NR	N: 463 Mean:1.14 SE: 0.08	No
Kattan,2007[6]	Arm B- Decision support	Emergency department visits	mean # visits per year	NR	No	No	N: 471 Mean:3	NR	N: 466 Mean:0.87 SE: 0.07	No
Kattan,2007[6]	Arm A- Control (standard practice)	hospitalizations	mean # per year		No	No	N: 466 Mean:0.8	NR	N: 463 Mean:0.24 SE: 0.03	No
Kattan,2007[6]	Arm B- Decision	hospitalizations	mean # per year	NR	No	No	N: 471,(1.1)	NR	N: 466 Mean:0.22	No

Author, Year	Arm	Clinical Outcome	Definition of Scale	Range of Scale	Were outcomes measured over a period of at least 12 months?	Is there enough information to determine seasonality?	Measurement at Baseline N n (%) mean SD	Measurement at end of treatment N n (%) mean SD	Measurement at last follow-up N n (%) mean SD	Were outcomes adjusted?
	n support								SE: 0.03	
Kattan,2007	Arm A-Control (standard practice)	Missed days of school	Mean # days per 2 weeks	NR	No	No	N: 466 Mean:1.1	NR	N: 463, Mean:0.72 SE: 0.04	No
Kattan,2007	Arm B-Decision support	Missed days of school	Mean # days per 2 weeks	NR	No	No	N: 471 Mean:0.9	NR	N: 466, Mean:0.67 SE: 0.04	No
Kattan,2007	Arm A-Control (standard practice)	Symptom Days	mean # per 2 weeks	NR	No	No	N: 466 Mean:2.1	NR	N: 463 Mean:1.6 SE: 0.08	No
Kattan,2007	Arm B-Decision support	Symptom Days	mean # per 2 weeks	NR	No	No	N: 471 Mean:2	NR	N: 466 Mean:1.42 SE: 0.07	No
Lesho,2005	Decision Support	Emergency department visits	NR	NR	NR	NR	n with events: 553	n with events: 193	NR	No
Lesho,2005	Decision Support	hospitalizations	NR	NR	NR	NR	N: NR n with events: 56	N: NR n with events: 23	NR	No
Lesho,2005	Decision Support	Lung function tests	NR	NR	NR	NR	N: 330,(65)	N: 334 (70)	NR	No
Lesho,2005	Decision Support	Rescue use of short-acting B2 agonists	NR	NR	NR	NR	N: NR n with events: 432	N: NR n with events: 203	NR	No
Lob S. H,	Longitu	Missed days	Caregivers	NR	Yes	No	N: 400	N: 400	N: 400	Yes.

Author, Year	Arm	Clinical Outcome	Definition of Scale	Range of Scale	Were outcomes measured over a period of at least 12 months?	Is there enough information to determine seasonality?	Measurement at Baseline N n (%) mean SD	Measurement at end of treatment N n (%) mean SD	Measurement at last follow-up N n (%) mean SD	Were outcomes adjusted?
2011[20]	dinal Evaluati on Group: Patient-level Intervie w Sample (T1-T3)	of work	missed any work in the past month because of the child's asthma				n with events: 87(21.8)	n with events: 39(9.8)	n with events: 24(6.0)	Variables included in initial models: size of the clinics' pediatric asthma population, percent of black patients, uninsured patients, children <5 years old, patients with moderate/ severe asthma.
Lob S, H, 2011[20]	Longitu dinal Evaluati on Group: Patient-level Intervie w Sample (T1-T3)	Quality of Life	Patients with "very good" quality of life (defined as a mean score ≥6). Includes children ≥7 years who completed quality of life interview.	NR	Yes	NR	N: 299 n with events: 127(42.5)	N: 299 n with events: 230(76.9)	N: 299 n with events: 252(84.3)	Yes. Variables included in initial models: size of the clinics' pediatric asthma population, percent of black patients, uninsured patients,

Author, Year	Arm	Clinical Outcome	Definition of Scale	Range of Scale	Were outcomes measured over a period of at least 12 months?	Is there enough information to determine seasonality?	Measurement at Baseline N n (%) mean SD	Measurement at end of treatment N n (%) mean SD	Measurement at last follow-up N n (%) mean SD	Were outcomes adjusted?
										children <5 years old, patients with moderate/ severe asthma.
Lob S, H., 2011[20]	Longitudinal Evaluation Group: Patient-level Interview Sample (T1-T3)	Missed days of school	Patients who missed any school in the past month because of asthma	NR	Yes	No	N: 537 n with events: 154(28.7)	N: 537 n with events: 78(14.5)	N: 537 n with events: 73(13.6)	Yes. Variables included in initial models: size of the clinics' pediatric asthma population, percent of black patients, uninsured patients, children <5 years old, patients with moderate/ severe asthma.
Lob S, H., 2011[20]	Longitudinal Evaluation Group:	Rescue use of short-acting B2 agonists.	Patients who used rescue medications frequently	NR	Yes	NR	N: 484 n with events: 149(20.8)	N: 484 n with events: 49(10.1)	N: 484 n with events: 38(7.9)	Yes. Variables included in initial models:

E-88

Author, Year	Arm	Clinical Outcome	Definition of Scale	Range of Scale	Were outcomes measured over a period of at least 12 months?	Is there enough information to determine seasonality?	Measurement at Baseline N n (%) mean SD	Measurement at end of treatment N n (%) mean SD	Measurement at last follow-up N n (%) mean SD	Were outcomes adjusted?
	Patient-level Interview Sample (T1-T3)		in last 2 weeks (more than twice per week)							size of the clinics' pediatric asthma population, percent of black patients, uninsured patients, children <5 years old, patients with moderate/severe asthma.
Lob S. H., 2011[20]	Longitudinal Evaluation Group: Patient-level Interview Sample (T1-T3)	Hospitalizations	Patients with any hospitalization attributed to asthma in the past 6 months.	0-100%	Yes	No	N: 761 n with events: 83(10.9)	N:761 n with events: 10(1.3)	N:761 n with events: 26(3.4)	Yes. Variables included in initial models: size of the clinics' pediatric asthma population, percent of black patients, uninsured patients, children <5 years old, patients

Author, Year	Arm	Clinical Outcome	Definition of Scale	Range of Scale	Were outcomes measured over a period of at least 12 months?	Is there enough information to determine seasonality?	Measurement at Baseline N n (%) mean SD	Measurement at end of treatment N n (%) mean SD	Measurement at last follow-up N n (%) mean SD	Were outcomes adjusted?
										with moderate/ severe asthma.
Lob. S. H., 2011[20]	Longitudinal Evaluation Group: Patient-level Interview Sample (T1-T3)	Emergency department visits	Patients with any ED visit attributed to asthma in past 6 months	NR	Yes	NR	N: 761 n with events: 225(29.6)	N: 761 n with events: 57(7.5)	N: 761 n with events: 71(9.3)	Yes. Variables included in initial models: size of the clinics' pediatric asthma population, percent of black patients, uninsured patients, children <5 years old, patients with moderate/ severe asthma.
Mahi-Taright,2004[39]	Education	Rescue use of short-acting B2 agonists	NR	NR	NR	NR	N: 137 n with outcomes: 6 (4)	N: 132 n with outcomes: 56 (43)	NR	No

Author, Year	Arm	Clinical Outcome	Definition of Scale	Range of Scale	Were outcomes measured over a period of at least 12 months?	Is there enough information to determine seasonality?	Measurement at Baseline N n (%) mean SD	Measurement at end of treatment N n (%) mean SD	Measurement at last follow-up N n (%) mean SD	Were outcomes adjusted?
Mangione-Smith,2005 [24]	Arm A-Control (standard practice)	Emergency department visits	Acute care service use (number of visits in last 6 mo)	NR	NR	NR	NR	NR	N: 126, Mean:0.5	Yes. Adjusted for child age, gender and race/ethnicity, parent education, household annual income, insurance type, severity of asthma and number of comorbidities.
Mangione-Smith,2005 [24]	Arm B-Learning collaborative	Emergency department visits	Acute care service use (number of visits in last 6 mo)	NR	NR	NR	NR	NR	N: 385,(0.8)	Yes. Adjusted for child age, gender and race/ethnicity, parent education, household annual income,

Author, Year	Arm	Clinical Outcome	Definition of Scale	Range of Scale	Were outcomes measured over a period of at least 12 months?	Is there enough information to determine seasonality?	Measurement at Baseline N n (%) mean SD	Measurement at end of treatment N n (%) mean SD	Measurement at last follow-up N n (%) mean SD	Were outcomes adjusted?
										insurance type, severity of asthma and number of comorbidities.
Mangione-Smith,2005 [24]	Arm A-Control (standard practice)	Missed days of school	School days missed in last mo due to child's asthma	NR	NR	NR	NR	NR	N: 126, Mean:1.6	Adjusted for child age, gender and race/ethnicity, parent education, household annual income, insurance type, severity of asthma an number of comorbidities.
Mangione-Smith,2005 [24]	Arm B-Learning collaborative	Missed days of school	School days missed in last mo due to child's asthma	NR	NR	NR	NR	NR	N: 385, Mean:1.4	Adjusted for child age, gender and race/ethnicity, parent education,

Author, Year	Arm	Clinical Outcome	Definition of Scale	Range of Scale	Were outcomes measured over a period of at least 12 months?	Is there enough information to determine seasonality?	Measurement at Baseline N n (%) mean SD	Measurement at end of treatment N n (%) mean SD	Measurement at last follow-up N n (%) mean SD	Were outcomes adjusted?
										household annual income, insurance type, severity of asthma and number of comorbidities.
Mangione-Smith, 2005 [24]	Arm A-Control (standard practice)	Quality of Life	Asthma Specific health related QOL-treatment problems	0-100	NR	NR	NR	NR	N: 126 Mean:85.3	Yes. Adjusted for child age, gender and race/ethnicity, parent education, household annual income, insurance type, severity of asthma and number of comorbidities.
Mangione-Smith, 2005 [24]	Arm B-Learning collabor	Quality of Life	Asthma Specific health related	0-100	NR	NR	NR	NR	N: 385 Mean:88.6	Yes. Adjusted for child age,

Author, Year	Arm	Clinical Outcome	Definition of Scale	Range of Scale	Were outcomes measured over a period of at least 12 months?	Is there enough information to determine seasonality?	Measurement at Baseline N n (%) mean SD	Measurement at end of treatment N n (%) mean SD	Measurement at last follow-up N n (%) mean SD	Were outcomes adjusted?
	ative		QOL-treatment problems							gender and race/ethnicity, parent education, household annual income, insurance type, severity of asthma and number of comorbidities.
Mangione-Smith, 2005[24]	Arm A-Standard practice	Quality of Life	General health-related quality of life (PedsQL 4.0 SF-15 scored on 0–100 scale)	0–100	NR	NR	NR	NR	N: 126 Mean:77	Yes. Adjusted for child age, gender and race/ethnicity, parent education, household annual income, insurance type, severity of asthma and number of comorbidit

Author, Year	Arm	Clinical Outcome	Definition of Scale	Range of Scale	Were outcomes measured over a period of at least 12 months?	Is there enough information to determine seasonality?	Measurement at Baseline N n (%) mean SD	Measurement at end of treatment N n (%) mean SD	Measurement at last follow-up N n (%) mean SD	Were outcomes adjusted?
										ies.
Mangione-Smith,2005 [24]	Arm B-Learning collaborative	Quality of Life	General health-related quality of life (PedsQL 4.0 SF-15 scored on 0–100 scale)	0-100	NR	NR	NR	NR	N: 385 Mean:80.2	Yes. Adjusted for child age, gender and race/ethnicity, parent education, household annual income, insurance type, severity of asthma and number of comorbidities.
Mangione-Smith,2005 [24]	Arm A - Control	Quality of Life	Asthma specific QOL-symptom scale (PedsQL 3.0 SF-22)	0-100	NR	NR	NR	NR	N: 126 Mean: 71.2	Yes. Adjusted for child age, gender and race/ethnicity, parent education, household annual income, insurance

Author, Year	Arm	Clinical Outcome	Definition of Scale	Range of Scale	Were outcomes measured over a period of at least 12 months?	Is there enough information to determine seasonality?	Measurement at Baseline N n (%) mean SD	Measurement at end of treatment N n (%) mean SD	Measurement at last follow-up N n (%) mean SD	Were outcomes adjusted?
										type, severity of asthma and number of comorbidities.
Mangione-Smith, 2005[24]	Arm B Intervention	Quality of Life	Asthma specific QOL – symptom scale (PedsQL 3.0 SF-22)	0-100	NR	NR	NR	NR	N: 385 Mean: 74.2	Yes. Adjusted for child age, gender and race/ethnicity, parent education, household annual income, insurance type, severity of asthma and number of comorbidities.

Author, Year	Arm	Clinical Outcome	Definition of Scale	Range of Scale	Were outcomes measured over a period of at least 12 months?	Is there enough information to determine seasonality?	Measurement at Baseline N n (%) mean SD	Measurement at end of treatment N n (%) mean SD	Measurement at last follow-up N n (%) mean SD	Were outcomes adjusted?
Mangione-Smith, 2005 [24]	Arm A - Control	Satisfaction	Parent satisfaction with provider communication (% satisfied)	0-100	NR	NR	NR	NR	N: 126 (55)	Yes. Adjusted for child age, gender and race/ethnicity, parent education, household annual income, insurance type, severity of asthma and number of comorbidities.

Author, Year	Arm	Clinical Outcome	Definition of Scale	Range of Scale	Were outcomes measured over a period of at least 12 months?	Is there enough information to determine seasonality?	Measurement at Baseline N n (%) mean SD	Measurement at end of treatment N n (%) mean SD	Measurement at last follow-up N n (%) mean SD	Were outcomes adjusted?
Mangione-Smith, 2005 [24]	Arm B Intervention	Satisfaction	Parent satisfaction with provider communication (% satisfied)	0-100	NR	NR	NR	NR	N: 385 (56)	Yes. Adjusted for child age, gender and race/ethnicity, parent education, household annual income, insurance type, severity of asthma and number of comorbidities.

Author, Year	Arm	Clinical Outcome	Definition of Scale	Range of Scale	Were outcomes measured over a period of at least 12 months?	Is there enough information to determine seasonality?	Measurement at Baseline N n (%) mean SD	Measurement at end of treatment N n (%) mean SD	Measurement at last follow-up N n (%) mean SD	Were outcomes adjusted?
Mangione-Smith, 2005 [24]	Arm A - Control	Satisfaction	Adolescent satisfaction with care	Scale score: 0-7	NR	NR	NR	NR	N: 126 Mean: 4.8	Yes. Adjusted for child age, gender and race/ethnicity, parent education, household annual income, insurance type, severity of asthma and number of comorbidities.

Author, Year	Arm	Clinical Outcome	Definition of Scale	Range of Scale	Were outcomes measured over a period of at least 12 months?	Is there enough information to determine seasonality?	Measurement at Baseline N n (%) mean SD	Measurement at end of treatment N n (%) mean SD	Measurement at last follow-up N n (%) mean SD	Were outcomes adjusted?
Mangione-Smith, 2005 [24]	Arm B Intervention	Satisfaction	Adolescent satisfaction with care	Scale score: 0-7	NR	NR	NR	NR	N: 385 Mean: 4.6	Yes. Adjusted for child age, gender and race/ethnicity, parent education, household annual income, insurance type, severity of asthma and number of comorbidities.

Author, Year	Arm	Clinical Outcome	Definition of Scale	Range of Scale	Were outcomes measured over a period of at least 12 months?	Is there enough information to determine seasonality?	Measurement at Baseline N n (%) mean SD	Measurement at end of treatment N n (%) mean SD	Measurement at last follow-up N n (%) mean SD	Were outcomes adjusted?
Mangione-Smith, 2005[24]	Arm A – Control	Work days missed	Parent lost work days in the last month due to child's asthma	NR	NR	NR	NR	NR	N: 126 Mean: 0.6	Yes. Adjusted for child age, gender and race/ethnicity, parent education, household annual income, insurance type, severity of asthma and number of comorbidities.

Author, Year	Arm	Clinical Outcome	Definition of Scale	Range of Scale	Were outcomes measured over a period of at least 12 months?	Is there enough information to determine seasonality?	Measurement at Baseline N n (%) mean SD	Measurement at end of treatment N n (%) mean SD	Measurement at last follow-up N n (%) mean SD	Were outcomes adjusted?
Mangione-Smith,2005[24]	Arm B - Intervention	Work days missed	Parent lost work days in the last month due to child's asthma	NR	NR	NR	NR	NR	N: 385 Mean: 0.6	Yes. Adjusted for child age, gender and race/ethnicity, parent education, household annual income, insurance type, severity of asthma and number of comorbidities.
McCowan,2 001[27]	Arm A- Control (standard practice)	Emergency department visits	Accident and emergency	NR	NR	NR	NR	NR	N: 330 n with events: 2, (1)	No
McCowan,2 001[27]	Arm B- Decision support	Emergency department visits	Accident and emergency	NR	NR	NR	NR	NR	N: 147 n with events: 0,(0)	No
McCowan,2 001[27]	Arm A- Control (standard practice	hospitalizations	Admissions	NR	No	No	NR	NR	N: 330 , n with events: 4 (1)	No.

Author, Year	Arm	Clinical Outcome	Definition of Scale	Range of Scale	Were outcomes measured over a period of at least 12 months?	Is there enough information to determine seasonality?	Measurement at Baseline N n (%) mean SD	Measurement at end of treatment N n (%) mean SD	Measurement at last follow-up N n (%) mean SD	Were outcomes adjusted?
McCowan,2 001[27]	Arm B-Decisio n support	hospitalizatio ns	Admissions	NR	No	No	NR	NR	N: 147 n with events: 0 (0)	No.
McCowan,2 001[27]	Arm A-Control (standar d practice)	Symptom Days	no time period noted	NR	No	No time period for symptom days.	NR	NR	N: 330 n with events: 44 (13)	No.
McCowan,2 001[27]	Arm B-Decisio n support	Symptom Days	no time period noted	NR	No	No time period for symptom days.	NR	NR	N: 147 n with events: 8 (5)	No.
Mitchell,20 05[8]	Arm A-Control (standar d practice)	Emergency department visits	# of attendance s at ED per patient week x 10^5.	NR	No	No	16.7 (14.6-18.8)	NR	10.9 (9.1-12.7)	No
Mitchell,20 05[8]	Arm B-Decisio n support	Emergency department visits	# of attendance s at ED per patient week x 10^5.	NR	No	No	14.7 (12.8-16.6)	NR	11.0 (9.4-12.6)	No
Mitchell,20 05[8]	Arm A-Control (standar d practice)	hospitalizatio ns	# of admissions per person week x 10^5	NR	No	No	N: NR 4.46 (CI: 3.18-5.75)	NR	N: NR 3.01 (CI: 2.08-3.94)	No
Mitchell,20 05[8]	Arm B-Decisio n	hospitalizatio ns	# of admissions per person	NR	No	No	N: NR 3.50 (CI: 2.34-4.66)	NR	N: NR 2.09 (CI: 1.35-2.81)	No

Author, Year	Arm	Clinical Outcome	Definition of Scale	Range of Scale	Were outcomes measured over a period of at least 12 months?	Is there enough information to determine seasonality?	Measurement at Baseline N n (%) mean SD	Measurement at end of treatment N n (%) mean SD	Measurement at last follow-up N n (%) mean SD	Were outcomes adjusted?
	support		week x 10^5							
Newton,2010[2]	Decision Support	Emergency department visits	NR	NR	NR	NR	N: NR, (10)	N: NR,(4)	NR	No
Newton,2010[2]	Decision Support	hospitalizations	NR	NR	NR	NR	N: NR,(4)	N: NR,(6)	NR	No
O'Laughlen,2008[33]	MSAGR group	Lung function tests	FEV1	NR	No	No	N: 24 Mean:99.88 SD:15.23	NR	N: 24, Mean:100.9 SD:12.54	No.
O'Laughlen,2008[33]	MSAGR group	Quality of Life	Physical health of child	NR	NR	NR	N: 24 Mean:70.97 SD:14.48	NR	N: 24, Mean:82.01 SD:16.59	No.
O'Laughlen,2008[33]	MSAGR group	Quality of Life	Activity of child	NR	NR	NR	N: 24 Mean:82.5 SD:16.75	NR	N: 24, Mean:91.04 SD:14.74	No.
O'Laughlen,2008[33]	MASGR group	Quality of Life	Activity of family	NR	NR	NR	N: 24 Mean:90.45 SD:11.27	NR	N: 24, Mean:98.26 SD:2.72	No.
O'Laughlen,2008[33]	MSAGR group	Quality of Life	Emotional health of child	NR	NR	NR	N: 24, Mean:77.71 SD:24.67	NR	N: 24, Mean:85.42 SD:20.95	No.
O'Laughlen,2008[33]	MSAGR group	Quality of Life	Emotional health of family	NR	NR	NR	N: 24, Mean:70.1, SD:19.08	NR	N: 24, Mean:74.45 SD:15.63	No.
Patel,2004[1]	Organizational change	Emergency department visits	Visits/1000 patients	NR	Yes	No	N: 451 n with outcomes: 148	N: 417 n with outcomes: 88	NR	No
Patel,2004[1]	Organizational Change	hospitalizations	Hospitalizations/1000 population	NR	Yes	No	N: 451 n with outcomes: 81	N: 427 n with outcomes: 37	NR	No
Ragazzi,2010[30]	Practice 1	Lung function tests	Spirometry	NR	NR	NR	N: 17,(6)	N: 24,(68)	NR	No
Ragazzi,20	Practice	Lung	Spirometry	NR	NR	NR	N: 26,(19)	N: 19,(27)	NR	No

Author, Year	Arm	Clinical Outcome	Definition of Scale	Range of Scale	Were outcomes measured over a period of at least 12 months?	Is there enough information to determine seasonality?	Measurement at Baseline N n (%) mean SD	Measurement at end of treatment N n (%) mean SD	Measurement at last follow-up N n (%) mean SD	Were outcomes adjusted?
10[30]	2	function tests								
Ragazzi,20 10[30]	Practice 3	Lung function tests	Spirometry	NR	NR	NR	N: 10,(0)	N: 21,(24)	NR	No
Richman,2 000[16]	Feedba ck	Emergency department visits	percent reporting no ED visits for asthma in last 6 months	0-100	No	No	N: 228 n with outcomes: 114 n with events: (82)	N: 317 n with outcomes: 158 n with events: (81)	NR	No.
Richman,2 000[16]	Feedba ck	hospitalizatio ns	percent reporting no admission for asthma in last 6 months	0-100	NR	NR	N: 228 n with outcomes: 114 n with events: (96)	N: 3-7 n with outcomes: 158 Mean: 94	NR	No.
Richman,2 000[16]	Feedba ck	Missed days of work	Percent reporting 0 parent work absence due to child's asthma in last 6 months	0-100	No	No	N: 228 n with outcomes: 114 n with events: NR (62)	N: 317 n with outcomes: 158 n with events: NR (62)	NR	No.
Richman,2 000[16]	Feedba ck	Parental perceptions	% reporting physician asthma care as excellent	0-100	No	No	N: 228 n with outcomes: 114 n with events: (50)	N:317 n with outcomes: 158 n with events:(50)	NR	No.
Richman,2 000[16]	Feedba ck	Urgent doctor visits	percent reporting no urgent	0-100	NR	NR	N: 228 n with outcomes: 114	N 317 n with outcomes: 158	NR	No.

E-105

Author, Year	Arm	Clinical Outcome	Definition of Scale	Range of Scale	Were outcomes measured over a period of at least 12 months?	Is there enough information to determine seasonality?	Measurement at Baseline N n (%) mean SD	Measurement at end of treatment N n (%) mean SD	Measurement at last follow-up N n (%) mean SD	Were outcomes adjusted?
			doctor visits for asthma last 6 months				n with events: (46)	n with events: (23)		
Ruoff, 2002[23]	Arm A- Before the flow sheet	Missed days of school	Days of school/work missed	NR	NR	NR	NR	NR	N: 122,(1.01)	No.
Ruoff, 2002[23]	Arm B- After implementation of the flow sheet	Missed days of school	Days of school/work missed	NR	NR	NR	NR	NR	N: 122,(73.68)	No.
Ruoff,2002[2][3]	Arm A- Before the flow sheet	Emergency department visits	Emergency room visits	NR	NR	NR	NR	NR	N: 122,(1.01)	No.
Ruoff,2002[2][3]	Arm B- After Implementation of the flow sheet	Emergency department visits	Emergency room visits	NR	NR	NR	NR	NR	N: 122,(73.68)	No.
Ruoff,2002[2][3]	Arm A- Before the flow sheet	hospitalizations	Hospitalizations	NR	NR	NR	NR	NR	N: 122,(2.02)	No.
Ruoff,2002[2][3]	Arm B- After implementation of the flow	hospitalizations	Hospitalizations	NR	NR	NR	NR	NR	N: 122,(73.68)	No.

Author, Year	Arm	Clinical Outcome	Definition of Scale	Range of Scale	Were outcomes measured over a period of at least 12 months?	Is there enough information to determine seasonality?	Measurement at Baseline N n (%) mean SD	Measurement at end of treatment N n (%) mean SD	Measurement at last follow-up N n (%) mean SD	Were outcomes adjusted?
Saini,2004[3][8]	sheet Arm A-Control 1	Quality of Life	Quality of life (0–80)	(0–80)	No	No	N: 22 Mean:44.7 SD:15.6	NR	N: 22, Mean:44.7 SD:15.6	No.
Saini,2004[3][8]	Arm B-Control 2	Quality of Life	Quality of life (0–80)	(0–80)	No	No	N: 28 Mean:32.3 SD:9.4	NR	N: 28 Mean:32.3 SD:9.4	No.
Saini,2004[3][8]	Arm C-Education	Quality of Life	Quality of life (0–80)	(0–80)	No	No	N: 52 Mean:40.6 SD:14.3	NR	N: 39 Mean:19 SD:13.5	No.
Schneider, 2008[6]	Arm A-Traditional quality circle	Emergency department visits	binary	Yes/No	Yes	NR	N: NR n with outcomes: 62 n with events: 13 (19.7)	NR	N: 62 n with outcomes: 62 n with events: 4 (6.1)	No
Schneider, 2008[6]	Arm B-Benchmark quality circle	Emergency department visits	binary	Yes/No	Yes	NR	N: NR n with outcomes: 113 n with events: 21 (17.6)	NR	N: 113 n with outcomes: 113 n with events: 13 (10.9)	No
Schneider, 2008[6]	Arm A-Traditional quality circle	hospitalizations	hospitalization in last 12 months	Yes/no	Yes	NR	N: NR n with outcomes: 62 n with events: 5 (7.6)	NR	N: 62 n with outcomes: 62 n with events: 3 (4.5)	No
Schneider, 2008[6]	Arm B-Benchmark quality circle	hospitalizations	hospitalization in last 12 months	Yes/no	Yes	NR	N: NR n with outcomes: 113 n with events: 9 (7.6)	NR	N: 113 n with outcomes: 113 n with events: 7 (5.9)	No
Schneider, 2008[6]	Arm A-Traditional quality circle	Symptom Days	Asthma step 1	1-4	Yes	NR	N: NR n with outcomes: 62 n with events: 15 (24.2)	NR	N: NR n with outcomes: 63 n with events: 15 (23.8)	No

Author, Year	Arm	Clinical Outcome	Definition of Scale	Range of Scale	Were outcomes measured over a period of at least 12 months?	Is there enough information to determine seasonality?	Measurement at Baseline N n (%) mean SD	Measurement at end of treatment N n (%) mean SD	Measurement at last follow-up N n (%) mean SD	Were outcomes adjusted?
Schneider, 2008[6]	Arm B-Benchmark quality circle	Symptom Days	Asthma step 1	1-4	Yes	NR	N: NR n with outcomes: 112 n with events: 31 (27.7)	NR	N: NR n with outcomes: 59 n with events: 13 (22)	No
Schneider, 2008[6]	Arm A-Traditional quality circle	Symptom Days	Asthma Step	Step 2	Yes	NR	N: NR n with outcomes: 62 n with events: 16 (25.8)	NR	N: NR n with outcomes: 63 n with events: 20 (31.7)	No
Schneider, 2008[6]	Arm B-Benchmark quality circle	Symptom Days	Asthma Step	Step 2	Yes	NR	N: NR n with outcomes: 112 n with events: 24 (21.4)	NR	N: NR n with outcomes: 59 n with events: 23 (39)	No
Schneider, 2008[6]	Arm A-Traditional quality circle	Symptom Days	Asthma Step	step 3	Yes	NR	N: NR n with outcomes: 62 n with events: 27 (43.5)	NR	N: NR n with outcomes: 63 n with events: 21 (33.3)	No
Schneider, 2008[6]	Arm B-Benchmark quality circle	Symptom Days	Asthma Step	step 3	Yes	NR	N: NR n with outcomes: 112 n with events: 46 (41.1)	NR	N: NR n with outcomes: 59 n with events: 19 (32.2)	No
Schneider, 2008[6]	Arm A-Traditional quality circle	Symptom Days	Asthma step	Step 4	Yes	NR	N: NR n with outcomes: 62 n with events: 4 (6.5)	NR	N: NR n with outcomes: 63 n with events: 7 (11.1)	No

Author, Year	Arm	Clinical Outcome	Definition of Scale	Range of Scale	Were outcomes measured over a period of at least 12 months?	Is there enough information to determine seasonality?	Measurement at Baseline N n (%) mean SD	Measurement at end of treatment N n (%) mean SD	Measurement at last follow-up N n (%) mean SD	Were outcomes adjusted?
Schneider, 2008[6]	Arm B-Benchmark quality circle	Symptom Days	Asthma step	Step 4	Yes	NR	N: NR n with outcomes: 112 n with events: 11 (9.8)	NR	N: NR n with outcomes: 59 n with events: 4 (6.8)	No
Schneider, 2008[6]	Arm A-Traditional quality circle	urgent doctor visits	"number of unscheduled visits"	integer values	Yes	NR	N: NR n with outcomes: 62 # visits: 14	NR	N: 62 n with outcomes: 62 # visits: 20	No
Schneider, 2008[6]	Arm B-Benchmark quality circle	urgent doctor visits	"number of unscheduled visits"	integer values	Yes	NR	N: NR n with outcomes: 113 # visits: 51	NR	N: 113 n with outcomes: 113 # visits: 20	No
Shah, 2011[3] [5]	Arm A-Control	Missed days of school	NR	NR	NR	NR	N: 108 n with outcomes: 89 (82)	N: 106 n with outcomes: 68 (64)	NR	No
Shah, 2011[3] [5]	Arm B-Practitioner Asthma Communication and Education (PACE)	Missed days of school	NR	NR	NR	NR	N: 110 n with outcomes: 73 (66)	N: 101 n with outcomes: 61 (60)	NR	No
Shah, 2011[3] [5]	Arm A-Control	Missed days of work	NR	NR	NR	NR	N: 108 n with outcomes: 45 (42)	N: 104 n with outcomes: 37 (36)	NR	No
Shah, 2011[3] [5]	Arm B-Practitioner	Missed days of work	NR	NR	NR	NR	N: 110 n with outcomes: 33 (30)	N: 101 n with outcomes: 26 (26)	NR	No

Author, Year	Arm	Clinical Outcome	Definition of Scale	Range of Scale	Were outcomes measured over a period of at least 12 months?	Is there enough information to determine seasonality?	Measurement at Baseline N n (%) mean SD	Measurement at end of treatment N n (%) mean SD	Measurement at last follow-up N n (%) mean SD	Were outcomes adjusted?
	Asthma Communication and Education (PACE)									
Shah,2011[3] [5]	Arm A-Control	urgent doctor visits	NR	NR	NR	NR	N: 108 n with outcomes: 34 (31)	N: 106 n with outcomes: 13 (12)	NR	No
Shah,2011[3] [5]	Arm B-Practitioner Asthma Communication and Education (PACE)	urgent doctor visits	NR	NR	NR	NR	N: 110 n with outcomes: 30 (27)	N: 101 n with outcomes: 18 (18)	NR	No
Shapiro,2011[1]	SBHC	Emergency department visits	Documentation during any visit	NR	No	No	N: 200, (26)	N: 200,(88)	NR	No
Shapiro,2011[1]	NYCHP	Emergency department visits	Documentation during any visit	NR	No	No	N: 197, (27.4)	N: 249,(90)	NR	No
Shapiro,2011[1]	SBHC	hospitalizations	Documentation during any visit	NR	No	No	N: 200,(51)	N: 200,(88)	NR	No
Shapiro,2011[1]	NYCHP	hospitalizations	Documentation during any visit	NR	No	No	N: 197,(41.1)	N: 249,(89.2)	NR	No
Shiffman,2000[17]	Arm A-Pre	Emergency department visits	Proportion of children with ED visit at 1	n, %	No	See prior comments	N: 91 n with outcomes: 84 n with events: 5	NR	NR	No.

Author, Year	Arm	Clinical Outcome	Definition of Scale	Range of Scale	Were outcomes measured over a period of at least 12 months?	Is there enough information to determine seasonality?	Measurement at Baseline N n (%) mean SD	Measurement at end of treatment N n (%) mean SD	Measurement at last follow-up N n (%) mean SD	Were outcomes adjusted?
			week follow up				(6)			
Shiffman,2000[17]	Arm B-Post	Emergency department visits	Proportion of children with ED visit at 1 week follow up	n, %	No	See prior comments	N: 74 n with outcomes: 69 n with events: 0 (0)	NR	NR	No.
Shiffman,2000[17]	Arm A-Pre	hospitalizations	proportion of children hospitalized	NR	No	See prior notes	N: 91 n with outcomes: 84 n with events: 4	NR	NR	No.
Shiffman,2000[17]	Arm B-Post	hospitalizations	proportion of children hospitalized	NR	No	See prior notes	N: 74 n with outcomes: 69 n with events: 0,(0)	NR	NR	No.
Shiffman,2000[17]	Arm A-Pre	Missed days of school	Missed days of school at one week follow up, yes no, then mean number	yes/no, and then integers for mean days	No	see prior comments	N: 91, n with outcomes: 84 n with events: 37 (44) Mean:1.29	NR	NR	No.
Shiffman,2000[17]	Arm B-Post	Missed days of school	Missed days of school at one week follow up, yes no, then mean number	yes/no, and then integers for mean days	No	see prior comments	N: 74 n with outcomes: 69 n with events: 33(48) Mean:1.04 SD:NR	NR	NR	No.
Shiffman,2000[17]	Arm A-Pre	Missed days of work	Missed days of work at one	yes/no, then integers	No	See prior comments	N: 91 n with outcomes: 84	NR	NR	No.

Author, Year	Arm	Clinical Outcome	Definition of Scale	Range of Scale	Were outcomes measured over a period of at least 12 months?	Is there enough information to determine seasonality?	Measurement at Baseline N n (%) mean SD	Measurement at end of treatment N n (%) mean SD	Measurement at last follow-up N n (%) mean SD	Were outcomes adjusted?
			week follow up, yes no, and then mean number	for number of days			n with events: 20 (24) Mean:0.56			
Shiffman, 2000[17]	Arm B-Post	Missed days of work	Missed days of work at one week follow up, yes no, and then mean number	yes/no, then integers for number of days	No	See prior comments	N: 74 n with outcomes: 69 n with events: 16 (23) Mean:0.46	NR	NR	No.
Stargachs, 2002[34]	Arm A-Control (standard practice)	Missed days of school	NR	NR	NR	NR	N: 177	N: 177 Mean:1.7 SD:0.4	NR	No.
Stargachs, 2002[34]	Arm B-Education	Missed days of school	NR	NR	NR	NR	N: 153	N: 153 Mean:1.1 SD:0.2	NR	No.
Stergachis, 2002[34]	Arm A-Control (standard practice)	Lung function tests	Mean number of days with peak flow >80% of personal best	NR	NR	NR	N: 177, Mean:0.74, SD:0.02	N: 177, Mean:0.79, SD:0.02	NR	No.
Stergachis, 2002[34]	Arm B-Education	Lung function tests	Mean number of days with peak flow >80% of personal best	NR	NR	NR	N: 153 Mean:0.71 SD:0.03	N: 153 Mean:0.76 SD:0.02	NR	No.

Author, Year	Arm	Clinical Outcome	Definition of Scale	Range of Scale	Were outcomes measured over a period of at least 12 months?	Is there enough information to determine seasonality?	Measurement at Baseline N n (%) mean SD	Measurement at end of treatment N n (%) mean SD	Measurement at last follow-up N n (%) mean SD	Were outcomes adjusted?
Suh,2001[13]	Intermittent	Emergency department visits	number of ED visits per patient	NR	NR	NR	N: 566 n with outcomes: 566 Mean: 0 SD:NR	N: 566 Mean:0.06 SD:0.32	NR	No.
Suh,2001[13]	Persistent	Emergency department visits	number of ED visits per patient	NR	NR	NR	N: 1050 Mean:0.2 SD:0.63	N: 1050 Mean:0.09 SD:0.4	NR	No.
Suh,2001[13]	Intermittent	hospitalizations	number of hospitalizations per patient	NR	No	Yes. Same 9 months of the year Jan-Sept for all study outcomes	N: 566 n with outcomes: 566 Mean: 0	N: 566 n with outcomes: 566 Mean: 0.02 SD:0.14	NR	No.
Suh,2001[13]	Persistent	hospitalizations	number of hospitalizations per patient	NR	No	Yes. Same 9 months of the year Jan-Sept for all study outcomes	N: 1050 Mean:0.08 SD:0.32	N: 1050 Mean:0.05 SD:0.24	NR	No.
Suh,2001[13]	Intermittent	Rescue use of short-acting B2 agonists	number of prescriptions for inhaled beta agonists	NR	No	Yes. Same time period	N: 566 n with outcomes: 566 total 257	NR	NR	No.
Suh,2001[13]	Persistent	Rescue use of short-acting B2 agonists	number of prescriptions for inhaled beta agonists	NR	No	Yes. Same time period	N: 1050 n with outcomes: 1050 n with events: 4543 (47.3) total 4543	N: 1050 n with events: 4206 (49.2) total 4206	NR	No.
Suh,2001[13]	Intermittent	Rescue use of short-acting B2 agonists	precriptions for oral beta agonists	NR	No	Yes. Same time period	N: 566 n with outcomes: 566 total 149	N:566 total 88	NR	No.
Suh,2001[13]	Persistent	Rescue use of short-	prescriptions for oral	NR	No	Yes. Same time period	N: 1050 n with events:	N: 1050 n with events: 289	NR	No.

Author, Year	Arm	Clinical Outcome	Definition of Scale	Range of Scale	Were outcomes measured over a period of at least 12 months?	Is there enough information to determine seasonality?	Measurement at Baseline N n (%) mean SD	Measurement at end of treatment N n (%) mean SD	Measurement at last follow-up N n (%) mean SD	Were outcomes adjusted?
		acting B2 agonists	beta agonists				522 (5.4) total 522	(3.4) total 289		
Sulaiman, 2010[3]	Arm A- ENT education	Emergency department visits	NR	NR	NR	NR	N: 97 n with outcomes: 3 (3.1)	N: 100 n with outcomes: 8 (8)	NR	No
Sulaiman, 2010[3]	Arm B- Asthma education and guidelines	Emergency department visits	NR	NR	NR	NR	N: 125 n with outcomes: 3 (2.4)	N: 125 n with outcomes: 10 (8)	NR	No
Sulaiman, 2010[3]	Arm C- Asthma guidelines only	Emergency department visits	NR	NR	NR	NR	N: 108 n with outcomes: 5 (4.6)	N: 108 n with outcomes: 3 (2.8)	NR	No
Sulaiman, 2010[3]	Arm A- ENT education	urgent doctor visits	NR	NR	NR	NR	N: 92 n with outcomes: 33 (35.9)	N: 93 n with outcomes: 34 (35.8)	NR	No
Sulaiman, 2010[3]	Arm B- Asthma education and guidelines	urgent doctor visits	NR	NR	NR	NR	N: 121 n with outcomes: 25 (20.7)	N: 123 n with outcomes: 31 (25.2)	NR	No
Sulaiman, 2010[3]	Arm C- Asthma guidelines	urgent doctor visits	NR	NR	NR	NR	N: 104 n with outcomes: 18 (17.3)	N: 107 n with outcomes: 28 (26.2)	NR	No
Thyne, 2007[29]	Arm A- Control	hospitalizations	NR	NR	No	No	NR	NR	NR	No.
Thyne, 2007[29]	Arm B- Time 1, 2002-2003	hospitalizations	NR	NR	No	No	N: NR n with events: (18)	N: NR n with events: (16)	N: NR n with events: (14)	No.

Author, Year	Arm	Clinical Outcome	Definition of Scale	Range of Scale	Were outcomes measured over a period of at least 12 months?	Is there enough information to determine seasonality?	Measurement at Baseline N n (%) mean SD	Measurement at end of treatment N n (%) mean SD	Measurement at last follow-up N n (%) mean SD	Were outcomes adjusted?
Weinberger ,2002[25]	Arm A- Usual care control group	Emergency department visits	Hospital or emergency department visit in past month (Admission)	NR	Yes	No	NR	NR	N: 246,(7.3)	No.
Weinberger ,2002[25]	Arm B- Peak flow meter monitoring control group	Emergency department visits	Hospital or emergency department visit in past month (Admission)	NR	Yes	No	NR	NR	N: 296,(14.6)	No.
Weinberger ,2002[25]	Arm C- Pharmaceutical care program (education, feedback, pay-for-performance)	Emergency department visits	Hospital or emergency department visit in past month (Admission)	NR	Yes	No	NR	NR	N: 356,(15.7)	No.
Weinberger ,2002[25]	Arm A- Usual care control group	Quality of Life	Overall HPQOL	1(worst) to 7 (best)	NR	NR	N: 165 Mean:4.4 SD:1.2	N: 142 Mean:4.9 SD:1.2	N: 2135 Mean:4.9 SD:1.3	No.
Weinberger ,2002[25]	Arm B- Peak Flow Meter	Quality of Life	Overall HPQOL	1(worst) to 7 (best)	NR	NR	N: 233 Mean:4.3 SD:1.1	N: 204 Mean:4.8 SD:1.2	N: 191 Mean:5 SD:1.2	No.

Author, Year	Arm	Clinical Outcome	Definition of Scale	Range of Scale	Were outcomes measured over a period of at least 12 months?	Is there enough information to determine seasonality?	Measurement at Baseline N n (%) mean SD	Measurement at end of treatment N n (%) mean SD	Measurement at last follow-up N n (%) mean SD	Were outcomes adjusted?
	Monitoring group									
Weinberger, 2002[25]	Arm C-Pharmaceutical Care Program (education, feedback, pay-for-performance)	Quality of Life	Overall HPQOL	1(worst) to 7 (best)	NR	NR	N: 262 Mean:4.5 SD:1.2	N: 225 Mean:5, SD:1.3	N: 207 Mean:5 SD:1.2	No.
Yawn, 2010[36]	Education and feedback	non urgent asthma care visits	NR	NR	NR	NR	N: 840,(4)	N: 850,(21)	NR	No.

ENT = ear nose throat; ER = Emergency Room; HCSD = Health Care Services Division; HPQOL = Health Profile Quality of Life; NR = Not Reported; NYCHP = New York Children's Health Project; SBHC = South Bronx Health Center; TOM = Therapeutic Outcomes Monitoring; QOL = Quality of Life

References

1. Shapiro A, Gracy D, Quinones W, Applebaum J, Sarmiento A. Arch Pediatr Adolesc Med: Putting guidelines into practice: improving documentation of pediatric asthma management using a decision-making tool. 2011; 165:412-8.

2. Newton WP, Lefebvre A, Donahue KE, Bacon T, Dobson A. J Contin Educ Health Prof: Infrastructure for large-scale quality-improvement projects: early lessons from North Carolina Improving Performance in Practice. 2010; 30:106-13.

3. Sulaiman ND, Barton CA, Liaw ST *et al.* Fam Pract: Do small group workshops and locally adapted guidelines improve asthma patients' health outcomes? A cluster randomized controlled trial. 2010; 27:246-54.

4. Horswell R, Butler MK, Kaiser M *et al.* Dis Manag: Disease management programs for the underserved. 2008; 11:145-52.

6. Schneider A, Wensing M, Biessecker K, Quinzler R, Kaufmann-Kolle P, Szecsenyi J. J Eval Clin Pract: Impact of quality circles for improvement of asthma care: results of a randomized controlled trial. 2008; 14:185-90.

7. Kattan M, Crain EF, Steinbach S *et al.* Pediatrics: A randomized clinical trial of clinician feedback to improve quality of care for inner-city children with asthma. 2006; 117:e1095-103.

8. Mitchell EA, Didsbury PB, Kruithof N *et al.* Acta Paediatr: A randomized controlled trial of an asthma clinical pathway for children in general practice. 2005; 94:226-33.

9. Lesho EP, Myers CP, Ott M, Winslow C, Brown JE. Mil Med: Do clinical practice guidelines improve processes or outcomes in primary care? 2005; 170:243-6.

10. Patel PH, Welsh C, Foggs MB. Dis Manag: Improved asthma outcomes using a coordinated care approach in a large medical group. 2004; 7:102-11.

11. Glasgow NJ, Ponsonby AL, Yates R, Beilby J, Dugdale P. BMJ: Proactive asthma care in childhood: general practice based randomised controlled trial. 2003; 327:659.

12. Coleman CI, Reddy P, Laster-Bradley NM, Dorval S, Munagala B, White CM. Ann Pharmacother: Effect of practitioner education on adherence to asthma treatment guidelines. 2003; 37:956-61.

13. Suh DC, Shin SK, Okpara I, Voytovich RM, Zimmerman A. Am J Manag Care: Impact of a targeted asthma intervention program on treatment costs in patients with asthma. 2001; 7:897-906.

14. Herborg H, Soendergaard B, Jorgensen T *et al.* J Am Pharm Assoc (Wash): Improving drug therapy for patients with asthma-part 2: Use of antiasthma medications. 2001; 41:551-9.

15. Cowie RL, Underwood MF, Mack S. Can Respir J: The impact of asthma management guideline dissemination on the control of asthma in the community. 2001 ; 8 Suppl A:41A-5A.

16. Richman MJ, Poltawsky JS. Stud Health Technol Inform: Partnership for excellence in asthma care: evidence-based disease management. 2000; 76:107-21.

17. Shiffman RN, Freudigman M, Brandt CA, Liaw Y, Navedo DD. Pediatrics: A guideline implementation system using handheld computers for office management of asthma: effects on adherence and patient outcomes. 2000; 105:767-73.

18. Cloutier MM, Grosse SD, Wakefield DB, Nurmagambetov TA, Brown CM. American Journal of Managed Care: The economic impact of an urban asthma management program. 2009; 15:345-51.

19. Halterman JS, McConnochie KM, Conn KM *et al.* Archives of Pediatrics and Adolescent Medicine: A randomized trial of primary care provider prompting to enhance preventive asthma therapy. 2005; 159:422-7.

20. Clark N, Gong M, Schork M, et al. Impact of education for physicians on patient outcomes. Pediatrics 1998; 101(5):831-6.

21. Brown R, Bratton SL, Cabana MD, Kaciroti N, Clark NM. Chest: Physician asthma education program improves outcomes for children of low-income families. 2004; 126:369-74.

22. Homer CJ, Forbes P, Horviz L, Peterson LE, Wypij D, Heinrich P. Archives of Pediatrics and Adolescent Medicine: Impact of a quality improvement program on care and outcomes for children with asthma. 2005; 159:464-9.

23. Ruoff G. Family Medicine: Effects of flow sheet implementation on physician performance in the management of asthmatic patients.

2002; 34:514-7.

24. Mangione-Smith R, Schonlau M, Chan KS *et al.* Ambulatory Pediatrics: Measuring the effectiveness of a collaborative for quality improvement in pediatric asthma care: Does implementing the chronic care model improve processes and outcomes of care? 2005; 5:75-82.

25. Weinberger M, Murray MD, Marrero DG *et al.* Journal of the American Medical Association: Effectiveness of pharmacist care for patients with reactive airways disease: A randomized controlled trial. 2002; 288:1594-602.

26. Bryce FP, Neville RG, Crombie IK, Clark RA, McKenzie P. British Medical Journal: Controlled trial of an audit facilitator in diagnosis and treatment of childhood asthma in general practice. 1995; 310:838-42.

27. McCowan C, Neville RG, Ricketts IW, Warner FC, Hoskins G, Thomas GE. Medical Informatics and the Internet in Medicine: Lessons from a randomized controlled trial designed to evaluate computer decision support software to improve the management of asthma. 2001; 26:191-201.

28. Finkelstein JA, Lozano P, Fuhlbrigge AL *et al.* Health Serv Res: Practice-level effects of interventions to improve asthma care in primary care settings: the Pediatric Asthma Care Patient Outcomes Research Team. 2005; 40:1737-57.

29. Thyne SM, Marmor AK, Madden N, Herrick G. Paediatric and Perinatal Epidemiology: Comprehensive asthma management for underserved children. 2007; 21:29-34.

30. Ragazzi H, Keller A, Ehrensberger R, Irani AM. J Urban Health: Evaluation of a practice-based intervention to improve the management of pediatric asthma. 2011; 88 Suppl 1:38-48.

31. Hagmolen of ten Have W, van den Berg NJ, van der Palen J, van Aalderen WM, Bindels PJ. Prim Care Respir J: Implementation of an asthma guideline for the management of childhood asthma in general practice: a randomised controlled trial. 2008; 17:90-6.

32. Bell LM, Grundmeier R, Localio R *et al.* Pediatrics: Electronic health record-based decision support to improve asthma care: a cluster-randomized trial. 2010; 125:e770-7.

33. O'Laughlen MC, Hollen PJ, Rakes G, Ting S. Pediatric Asthma, Allergy and Immunology: Improving pediatric asthma by the MSAGR algorithm: A multicolored, simplified, asthma guideline reminder. 2008; 21:119-27.

34. Stergachis A , Gardner JS, Anderson MT, Sullivan SD. Journal of the American Pharmaceutical Association (Washington,D.C. : 1996): Improving pediatric asthma outcomes in the community setting: does pharmaceutical care make a difference? 2002; 42:743-52.

35. Shah S, Sawyer SM, Toelle BG *et al.* Med J Aust: Improving paediatric asthma outcomes in primary health care: a randomised controlled trial. 2011; 195:405-9.

36. Yawn BP, Bertram S, Wollan P. Journal of Asthma and Allergy: Introduction of asthma APGAR tools improve asthma management in primary care practices. 2008; 1-10.

37. Baker R, Fraser RC, Stone M, Lambert P, Stevenson K, Shiels C. Br J Gen Pract: Randomised controlled trial of the impact of guidelines, prioritized review criteria and feedback on implementation of recommendations for angina and asthma. 2003; 53:284-91.

38. Saini B, Krass I, Armour C. Annals of Pharmacotherapy: Development, implementation, and evaluation of a community pharmacy-based asthma care model. 2004; 38:1954-60.

39. Mahi-Taright S, Belhocine M, Ait-Khaled N. Int J Tuberc Lung Dis: Can we improve the management of chronic obstructive respiratory disease? The example of asthma in adults. 2004; 8:873-81.

40. Cloutier MM, Wakefield DB, Carlisle PS, Bailit HL, Hall CB. Arch Pediatr Adolesc Med: The effect of Easy Breathing on asthma management and knowledge. 2002; 156:1045-51.

41. Hoskins G, Neville RG, Smith B, Clark RA. Health Bull (Edinb): Does participation in distance learning and audit improve the care of patients with acute asthma attacks? The General Practitioners in Asthma Group. 1997; 55:150-5.

42. Gorton TA, Cranford CO, Golden WE, Walls RC, Pawelak JE. Arch Fam Med: Primary care physicians' response to dissemination of practice guidelines. 1995; 4:135-42.

Evidence Table 6. Healthcare process outcomes: Baseline and end of treatment

Author, Year	Health Care Process Outcomes	Arm	Definition of Scale	Range of Scale	Were outcomes measured over a period of at least 12 months?	Is there enough information to determine seasonality?	Measurement at Baseline n (%) mean SD	Measurement at end of treatment n (%) mean SD	Measurement at last follow-up n (%) mean SD	Were outcomes adjusted?
Ables,2002[19]	Documentation of level of asthma control/severity	Education and reminders	NR	NR	NR	NR	N: 126 (8.5)	N: 175 (51)	NR	No.
Ables,2002[19]	Documentation of level of asthma control/severity	Education and Reminders	NR	NR	NR	NR	N: 126 (8.5)	N: 175 (51)	NR	No.
Armour,2007[18]	Documentation of asthma control/severity	Arm A-Control	Proportion of patients classified as severe	NR	No	NR	N: 205 n with events: (71.2)	N: 186 n with events: (67.9)	NR	Yes.
Armour,2007[18]	Documentation of asthma control/severity	Arm B-Pharmacy Asthma Care Program (PACP)	Proportion of patients classified as severe	NR	No (time: 9 months)	NR	N: 191 n with events: (87.9)	N: 165 n with events: (52.7)	NR	Yes.
Baker,2003[26]	Environmental control practice recommendations	Arm A-Guidelines only	patient's current smoking status has been established and recorded (past 12 months)	NR	NR	NR	N: 428 n with outcomes: 120 (28)	NR	N: 490 n with outcomes: 146 (29.8)	No.
Baker,2003[26]	Environmental control practice recommendations	Arm B-Guidelines with audit criteria	patient's current smoking status has been	NR	NR	NR	N: 451 n with outcomes: 114 (25.3)	NR	N: 480 n with outcomes: 158 (32.9)	No.

Author, Year	Health Care Process Outcomes	Arm	Definition of Scale	Range of Scale	Were outcomes measured over a period of at least 12 months?	Is there enough information to determine seasonality?	Measurement at Baseline n (%) mean SD	Measurement at end of treatment n (%) mean SD	Measurement at last follow-up n (%) mean SD	Were outcomes adjusted?
			established and recorded (past 12 months)							
Baker,2003[26]	Environmental control practice recommendations	Arm C- Guidelines with audit criteria and feedback	patient's current smoking status has been established and recorded (past 12 months)	NR	NR	NR	N: 400 n with outcomes: 110 (27.5)	NR	N: 473 n with outcomes: 165 (35.2)	No.
Baker,2003[26]	Environmental control practice recommendations	Arm A- Guidelines only	patients have been advised to avoid passive smoking	NR	NR	NR	N: 428 n with outcomes: 97 (22.7)	NR	N: 490 n with outcomes: 105 (21.4)	No.
Baker,2003[26]	Environmental control practice recommendations	Arm B- Guidelines with audit criteria	patients have been advised to avoid passive smoking	NR	NR	NR	N: 451 n with outcomes: 76 (16.8)	NR	N: 480 n with outcomes: 82 (17.1)	No.
Baker,2003[26]	Environmental control practice recommendations	Arm C- Guidelines with audit criteria and feedback	patients have been advised to avoid passive smoking	NR	NR	NR	N: 400 n with outcomes: 73 (18.2)	NR	N: 473 n with outcomes: 95 (20.1)	No.
Baker,2003[26]	Prescriptions for controller medicine	Arm A- Guidelines only	In patients using beta-2 agonists, compliance has been checked	NR	NR	NR	N: 347 n with outcomes: 285 n with events: 285 (82.1)	N: 396 n with outcomes: 324 n with events: 324 (81.8)	NR	No.
Baker,2003[26]	Prescriptions for	Arm B- Guidelines	In patients using beta-2	NR	NR	NR	N: 386 n with	N: 403 n with	NR	No.

Author, Year	Health Care Process Outcomes	Arm	Definition of Scale	Range of Scale	Were outcomes measured over a period of at least 12 months?	Is there enough information to determine seasonality?	Measurement at Baseline n (%) mean SD	Measurement at end of treatment n (%) mean SD	Measurement at last follow-up n (%) mean SD	Were outcomes adjusted?
	controller medicine	with audit criteria	agonists compliance has been checked				outcomes: 335 n with events: 335 (86.8)	outcomes: 328 n with events: 328 (81.4)		
Baker,2003[26]	Prescriptions for controller medicine	Arm C- Guidelines with audit criteria and feedback	In patients using beta-2 agonists compliance has been checked	NR	NR	NR	N: 349 n with outcomes: 300 n with events: 300 (86)	N: 405 n with outcomes: 345 n with events: 345 (85.2)	NR	No.
Baker,2003[26]	Prescriptions for controller medicine	Arm A- Guidelines only	patients have been treated with cheapest inhaled steroid (beclomethas one)	NR	NR	NR	N: 301 n with outcomes: 134 (44.5)	NR	N: 334 n with outcomes: 149 (44.6)	No.
Baker,2003[26]	Prescriptions for controller medicine	Arm B- Guidelines with audit criteria	patients have been treated with cheapest inhaled steroid (beclomethas one)	NR	NR	NR	N: 334 n with outcomes: 117 (35)	NR	N: 353 n with outcomes: 163 (46.2)	No.
Baker,2003[26]	Prescriptions for controller medicine	Arm C- Guidelines with audit criteria and feedback	patients have been treated with cheapest inhaled steroid (beclomethas one)	NR	NR	NR	N: 298 n with outcomes: 128 (43)	NR	N: 358 n with outcomes: 211 (58.9)	No.
Baker,2003[26]	Self-management education	Arm A- Guidelines only	patient's inhaler technique has been checked and recorded	NR	NR	NR	N: 412 n with outcomes: 53 (12.9)	NR	N: 488 n with outcomes: 66 (13.5)	No.
Baker,2003	Self-	Arm B-	patient's	NR	NR	NR	N: 442	NR	N: 479	No.

Author, Year	Health Care Process Outcomes	Arm	Definition of Scale	Range of Scale	Were outcomes measured over a period of at least 12 months?	Is there enough information to determine seasonality?	Measurement at Baseline n (%) mean SD	Measurement at end of treatment n (%) mean SD	Measurement at last follow-up n (%) mean SD	Were outcomes adjusted?
3[26]	management education	Guidelines with audit criteria	inhaler technique has been checked and recorded				n with outcomes: 61 (13.8)		n with outcomes: 54 (11.3)	
Baker,2003[26]	Self-management education	Arm C-Guidelines with audit criteria and feedback	patient's inhaler technique has been checked and recorded	NR	NR	NR	N: 385 n with outcomes: 93 (24.2)	NR	N: 471 n with outcomes: 97 (20.6)	No.
Bell,2009[8]	Prescriptions for controller medicine	Arm A-Control UP	Controller medication prescribed (Patients with persistent asthma)	NR	NR	NR	NR	NR	N: 1193 n with outcomes: 947 (79)	No.
Bell,2009[8]	Prescriptions for controller medicine	Arm A-UP Control	Controller medication prescribed	NR	Yes	The education period was from October 13, 2006, to April 15, 2007, and the intervention 2 (follow up) period was from October 16, 2007, to April 15, 2008.	N: 1193 n with outcomes: 947 (79)	N 1328 n with outcomes: 1068 (80)	NR	No.
Bell,2009[8]	Prescriptions for controller medicine	Arm B-UP Intervention	Controller medication prescribed	NR	Yes	The education period was from October 13, 2006, to April 15, 2007, and the intervention 2 (follow up) period was	N: 1123 n with outcomes: 798 (71)	NR	N: 1205 n with outcomes: 943 (78)	No.

Author, Year	Health Care Process Outcomes	Arm	Definition of Scale	Range of Scale	Were outcomes measured over a period of at least 12 months?	Is there enough information to determine seasonality?	Measurement at Baseline n (%) mean SD	Measurement at end of treatment n (%) mean SD	Measurement at last follow-up n (%) mean SD	Were outcomes adjusted?
						from October 16, 2007, to April 15, 2008.				
Bell,2009[8]	Prescriptions for controller medicine	Arm B-UP intervention	Controller medication prescribed	NR	NR	NR	N: 1123 n with outcomes: 798 (71)	N: 1205 n with outcomes: 943 (78)	NR	No.
Bell,2009[8]	Prescriptions for controller medicine	Arm C-	Controller medication prescribed	NR	Yes	The education period was from October 13, 2006, to April 15, 2007, and the intervention 2 (follow up) period was from October 16, 2007, to April 15, 2008.	N: 347 n with outcomes: 168 (48)	NR	N: 409 n with outcomes: 209 (51)	No.
Bell,2009[8]	Prescriptions for controller medicine	Arm C-SP Control	Controller medication prescribed	NR	NR	NR	N: 347 n with outcomes: 168 (48)	N: 409 n with outcomes: 209 (51)	NR	No.
Bell,2009[8]	Prescriptions for controller medicine	Arm D-SP intervention	Controller medication prescribed	NR	Yes	The education period was from October 13, 2006, to April 15, 2007, and the intervention 2 (follow up) period was from October 16, 2007, to April 15, 2008.	N: 782 n with outcomes: 527 (67)	NR	N: 926 n with outcomes: 682 (74)	No.
Bell,2009[8]	Prescriptions for	Arm D-SP Intervention	Controller medication	NR	NR	NR	N: 782 n with	N: 926 n with	NR	No.

Author, Year	Health Care Process Outcomes	Arm	Definition of Scale	Range of Scale	Were outcomes measured over a period of at least 12 months?	Is there enough information to determine seasonality?	Measurement at Baseline n (%) mean SD	Measurement at end of treatment n (%) mean SD	Measurement at last follow-up n (%) mean SD	Were outcomes adjusted?
	controller medicine	n	prescribed				outcomes: 527 (68)	outcomes: 682 (74)		
Bender, 2011[1]	Asthma action plans	Education, coaching, and toolkit	NR	NR	NR	NR	N: (0) IQR: 10	N: (20) IQR: 47.5	NR	No.
Bender, 2011[1]	Prescriptions for controller medicine	Education, coaching, and toolkit	NR	NR	NR	NR	N: NR (25) IQR: 70	N: NR (50) IQR: 65	NR	No.
Bryce, 1995[35]	Prescription of peak flow meter	Arm A- Arm A- Control (standard practice)	Peak flow meters	NR	NR	NR	N: 1563 n with events: 12	IQR	N: 1563 n with events: 38	No.
Bryce, 1995[35]	Prescription of peak flow meter	Arm B- Reminders and tools	Peak flow meters	NR	NR	NR	N: 1585 n with events: 16	IQR	N: 1585 n with events: 101	No.
Bryce, 1995[35]	Prescriptions for controller medicine	Arm A- Arm A- Control (standard practice)	Prophylactic agents cromoglycate	NR	NR	NR	N: 1563 n with events: 99	IQR	N: 1585 n with events: 78	No.
Bryce, 1995[35]	Prescriptions for controller medicine	Arm B- Reminders and tools	Prophylactic agents cromoglycate	NR	NR	NR	N: 1585 n with events: 103	IQR	N: 1585 n with events: 123	No.
Bryce, 1995[35]	Prescriptions for controller medicine	Arm A- Arm A- Control (standard practice)	Prophylactic agents:Inhaled steroids	NR	NR	NR	N: 1563 n with events: 94	IQR	N: 1585 n with events: 150	No.
Bryce, 1995[35]	Prescriptions for controller medicine	Arm B- Reminders and tools	Prophylactic agents:Inhaled steroids	NR	NR	NR	N: 1585 n with events: 93	IQR	N: 1585 n with events: 151	No.
Bryce, 199	Prescription	Arm A-	Bronchodilato	NR	Yes	No	N: 1563	IQR	N: 1563	No.

Author, Year	Health Care Process Outcomes	Arm	Definition of Scale	Range of Scale	Were outcomes measured over a period of at least 12 months?	Is there enough information to determine seasonality?	Measurement at Baseline n (%) mean SD	Measurement at end of treatment n (%) mean SD	Measurement at last follow-up n (%) mean SD	Were outcomes adjusted?
5[35]	s for controller medicine	Arm A- Control (standard practice)	rs Inhaled				n with events: 285		n with events: 310	
Bryce, 199 5[35]	Prescriptions for controller medicine	Arm B- Reminders and tools	Bronchodilators Inhaled	NR	Yes	No	N: 1585 n with events: 297	NR	N: 1585 n with events: 386	No.
Bryce, 199 5[35]	Prescriptions for controller medicine	Arm A- Control (standard practice)	Bronchodilators Oral	NR	NR	NR	N: 1563 n with events: 239	NR	N: 1585 n with events: 108	No.
Bryce, 199 5[35]	Prescriptions for controller medicine	Arm B- Reminders and tools	Bronchodilators Oral	NR	NR	NR	N: 1585 with events: 256	NR	N: 1585 with events: 166	No.
Cho, 2010[3][9]	Prescriptions for controller medicine	Decision Support	NR	NR	No	NR	N: 100 (39)	N: 96 (73)	NR	No.
Clark, 200 2[2]	Asthma action plans	Arm A-	NR	NR	NR	NR	NR	(16)	NR	No.
Clark, 200 2[2]	Asthma action plans	Arm B- Education	NR	NR	NR	NR	NR	(26)	NR	No.
Clark, 200 2[2]	Follow-up visits	Arm A-	Scheduled	NR	NR	NR	NR	Mean:2.25	NR	Yes. Baseline scores and group assignment
Clark, 200 2[2]	Follow-up visits	Arm A-	After an episode of symptoms	NR	NR	NR	NR	Mean:1.61	NR	No.
Clark, 200	Follow-up	Arm B-	Scheduled	NR	NR	NR	NR	Mean:1.24	NR	Yes.

Author, Year	Health Care Process Outcomes	Arm	Definition of Scale	Range of Scale	Were outcomes measured over a period of at least 12 months?	Is there enough information to determine seasonality?	Measurement at Baseline n (%) mean SD	Measurement at end of treatment n (%) mean SD	Measurement at last follow-up n (%) mean SD	Were outcomes adjusted?
2²	visits	Education								Baseline scores and group assignment
Clark,200 2²	Follow-up visits	Arm B-Education	After an episode of symptoms	NR	NR	NR	NR	Mean:0.94	NR	No.
Clark,200 2²	Prescriptions for controller medicine	Arm A-	NR	NR	NR	NR	NR	70.3)	NR	No.
Clark,200 2²	Prescriptions for controller medicine	Arm B-Education	NR	NR	NR	NR	NR	82.7)	NR	No.
Cloutier,2 002[40]	Prescriptions for controller medicine	Mild, intermittant	no. of inhaled corticosteroid prescriptions per child per year (on claims)	NR	Yes	NR	N: NR n with outcomes: NR n with events: NR (NR) Mean:0.05	NR	N: NR n with outcomes: NR n with events: NR,(NR) Mean:0.3	No.
Cloutier,2 002[40]	Prescriptions for controller medicine	Mild, persistant	no. of inhaled corticosteroid prescriptions per child per year (on claims)	NR	Yes	NR	N: NR Mean:0.33	NR	N: NR Mean:1.15, SD:0	No.
Cloutier,2 002[40]	Prescriptions for controller medicine	Moderate	no. of inhaled corticosteroid prescriptions per child per year (on claims)	NR	Yes	NR	N: NR Mean:1.25	NR	N: NR Mean:2.46	No.
Cloutier,2 002[40]	Prescriptions for controller	Severe persistant	no. of inhaled corticosteroid prescriptions	NR	Yes	NR	N: NR Mean:1.61	NR	N: NR Mean:5.7	No.

Author, Year	Health Care Process Outcomes	Arm	Definition of Scale	Range of Scale	Were outcomes measured over a period of at least 12 months?	Is there enough information to determine seasonality?	Measurement at Baseline n (%) mean SD	Measurement at end of treatment n (%) mean SD	Measurement at last follow-up n (%) mean SD	Were outcomes adjusted?
	medicine		per child per year (on claims)							
Cloutier,2 002[40]	Prescriptions for controller medicine	Mild, intermittent	no oral steroid RXs per child per year	NR	Yes	NR	N: NR Mean:0.37	NR	N: NR Mean:0.1	No.
Cloutier,2 002[40]	Prescriptions for controller medicine	Mild, persistent	no oral steroid RXs per child per year	NR	Yes	NR	N: NR Mean:0.49	NR	N: NR Mean:0.43	No.
Cloutier,2 002[40]	Prescriptions for controller medicine	Moderate	no oral steroid RXs per child per year	NR	Yes	NR	N: NR Mean:1.07 SD:NR	NR	N: NR Mean:0.16 SD:NR	No.
Cloutier,2 002[40]	Prescriptions for controller medicine	Severe, persistent	no oral steroid RXs per child per year	NR	Yes	NR	N: NR Mean:2.06	NR	N: NR Mean:0 SD:NR	No.
Cloutier,2 002[40]	Prescriptions for controller medicine	Mild, intermittent	Prescriptions of nonsteroidal inhaled anti-inflammatory Rxs per child per year	NR	Yes	NR	N: NR Mean:0.14	NR	N: NR Mean:0.13	No.
Cloutier,2 002[40]	Prescriptions for controller medicine	Mild, persistent	Prescriptions of nonsteroidal inhaled anti-inflammatory Rxs per child per year	NR	Yes	NR	N: NR Mean:0.49	NR	N: NR Mean:0.43	No.
Cloutier,2 002[40]	Prescriptions for controller medicine	Moderate, persistent	Prescriptions of nonsteroidal inhaled anti-	NR	Yes	NR	N: NR Mean:1.07	NR	N: NR Mean:0.16	No.

Author, Year	Health Care Process Outcomes	Arm	Definition of Scale	Range of Scale	Were outcomes measured over a period of at least 12 months?	Is there enough information to determine seasonality?	Measurement at Baseline n (%) mean SD	Measurement at end of treatment n (%) mean SD	Measurement at last follow-up n (%) mean SD	Were outcomes adjusted?
			inflammatory Rxs per child per year							
Cloutier, 2002[40]	Prescriptions for controller medicine	Severe, persistent	Prescriptions of nonsteroidal inhaled anti-inflammatory Rxs per child per year	NR	Yes	NR	N: NR Mean:1.72	NR	N: NR, Mean:0.5	No.
Cloutier, 2009[41]	Prescriptions for controller medicine	Decision support	NR	NR	Yes	NR	280.8 per 100 children	NR	272.8 per 100 children	Yes. Controlled for asthma severity, sex, linic, chronological time, and race/ethnicity.
Cloutier, 2009[41] ii	Prescriptions for controller medicine	Decision support	NR	NR	Yes	NR	32.1 per 100 children	NR	10.8 per 100 children	Yes. Controlled for asthma severity, sex, linic, chronological time, and race/ethnicity.
Cloutier, 2009[41] ii	Prescriptions for controller medicine	Decision support	NR	NR	NR	NR	120.5 per 100 children	NR	128.1 per 100 children	Yes. Controlled for asthma severity, sex, linic, chronological time,

Author, Year	Health Care Process Outcomes	Arm	Definition of Scale	Range of Scale	Were outcomes measured over a period of at least 12 months?	Is there enough information to determine seasonality?	Measurement at Baseline n (%) mean SD	Measurement at end of treatment n (%) mean SD	Measurement at last follow-up n (%) mean SD	Were outcomes adjusted?
										and race/ethnicity.
Cloutier,2 009[41] ii	Prescription s for controller medicine	Decision support	NR	NR	Yes	NR	280.8 per 100 children	NR	272.8 per 100 children	Yes. Controlled for asthma severity, sex, linic, chronological time, and race/ethnicity.
Cloutier,2 009[41] ii	Prescription s for controller medicine	Decision support	NR	NR	Yes	NR	78.4 per 100 children	NR	123.6 per 100 children	Yes. Controlled for asthma severity, sex, linic, chronological time, and race/ethnicity.
Cloutier,2 009[41] ii	Prescription s for controller medicine	Decision support	NR	NR	Yes	NR	32.1 per 100 children	NR	10.8 per 100 children	Yes. Controlled for asthma severity, sex, linic, chronological time, and race/ethnicity.
Cloutier,2 009[41] ii	Prescription s for controller medicine	Decision support	NR	NR	NR	NR	120.5 per 100 children	NR	128.1 per 100 children	Yes. Controlled for asthma severity,

Author, Year	Health Care Process Outcomes	Arm	Definition of Scale	Range of Scale	Were outcomes measured over a period of at least 12 months?	Is there enough information to determine seasonality?	Measurement at Baseline n (%) mean SD	Measurement at end of treatment n (%) mean SD	Measurement at last follow-up n (%) mean SD	Were outcomes adjusted?
										sex, linic, chronologi cal time, and race/ethni city.
Cloutier,2 009[41 ii]	Prescription s for controller medicine	Decision support	NR	NR	Yes	NR	44.0 per 100 children	NR	30.4 per 100 children	Yes. Controlled for asthma severity, sex, linic, chronologi cal time, and race/ethni city.
Cloutier,2 009[41 ii]	Prescription s for controller medicine	Decision support	NR	NR	Yes	NR	44.0 per 100 children	NR	30.4 per 100 children	Yes. Controlled for asthma severity, sex, linic, chronologi cal time, and race/ethni city.
Cloutier,2 009[41 ii]	Prescription s for controller medicine	Decision support	NR	NR	Yes	NR	78.4 per 100 children	NR	123.6 per 100 children	Yes. Controlled for asthma severity, sex, linic, chronologi cal time, and race/ethni city.
Coleman,	Prescription	Arm A-	Claim	NR	NR	NR	N: 510	NR	N: 510	No.

Author, Year	Health Care Process Outcomes	Arm	Definition of Scale	Range of Scale	Were outcomes measured over a period of at least 12 months?	Is there enough information to determine seasonality?	Measurement at Baseline n (%) mean SD	Measurement at end of treatment n (%) mean SD	Measurement at last follow-up n (%) mean SD	Were outcomes adjusted?
2003[36]	of peak flow meter	Comparison	submitted				n with outcomes: 510 n with events: 4 (1)		n with outcomes: 510 n with events: 11 (2)	
Coleman, 2003[36]	Prescription of peak flow meter	Arm B-Intervention	Claim submitted	NR	NR	NR	N: 135 n with outcomes: 135 n with events: 0 (0)	NR	N: 135 n with outcomes: 135 n with events: 0 (0)	No.
Cowie, 2001[42]	Prescriptions for controller medicine	Arm A: Basic Education	"using inhaled steroid"	Yes/No	Yes	NR	NR	N: NR n with outcomes: 174 n with events: NR (55)	NR	No.
Cowie, 2001[42]	Prescriptions for controller medicine	Arm B: Intermediate Education	"using inhaled steroid"	Yes/No	Yes	NR	NR	N: NR n with outcomes: 55 n with events: NR (67)	NR	No.
Cowie, 2001[42]	Prescriptions for controller medicine	Arm C: Intensive Education	"using inhaled steroid"	Yes/No	Yes	NR	NR	N: NR n with outcomes: 98 n with events: NR (72)	NR	No.
Daniels, 2005[3]	Asthma action plans	Arm A-Control	% of chart reviews	0-100%	NR	NR	N: 136079 (32.6)	NR	(23.3)	No.
Daniels, 2005[3]	Asthma action plans	Arm B-Education	% of chart reviews	0-100%	NR	NR	N: 90555 (18.7)	NR	N: NR (25.7)	No.
Daniels, 2005[3]	Self-management education	Arm A-Control	% of chart reviews	0-100%	NR	NR	N: 136079	NR	NR	No.
Davis, 2004[43]	Prescriptions for controller	Arm A-Cotrol (guideline	ICS prescriptions/month	NR	No	No	N: 34 Mean:2.64	N: 34 Mean:3.28	NR	No.

Author, Year	Health Care Process Outcomes	Arm	Definition of Scale	Range of Scale	Were outcomes measured over a period of at least 12 months?	Is there enough information to determine seasonality?	Measurement at Baseline n (%) mean SD	Measurement at end of treatment n (%) mean SD	Measurement at last follow-up n (%) mean SD	Were outcomes adjusted?
	medicine	s only)								
Davis, 2004[43]	Prescriptions for controller medicine	Arm B-Education and toolkit	ICS prescriptions/ month	NR	No	No	N: 20 Mean:2.54 Range: 0-9.5	N: 20 Mean:7.76 Range:2.83-12.33	NR	No.
Davis, 2010[20]	Documentation of level of asthma control/severity	Decision Support	NR	NR	Yes	No	N: 180 n with outcomes: 43 (24)	N: 180 n with outcomes: 79 (44)	NR	No.
Davis, 2010[20]	Prescriptions for controller medicine	Decision support	ICS	NR	NR	NR	N: 180 n with outcomes: 71 (39.4)	N: 180 n with outcomes: 92 (51.1)	NR	No.
de Vries, 1995[44]	Prescriptions for controller medicine	Arm A-Reference 2007	Proportion with no inhaled corticosteroid (ICS) Rx while on long-acting betamimetics.	0-100%	Yes	NR	NR	NR	N: 477 n with outcomes: 41 n with events: NR (8.6)	No.
de Vries, 1995[44]	Prescriptions for controller medicine	Arm B-Intervention 2007	Proportion with no inhaled corticosteroid (ICS) Rx while on long-acting betamimetics.	0-100%	Yes	NR	NR	NR	N: 219 n with outcomes: 6 n with events: NR (2.7)	No.
de Vries, 1995[44]	Prescriptions for controller medicine	Arm A-Reference 2007	Proportion with more than one type of inhaler (failure to adhere to guidelines)	0-100%	NR	NR	NR	NR	N: 2311 n with outcomes: 119 n with events: NR (5.1)	No.

Author, Year	Health Care Process Outcomes	Arm	Definition of Scale	Range of Scale	Were outcomes measured over a period of at least 12 months?	Is there enough information to determine seasonality?	Measurement at Baseline n (%) mean SD	Measurement at end of treatment n (%) mean SD	Measurement at last follow-up n (%) mean SD	Were outcomes adjusted?
de Vries, 1995 [44]	Prescriptions for controller medicine	Arm B- Intervention 2007	Proportion with more than one type of inhaler (failure to adhere to guidelines)	0-100%	NR	NR	NR	NR	N: 849 n with outcomes: 43 n with events: NR (5.1)	No.
de Vries, 1995 [44]	Prescriptions for controller medicine	Arm C-2002	Proportion with more than one type of inhaler (failure to adhere to guidelines)	0-100%	NR	NR	NR	NR	N: 3217 n with outcomes: 239 n with events: NR (7.4)	No.
de Vries, 1995 [44]	Prescriptions for controller medicine	Arm A- Reference 2007	Proportion having no short-acting betamimetics Rx	0-100%	NR	NR	NR	NR	N: 3527 n with outcomes: 534 n with events: NR (15.4)	No.
de Vries, 1995 [44]	Prescriptions for controller medicine	Arm B- Intervention 2007	Proportion having no short-acting betamimetics Rx	0-100%	NR	NR	NR	NR	N: 1447 n with outcomes: 176 n with events: NR (12.1)	No.
de Vries, 1995 [44]	Prescriptions for controller medicine	Arm C-2002	Proportion having no short-acting betamimetics Rx	0-100%	NR	NR	NR	NR	N: 3612 n with outcomes: 559 n with events: NR (15.5)	No.
Eccles, 2002 [27]	Environmental control practice recommendations	Arm A- Angina	n(%) with known smoking status	%:0-100	Yes	NR	N: NR n with outcomes: 1163 n with events: 305 (26)	N: NR n with outcomes: 1163 n with events: 367 (32)	NR	No.
Eccles, 2002 [27]	Environmental control practice	Arm A- Angina	n (%) of patients with documented	%:0-100	Yes	NR	N: NR n with outcomes: 1163	N: NR n with outcomes: 1163	NR	No.

Author, Year	Health Care Process Outcomes	Arm	Definition of Scale	Range of Scale	Were outcomes measured over a period of at least 12 months?	Is there enough information to determine seasonality?	Measurement at Baseline n (%) mean SD	Measurement at end of treatment n (%) mean SD	Measurement at last follow-up n (%) mean SD	Were outcomes adjusted?
	recommend ations		smoking cessation advice or nicotine replacement therapy				n with events: 68 (6)	n with events: 103 (9)		
Eccles,20 02[27]	Environme ntal control practice recommend ations	Arm B-Asthma	n (%) of patients with documented smoking cessation advice or nicotine replacement therapy	%:0-100	Yes	NR	N: NR n with outcomes: 1129 n with events: 57 (5)	N: NR n with outcomes: 1129 n with events: 81 (7)	NR	No.
Eccles,20 02[27]	Environme ntal control practice recommend ations	Arm A-Angina	n (%) with known smoking status	%:0-100	Yes	NR	N: NR n with outcomes: 1163 n with events: 305 (26)	N: NR n with outcomes: 1163 n with events: 367 (32)	NR	No.
Eccles,20 02[27]	Environme ntal control practice recommend ations	Arm B-Asthma	n(%) with known smoking status	%:0-100	Yes	NR	N: NR n with outcomes: 1200 n with events: 285 (24)	N: NR n with outcomes: 1200 n with events: 370 (32)	NR	No.
Eccles,20 02[27]	Prescription s for controller medicine	Arm A-Angina	n (%) of patients prescribed long acting beta 2 agonists	%:0-100	Yes	NR	N: NR n with outcomes: 1385 n with events: 164 (12)	N: NR n with outcomes: 1385 n with events: 183 (13)	NR	No.
Eccles,20 02[27]	Prescription s for controller medicine	Arm B-Asthma	n (%) of patients prescribed long acting beta 2 agonists	%:0-100	Yes	NR	N: NR n with outcomes: 1391 n with events: 181 (13)	N: NR n with outcomes: 1391 n with events: 198 (14)	NR	No.

E-135

Author, Year	Health Care Process Outcomes	Arm	Definition of Scale	Range of Scale	Were outcomes measured over a period of at least 12 months?	Is there enough information to determine seasonality?	Measurement at Baseline n (%) mean SD	Measurement at end of treatment n (%) mean SD	Measurement at last follow-up n (%) mean SD	Were outcomes adjusted?
Eccles, 2002[27]	Prescriptions for controller medicine	Arm A- Angina	number (%) of patients prescribed inhaled corticosteroids	%:0-100	Yes	NR	N: NR n with outcomes: 1385 n with events: 1004 (73)	N: NR n with outcomes: 1385 n with events: 975 (70)	NR	No.
Eccles, 2002[27]	Prescriptions for controller medicine	Arm B- Asthma	number (%) of patients prescribed inhaled corticosteroids	%:0-100	Yes	NR	N: NR n with outcomes: 1391 n with events: 1065 (77)	N: NR n with outcomes: 1391 n with events: 1001 (72)	NR	No.
Eccles, 2002[27]	Self-management education	Arm A- Angina	n(%) who received asthma education, action plan, or both	%:0-100	Yes	NR	N: NR n with outcomes: 1163 n with events: 108 (9)	N: NR n with outcomes: 1163 n with events: 78 (7)	NR	No.
Eccles, 2002[27]	Self-management education	Arm B- Asthma	n(%) who received asthma education, action plan, or both	%:0-100	Yes	NR	N: NR n with outcomes: 1200 n with events: 79 (7)	N: NR n with outcomes: 1200 n with events: 60 (5)	NR	No.
Fairall, 2010[28]	Environmental control practice recommendations	Arm A- Control (standard practice)	patients receiving counseling on smoking cessation, among those self-identified as current smokers	0-100%	No	No	N: 193	NR	n with outcomes: 127 (65.8)	No.
Fairall, 2010[28]	Environmental control practice recommend	Arm B- Decision support outreach	patients receiving counseling on smoking	0-100%	No	No	N: 164	NR	n with outcomes: 112 (65.8)	No.

Author, Year	Health Care Process Outcomes	Arm	Definition of Scale	Range of Scale	Were outcomes measured over a period of at least 12 months?	Is there enough information to determine seasonality?	Measurement at Baseline n (%) mean SD	Measurement at end of treatment r (%) mean SD	Measurement at last follow-up n (%) mean SD	Were outcomes adjusted?
	ations	group	cessation, among those self-identified as current smokers							
Fairall,2010[28]	Prescriptions for controller medicine	Arm A- Control (standard practice)	Mean use of health care resources (inhaled corticosteroids [No. units])	NR	No	No	NR	NR	N: 926 Mean:0.08	No.
Fairall,2010[28]	Prescriptions for controller medicine	Arm B- Decision support outreach group	Mean use of health care resources (Beta-agonists [No. units])	NR	No	No	N: 1000	NR	N: 930	No.
Fairall,2010[28]	Prescriptions for controller medicine	Arm A- control (standard practice)	prescriptions for inhaled corticosteroids filled among patients in each study arm during the study period	0-100%	No	NR	N: NR	NR	N: 926 n with outcomes: 77 (7.7)	No.
Fairall,2010[28]	Prescriptions for controller medicine	Arm B- Decision support outreach group	prescriptions for inhaled corticosteroids filled among patients in each study arm during the study period	0-100%	No	NR	N: 1000	NR	N: 930 n with events: 137 (13.7)	No.
Feder,1995[32]	Follow-up visits	Arm A- Diabetes	Consultation rates for	NR	Yes	NR	Mean:1.2	Mean:1.4	NR	No.

Author, Year	Health Care Process Outcomes	Arm	Definition of Scale	Range of Scale	Were outcomes measured over a period of at least 12 months?	Is there enough information to determine seasonality?	Measurement at Baseline n (%) mean SD	Measurement at end of treatment n (%) mean SD	Measurement at last follow-up n (%) mean SD	Were outcomes adjusted?
		education	asthma: per patient per year							
Feder, 1995[32]	Follow-up visits	Arm B-Education, reminders, and audit	Consultation rates for asthma: per patient per year	NR	Yes	NR	Mean:1	Mean:1.5	NR	No.
Finkelstein, 2005[33ii]	Follow-up visits	Arm A-Control (standard practice)	Mean	NR	Yes	NR	N: 1531 Mean:2 0.44	NR	NR	No.
Finkelstein, 2005[33i]	Follow-up visits	Arm B-PLE Intervention	Mean	NR	Yes	NR	N: 2003 Mean:1.75 SD:0.45	NR	NR	No.
Finkelstein, 2005[33i]	Follow-up visits	Arm C-Planned Care Intervention	Mean	NR	Yes	NR	N: 1635 Mean:1.79 SD:0.21	NR	NR	No.
Finkelstein, 2005[33i]	Prescriptions for controller medicine	Arm A-Control (standard practice)	Mean	NR	Yes	NR	N: 1531 Mean:0.76 SD:0.14	NR	NR	No.
Finkelstein, 2005[33i]	Prescriptions for controller medicine	Arm A-Control (standard practice)	Mean	NR	Yes	NR	N: 1531 Mean:0.43 SD:0.15	NR	NR	No.
Finkelstein, 2005[33i]	Prescriptions for controller medicine	Arm A-Control (standard practice)	Mean	NR	Yes	NR	N: 1531 Mean:0.31 SD:0.04	NR	NR	No.
Finkelstein, 2005[33i]	Prescriptions for controller medicine	Arm B-PLE Intervention	Mean	NR	Yes	NR	N: 2003 Mean:0.68 SD:0.15	NR	NR	No.

Author, Year	Health Care Process Outcomes	Arm	Definition of Scale	Range of Scale	Were outcomes measured over a period of at least 12 months?	Is there enough information to determine seasonality?	Measurement at Baseline n (%) mean SD	Measurement at end of treatment n (%) mean SD	Measurement at last follow-up n (%) mean SD	Were outcomes adjusted?
Finkelstein ,2005[33i]	Prescription s for controller medicine	Arm B-PLE Interventio n	Mean	NR	Yes	NR	N: 2003 Mean:0.39 SD:0.12	NR	NR	No.
Finkelstein ,2005[33i]	Prescription s for controller medicine	Arm B-PLE Interventio n	Mean	NR	Yes	NR	N: 2003 Mean:0.33 SD:0.1	NR	NR	No.
Finkelstein ,2005[33i]	Prescription s for controller medicine	Arm C-Planned Care Interventio n	Mean	NR	Yes	NR	N: 1635 Mean:0.77 SD:0.13	NR	NR	No.
Finkelstein ,2005[33i]	Prescription s for controller medicine	Arm C-Planned Care Interventio n	Mean	NR	Yes	NR	N: 1635 Mean:0.44 SD:0.13	NR	NR	No.
Finkelstein ,2005[33i]	Prescription s for controller medicine	Arm C-Planned Care Interventio n	Mean	NR	Yes	NR	N: 1635 Mean:0.26 SD:0.07	NR	NR	No.
Fox, 2007[21]	Asthma action plans	Quality improvem ent	Documentatio n at the last visit that a written action plan was created or existing plan updated or reviewed.	0-100	Yes	NR	N: 280, (15.0)	N: 280, (43.2)	NR	No.
Fox,2007[2] [1]	Documenta tion of level of asthma control/sev erity	Quality Improvem ent	Documentatio n at the last visit of severity classification.	0-100	Yes	No	N: 280 (37.1)	N: 280 (69.3)	NR	No.

E-139

Author, Year	Health Care Process Outcomes	Arm	Definition of Scale	Range of Scale	Were outcomes measured over a period of at least 12 months?	Is there enough information to determine seasonality?	Measurement at Baseline n (%) mean SD	Measurement at end of treatment n (%) mean SD	Measurement at last follow-up n (%) mean SD	Were outcomes adjusted?
Frankowski,2006[4]	Asthma action plans	Arm B- Multicomponent: Education and feedback	NR	NR	NR	NR	N: 150 n with outcomes: 34 (22.7)	N: 150 n with outcomes: 100 (66.7)	NR	No.
Glasgow,2003[5]	Asthma action plans	Arm A- Control	Have a written asthma action plan	NR	Yes	No	N: 73 n with outcomes: 20 (28)	NR	N: 71 n with outcomes: 24 (34)	No.
Glasgow,2003[5]	Asthma action plans	Arm B- Decision support	Have a written asthma action plan	NR	Yes	No	N: 101 n with outcomes: 23 (23)	NR	N: 95 n with outcomes: 42 (44)	No.
Glasgow,2003[5]	Prescriptions for controller medicine	Arm A- Control	Uses nebuliser	NR	NR	NR	N: 73 n with outcomes: 29 (40)	NR	N: 71, n with outcomes: 24,(34)	No.
Glasgow,2003[5]	Prescriptions for controller medicine	Arm B- Decision support	Uses nebuliser	NR	NR	NR	N: 101 n with outcomes: 36 (36)	NR	N: 95, n with outcomes: 20,(21)	No.
Gorton,1995[37]	Prescription of peak flow meter	Arm A- Control comparison site	NR	NR	NR	NR	NR	NR	Mean: 0.05 SD:1.08	No.
Gorton,1995[37]	Prescription of peak flow meter	Arm B- Site A	NR	NR	NR	NR	NR	NR	Mean:0.73 SD:1.22	No.
Gorton,1995[37]	Prescription of peak flow meter	Arm C-	NR	NR	NR	NR	NR	NR	Mean:0.88 SD:1.02	No.
Hagmolen,2008[45]	Prescriptions for controller medicine	Arm A- guideline	Prescribed regular ICS treatment with mean ≥ 1 puff per day	0-100	Yes	NR	N: 114 n with events: NR (11)	NR	N: 98, n with events: NR,(9)	Yes. Baseline adjusted

Author, Year	Health Care Process Outcomes	Arm	Definition of Scale	Range of Scale	Were outcomes measured over a period of at least 12 months?	Is there enough information to determine seasonality?	Measurement at Baseline n (%) mean SD	Measurement at end of treatment n (%) mean SD	Measurement at last follow-up n (%) mean SD	Were outcomes adjusted?
Hagmolen, 2008[45]	Prescriptions for controller medicine	Arm B- guideline extract plus education	Prescribed regular ICS treament with mean > 1 puff per day	0-100	Yes	NR	N: 143 n with events: NR (11)	NR	N: 133 n with events: NR (13)	Yes. Baseline adjusted
Hagmolen, 2008[45]	Prescriptions for controller medicine	Arm C-	Prescribed regular ICS treament with mean > 1 puff per day	0-100	Yes	NR	N: 147 n with events: NR (16)	NR	N: 131 n with events: NR (25)	Yes. Baseline adjusted
Halterman, 2005[46]	Prescriptions for controller medicine	Arm A- Control (standard practice)	NR	NR	No	No	N: 77	NR	N: 77 n with outcomes: 20 n with events: NR (26)	No.
Halterman, 2005[46]	Prescriptions for controller medicine	Arm B- Decision support	NR	NR	No	No	N: 73	NR	N: 73 n with outcomes: 16 n with events: NR (21.9)	No.
Halterman, 2006[6]	Asthma action plans	Arm A- Control (standard practice)	NR	NR	Unable to determine	NR	N: 124	NR	N: 114 n with outcomes: 27 n with events: (23.7)	No.
Halterman, 2006[6]	Asthma action plans	Arm B- Decision support	NR	NR	Unable to determine	NR	N: 122	NR	N: 112 n with outcomes: 56 n with events: (50)	No.
Halterman, 2006[6]	Prescriptions for controller medicine	Arm A- Control (standard practice)	NR	NR	NR	NR	N: 124	NR	N: 114 n with outcomes: 38 n with events: NR (33.3)	No.
Halterman, 2006[6]	Prescriptions for	Arm B- Decision	NR	NR	NR	NR	N: 122	NR	N: 112 n with	No.

Author, Year	Health Care Process Outcomes	Arm	Definition of Scale	Range of Scale	Were outcomes measured over a period of at least 12 months?	Is there enough information to determine seasonality?	Measurement at Baseline n (%) mean SD	Measurement at end of treatment n (%) mean SD	Measurement at last follow-up n (%) mean SD	Were outcomes adjusted?
	controller medicine	support	controller medicine						outcomes: 46 n with events: NR (41.1)	
Herborg,2001[47iii]	Prescriptions for controller medicine	Arm A-control (standard practice)	proportion of patients using short acting beta agonists who were prescribed ICS	0-100	Yes	NR	N: NR n with outcomes: NR (68)	N: NR n with outcomes: NR (70.4)	NR	No.
Herborg,2001[47iii]	Prescriptions for controller medicine	Arm B-TOM	proportion of patients using short acting beta agonists who were prescribed ICS	0-100	Yes	NR	N: NR n with outcomes: NR n with events: NR (68)	N: NR n with outcomes: NR n with events: NR (84.3)	NR	No.
Homer,2005[7]	Asthma action plans	Arm A-Control (standard practice)	NR	NR	NR	NR	N: 337 (37)	N: 254 (41)	NR	No.
Homer,2005[7]	Asthma action plans	Arm B-Learning collaborative	NR	NR	NR	NR	N: 294 (53)	N: 236 (54)	NR	No.
Horswell,2008[8]	Asthma action plans	HCSD's DM program	Proportion of clinic visitors in past ? months with current action plan	0-100%	NR	NR	(60)	NR	N: 2199 (84)	No.
Horswell,2008[8]	Documentation of level of asthma control/severity	HCSD's DM program	% of clinic visitors in past 3 months with current severity assessment	0-100%	NR	NR	N: NR (71)	NR	N: 2199 (89)	No.

Author, Year	Health Care Process Outcomes	Arm	Definition of Scale	Range of Scale	Were outcomes measured over a period of at least 12 months?	Is there enough information to determine seasonality?	Measurement at Baseline n (%) mean SD	Measurement at end of treatment n (%) mean SD	Measurement at last follow-up n (%) mean SD	Were outcomes adjusted?
Horswell,2008[8]	Prescriptions for controller medicine	Arm B-HCSD's DM program intervention	Proportion of patients on a corticosteroid.	0-100%	NR	NR	(73)	NR	N: 2199 (81)	No.
Horswell,2008[8]	Prescriptions for controller medicine	Arm B-HCSD's DM program intervention	% of patients on a beta agonist	0-100%	NR	NR	(79)	NR	N: 2199 (92)	No.
Hoskins,1997[48]	Prescriptions for controller medicine	Arm A- Step up in preventive care	Step up in preventive care	NR	NR	NR	N: 782 n with outcomes: 782, n with events: 402 (51)	N: 669 n with outcomes: 669 n with events: 382 (57)	NR	No.
Hoskins,1997[48]	Prescriptions for controller medicine	Arm A- Systemic steroids	Use of systemic steroids for acute attack	Yes or No	NR	NR	N: 782 n with outcomes: 782 n with events: 563 (72)	N: 669 n with outcomes: 669 n with events: 506 (76)	NR	No.
Hoskins,1997[48]	Prescriptions for controller medicine	Arm B- Education and feedback	Use of systemic steroids for acute attack	Yes or No	NR	NR	NR	NR	NR	No.
Kattan,2006[34]	Follow-up visits	Arm A- Control (standard practice)	# of visits per year	NR	NR	NR	N: 466 Mean:5.5	NR	N: 463 Mean:1.31 SE: 0.08	No.
Kattan,2006[34]	Follow-up visits	Arm B- Decision support, education, other guidelines	# of visits per year	NR	NR	NR	N: 471 Mean:5.6	NR	N: 466 Mean:1.14 SE: 0.08	No.
Lesho,200	Prescription	Decision	NR	NR	NR	NR	N: 330	N: 334	NR	No.

Author, Year	Health Care Process Outcomes	Arm	Definition of Scale	Range of Scale	Were outcomes measured over a period of at least 12 months?	Is there enough information to determine seasonality?	Measurement at Baseline n (%) mean SD	Measurement at end of treatment n (%) mean SD	Measurement at last follow-up n (%) mean SD	Were outcomes adjusted?
5[49]	s for controller medicine	Support					(66)	(67)		
Lesho,200 5[49]	Self-management education	Decision Support	NR	NR	Unable to determine	No	N: 330 (51)	N: 334 (65)	NR	No.
Liaw,2008 [9]	Asthma action plans	Arm A-Control (Group 2)	% who report that they "usually write an Asthma Action plan." (yes/no)	0-100%	NR	NR	N: 17 n with outcomes: 10 (58.8)	NR	N: 15 n with outcomes: 13 (86.7)	No.
Liaw,2008 [9]	Asthma action plans	Arm B-Control (unrelated education: Group 3)	% who report that they "usually write an Asthma Action plan." (yes/no)	0-100%	NR	NR	N: 15 n with outcomes: 12 (80)	NR	N: 9 n with outcomes: 6 (66.7)	No.
Liaw,2008 [9]	Asthma action plans	Arm C-Education and guidelines	% who report that they "usually write an Asthma Action plan." (yes/no)	0-100%	NR	NR	N: 18 n with outcomes: 11 (6.1)	NR	N: 17 n with outcomes: 15 (88.2)	No.
Lob S. H., 2011[20]	Asthma action plan	Longitudinal Evaluation Group - Patient-level Interview Sample	Any healthcare provider reviewed written asthma action plan with the patient at the last visit	NR	Yes	No	N: 761 n with events: 307(40.3)	N: 761 n with events: 512(67.3)	N: 761 n with events: 571(75.0)	Yes. Variables included in initial models: size of the clinics' pediatric asthma population; percent of black

E-144

Author, Year	Health Care Process Outcomes	Arm	Definition of Scale	Range of Scale	Were outcomes measured over a period of at least 12 months?	Is there enough information to determine seasonality?	Measurement at Baseline n (%) mean SD	Measurement at end of treatment n (%) mean SD	Measurement at last follow-up n (%) mean SD	Were outcomes adjusted?
										patients, uninsured patients, children <5 years old, patients with moderate/ severe asthma.
Lob S. H., 2011[20]	Self-management Education	Longitudinal Evaluation Group - Patient-level Interview Sample	Provider every provided trigger educaiton	NR	Yes	No	N: 713 n with events: 376(52.7)	N: 713 n with events: 639(96.6)	N: 713 n with events: 699(98.0)	Yes. Variables included in initial models: size of the clinics' pediatric asthma population; percent of black patients, uninsured patients, children <5 years old, patients with moderate/ severe asthma.
Lundborg, 1999[50]	Prescriptions for controller	Arm A- Control (standard	Ipratropium (R03BB) prescription	NR	NR	NR	n with outcomes: 67 n with events: 2	n with outcomes: 72 n with events: 2	NR	No.

E-145

Author, Year	Health Care Process Outcomes	Arm	Definition of Scale	Range of Scale	Were outcomes measured over a period of at least 12 months?	Is there enough information to determine seasonality?	Measurement at Baseline n (%) mean SD	Measurement at end of treatment n (%) mean SD	Measurement at last follow-up n (%) mean SD	Were outcomes adjusted?
	medicine	practice)								
Lundborg, 1999[50]	Prescriptions for controller medicine	Arm B- Education and feedback	Ipratropium (R03BE prescription)	NR	NR	NR	n with outcomes: 67 n with events: 2 (NR)	N: NR n with outcomes: 81 n with events: 2.5 (NR)	NR	No.
Lundborg, 1999[50]	Prescriptions for controller medicine	Arm A- Control (standard practice)	Sodiumcromoglycate (R03BC presciptions)	NR	NR	NR	n with outcomes: 47 n with events: 1.5	n with outcomes: 58 n with events: 1	NR	No.
Lundborg, 1999[50]	Prescriptions for controller medicine	Arm B- Education and feedback	Sodiumcromoglycate (R03BC presciptions)	NR	NR	NR	n with outcomes: 45 n with events: 1	n with outcomes: 29 n with events: 1	NR	No.
Lundborg, 1999[50]	Prescriptions for controller medicine	Arm A- Control (standard practice)	Selective -2 agonists, oral (R03CC prescri-ctions)	NR	NR	NR	n with outcomes: 101 n with events: 5.5	n with outcomes: 66 n with events: 3	NR	No.
Lundborg, 1999[50]	Prescriptions for controller medicine	Arm B- Education and feedback	Selective -2 agonists oral (R03CC prescri-ctions)	NR	NR	NR	n with outcomes: 84 n with events: 4	n with outcomes: 68 n with events: 2.5	NR	No.
Lundborg, 1999[50]	Prescriptions for controller medicine	Arm A- Control (standard practice)	Xantines (R03DA prescriptions)	NR	NR	NR	n with outcomes: 45 n with events: 1	n with outcomes: 38 n with events: 2	NR	No.
Lundborg, 1999[50]	Prescriptions for controller medicine	Arm B- Education and feedback	Xantines (R03DA prescriptions)	NR	NR	NR	n with outcomes: 41 n with events: 2	n with outcomes: 22 n with events: 0	NR	No.
Lundborg, 1999[50]	Prescriptions for controller medicine	Arm A- Control (standard practice)	Glucocorticoids, oral (H02AB) prescriptions	NR	NR	NR	n with outcomes: 105 n with events: 5	n with outcomes: 89 n with events: 4.5	NR	On with events = GP group median
Lundborg, 1999[50]	Prescriptions for controller	Arm B- Education and	Glucocorticoids, oral (H02AB)	NR	NR	NR	n with outcomes: 86 n with events: 1	n with outcomes: 95 n with events:	NR	On with events = GP group

Author, Year	Health Care Process Outcomes	Arm	Definition of Scale	Range of Scale	Were outcomes measured over a period of at least 12 months?	Is there enough information to determine seasonality?	Measurement at Baseline n (%) mean SD	Measurement at end of treatment n (%) mean SD	Measurement at last follow-up n (%) mean SD	Were outcomes adjusted?
	medicine	feedback	prescriptions					3.5		median
Lundborg, 1999[50]	Prescriptions for controller medicine	Arm A-Control (standard practice)	Glucocorticoids, inhaled(R03BA) prescriptions	NR	NR	NR	n with outcomes: 1152 n with events: 51	n with outcomes: 1247 n with events: 61	NR	No.
Lundborg, 1999[50]	Prescriptions for controller medicine	Arm B-Education and feedback	Glucocorticoids, inhaled(R03BA) prescriptions	NR	NR	NR	n with outcomes: 862 n with events: 42	n with outcomes: 1002 n with events: 52	NR	No.
Lundborg, 1999[50]	Prescriptions for controller medicine	Arm A-Control (standard practice)	Antibiotics for systemic use (J01) prescriptions	NR	NR	NR	n with outcomes: 597, n with events: 26.5	n with outcomes: 390, n with events: 17	NR	0n with events = GP group median
Lundborg, 1999[50]	Prescriptions for controller medicine	Arm B-Education and feedback	Antibiotics for systemic use (J01) prescriptions	NR	NR	NR	n with outcomes: 433 n with events: 27	n with outcomes: 384 n with events: 15.5	NR	0n with events = GP group median
Lundborg, 1999[50]	Prescriptions for controller medicine	Arm A-Control (standard practice)	Selective beta-2 agonists, inhaled (R03AC) prescriptions for asthma patients	NR	NR	NR	n with outcomes: 3174 n with events: 168.5	n with outcomes: 2343 n with events: 123	NR	No.
Lundborg, 1999[50]	Prescriptions for controller medicine	Arm B-Education and feedback	Selective beta-2 agonists, inhaled (R03AC) prescriptions for asthma patients	NR	NR	NR	n with outcomes: 1809 n with events: 105.5	n with outcomes: 1830 n with events: 88.5	NR	No.
Mahi-Taright	Prescriptions for	Education	Inhaled corticosteroid	NR	Unable to determine	No	N: 49 n with	N: 151 n with	NR	No.

Author, Year	Health Care Process Outcomes	Arm	Definition of Scale	Range of Scale	Were outcomes measured over a period of at least 12 months?	Is there enough information to determine seasonality?	Measurement at Baseline n (%) mean SD	Measurement at end of treatment n (%) mean SD	Measurement at last follow-up n (%) mean SD	Were outcomes adjusted?
,2003[51]	controller medicine		s				outcomes: 0 (0)	outcomes: 18 (11.9)		
Mangione-Smith,2005[10]	Asthma action plans	Arm A-control	All patients should have a written action plan in the medical record that is based on changes in symptoms or peak flow measurements	NR	NR	NR	N: 126	NR	N: 126,(22)	No.
Mangione-Smith,2005[10]	Asthma action plans	Arm B-intervention	All patients should have a written action plan in the medical record that is based on changes in symptoms or peak flow measurements	NR	NR	NR	N: 385	NR	N: 385,(41)	No.
Martens,2006[52]	Prescriptions for controller medicine	Arm A-control (standard practice)	Inhaled corticosteroids	NR	NR	NR	N: 54 Mean:19 CI:13,28	N: 54 Mean:21 CI:13,33	N: 54 Mean:18 CI:11,26	No.
Martens,2006[52]	Prescriptions for controller medicine	Arm B-Guidelines and involved in development	Inhaled corticosteroids	NR	NR	NR	N: 53 Mean:21 CI: 14,33	N: 53 Mean:19 CI:10,28	N: 53 Mean:14 CI:9,23	No.
Martens,2006[52]	Prescriptions for controller medicine	Arm C-Guidelines only	Inhaled corticosteroids	NR	NR	NR	N: 26 Mean:24 CI:13,28	N: 26 Mean:21 CI:12,33	N: 26 Mean:19 CI:13,28	No.
Martens,2	Prescription	Arm D-	Inhaled	NR	NR	NR	N: 27	N: 27	N: 27	No.

Author, Year	Health Care Process Outcomes	Arm	Definition of Scale	Range of Scale	Were outcomes measured over a period of at least 12 months?	Is there enough information to determine seasonality?	Measurement at Baseline n (%) mean SD	Measurement at end of treatment n (%) mean SD	Measurement at last follow-up n (%) mean SD	Were outcomes adjusted?
006[52]	s for controller medicine	Interevntion of intervention group	corticosteroids					Mean:22 CI:12,32	Mean:15 CI:10,29	
Martens,2 006[52]	Prescriptions for controller medicine	Arm A-control group (standard practice)	short term beta 2 sympatomimetics	NR	Yes	NR	N: 54 Mean:29 CI: 19, 35	N: 54 Mean:28 CI:19,14	Mean:27 CI: 20,38	No.
Martens,2 006[52]	Prescriptions for controller medicine	Arm B-intervention (overall)	short term beta 2 sympatomimetics	NR	Yes	NR	N: 53 Mean:28 CI: 21,44	N: 53 Mean:29 CI:18,39	N: 53 Mean:28 CI:9,36	No.
Martens,2 006[52]	Prescriptions for controller medicine	Arm C-Guidelines only	short term beta 2 sympatomimetics	NR	Yes	NR	N: 26 Mean:35 CI:23,47	N: 23 Mean:37 CI:25,49	N: 26 Mean:36 CI:24,48	No.
Martens,2 006[52]	Prescriptions for controller medicine	Arm D-interevntion of intervention	short term beta 2 sympatomimetics	NR	Yes	NR	N: 27 Mean:37 CI:26,48	N: 27 Mean:37 CI:26,48	N: 27 Mean:34 CI:24,44	No.
Martens,2 007[53]	Prescriptions for controller medicine	Arm A-Cholesterol	the ratio of # of prescriptions for inhaled steroids to # of all asthma prescriptions for mild persistent asthma among patients > 7 years old	0-100	No	Yes. Data collected over an entire year in both groups post start of intervention	NR	NR	N: NR , n with outcomes: NR , n with events: NR, (27) Confidence interval 14-47	No.
Martens,2 007[53]	Prescriptions for	Arm B-antibiotics,	the ratio of # of	0-100	No	Yes. Data collected over	NR	NR	N: NR , n with outcomes: NR ,	No.

Author, Year	Health Care Process Outcomes	Arm	Definition of Scale	Range of Scale	Were outcomes measured over a period of at least 12 months?	Is there enough information to determine seasonality?	Measurement at Baseline n (%) mean SD	Measurement at end of treatment n (%) mean SD	Measurement at last follow-up n (%) mean SD	Were outcomes adjusted?
	controller medicine	asthma/ COPD	prescriptions for inhaled steroids to # of all asthma prescriptions for mild persistent asthma among patients > 7 years old			an entire year in both groups post start of intervention			n with events: NR, (44) confidence interval 30-56	
Martens, 2007[53]	Prescriptions for controller medicine	Arm A- Cholesterol	number of inhaled corticosteroid prescriptions for mildly persistent asthma with maintenance treatment among patients >7 per GP per 1000 patients	0-1000	NR	NR	NR	NR	N: NR, see scale above 1.4, confidence interval 0.7-4.0	No.
Martens, 2007[53]	Prescriptions for controller medicine	Arm B- Antibiotics, asthma /COPD	number of inhaled corticosteroid prescriptions for mildly persistent asthma with maintenance treatment among patients >7 per GP per 1000 patients	0-1000	NR	NR	NR	NR	N: NR, see scale: 1.7, CI 1.0-2.6	No.

E-150

Author, Year	Health Care Process Outcomes	Arm	Definition of Scale	Range of Scale	Were outcomes measured over a period of at least 12 months?	Is there enough information to determine seasonality?	Measurement at Baseline n (%) mean SD	Measurement at end of treatment n (%) mean SD	Measurement at last follow-up n (%) mean SD	Were outcomes adjusted?
McCowan, 2001[11]	Asthma action plans	Arm A- Control (standard practice)	Use a self management plan	Yes or No	No	6 month follow-up	NR	NR	N: 330 n with events: 173 (52)	No.
McCowan, 2001[11]	Asthma action plans	Arm B- Decision support	Use a self management plan	Yes or No	No	6 month follow-up	NR	NR	N: 147 n with events: 74 (50)	No.
McCowan, 2001[11]	Prescription of peak flow meter	Arm A- Control (standard practice)	Primary care consultations (No. of patients):Issued peak flow meter	NR	No	6 month follow-up	NR	NR	N: 330 n with outcomes: 158 n with events: 158 (48)	No.
Mitchell, 2005[54]	Prescriptions for controller medicine	Arm A- Control (standard practice)	# inhalers or Rx's per 1000 patient months (95% CI's)	NR	NR	NR	N: NR 14.2 (13.8-14.6)	NR	N: NR 13.7 (13.3-14.1)	No.
Mitchell, 2005[54]	Prescriptions for controller medicine	Arm A- Control (standard practice)	# inhalers or Rx's per 1000 patient months (95% CI's)	NR	NR	NR	N: NR 15.0 (14.6-15.4)	NR	N: 13.2 (12.8-14.1)	No.
Mitchell, 2005[54]	Prescriptions for controller medicine	Arm A- Control (standard practice)	# inhalers or Rx's per 1000 patient months (95% CI's)	NR	NR	NR	N: NR 2.8 (2.6-3.0)	NR	N: NR 2.0 (1.8-2.2)	No.
Mitchell, 2005[54]	Prescriptions for controller medicine	Arm A- Control (standard practice)	# inhalers or Rx's per 1000 patient months (95% CI's)	NR	NR	NR	N: NR 0.49 (0.42-0.56)	NR	N: NR 0.45 (0.38-0.52)	No.
Mitchell, 2005[54]	Prescriptions for controller medicine	Arm A- Control (standard practice)	# inhalers or Rx's per 1000 patient months (95% CI's)	NR	NR	NR	N: NR 0.98 (0.88-1.08)	NR	N: NR 0.54 (0.46-0.62)	No.

Author, Year	Health Care Process Outcomes	Arm	Definition of Scale	Range of Scale	Were outcomes measured over a period of at least 12 months?	Is there enough information to determine seasonality?	Measurement at Baseline n (%) mean SD	Measurement at end of treatment n (%) mean SD	Measurement at last follow-up n (%) mean SD	Were outcomes adjusted?
Mitchell, 2005[54]	Prescriptions for controller medicine	Arm A- Control (standard practice)	# inhalers or Rx's per 1000 patient months (95% CI's)	NR	NR	NR	N: NR, 0.018 (0.004-0.032)	NR	N: NR, 0.003 (0-0.009)	No.
Mitchell, 2005[54]	Prescriptions for controller medicine	Arm B- Decision support	# inhalers or Rx's per 1000 patient months (95% CI's)	NR	NR	NR	N: NR, 13.5 (13.1-13.9)	NR	N: NR 13.2 (12.8-13.6)	No.
Mitchell, 2005[54]	Prescriptions for controller medicine	Arm B- Decision support	# inhalers or Rx's per 1000 patient months (95% CI's)	NR	NR	NR	N: NR, 15.3 (14.9-15.7)	NR	N: NR 14.0 (13.6-14.4)	No.
Mitchell, 2005[54]	Prescriptions for controller medicine	Arm B- Decision support	# inhalers or Rx's per 1000 patient months (95% CI's)	NR	NR	NR	N: NR 6.2 (5.9-6.5)	NR	N: NR 3.2 (3.0-3.4)	No.
Mitchell, 2005[54]	Prescriptions for controller medicine	Arm B- Decision support	# inhalers or Rx's per 1000 patient months (95% CI's)	NR	NR	NR	N: NR 0.46 (0.39-0.53)	NR	N: NR 0.35 (0.29-0.41)	No.
Mitchell, 2005[54]	Prescriptions for controller medicine	Arm B- Decision support	# inhalers or Rx's per 1000 patient months (95% CI's)	NR	NR	NR	N: NR 1.30 (1.08-1.42)	NR	N: NR 0.80 (0.71-0.89)	No.
Mitchell, 2005[54]	Prescriptions for controller medicine	Arm B- Decision support	# inhalers or Rx's per 1000 patient months (95% CI's)	NR	NR	NR	N: NR 0.029 (0.011-0.047)	NR	N: NR 0.020 (0.005-0.035)	No.
Newton, 20	Asthma	Decision	NR	NR	Yes	No	N: NR	N: NR	NR	No.

Author, Year	Health Care Process Outcomes	Arm	Definition of Scale	Range of Scale	Were outcomes measured over a period of at least 12 months?	Is there enough information to determine seasonality?	Measurement at Baseline n (%) mean SD	Measurement at end of treatment n (%) mean SD	Measurement at last follow-up n (%) mean SD	Were outcomes adjusted?
10[12]	action plans	Support					(48)	(57)		
Patel,2004[13]	Asthma action plans	Organizational Change	NR	NR	Yes	No	N: 451 (11.1)	N: 427 (25.4)	NR	No.
Patel,2004[13]	Self-management education	Organizational Change	NR	NR	NR	NR	N: 451 (15.7)	N: 427 (26.1)	NR	No.
Ragazzi,2010[14]	Asthma action plans	Practice 1	NR	NR	NR	NR	N: 17 (18)	N: 24 (38)	NR	No.
Ragazzi,2010[14]	Asthma action plans	Practice 2	NR	NR	NR	NR	N: 26 (0)	N: 19 (32)	NR	No.
Ragazzi,2010[14]	Asthma action plans	Practice 3	NR	NR	NR	NR	N: 10 (0)	N: 21 (48)	NR	No.
Ragazzi,2010[14]	Follow-up visits	Practice 1	NR	NR	NR	NR	N: 17 (76)	N: 24 (83)	NR	No.
Ragazzi,2010[14]	Follow-up visits	Practice 2	NR	NR	NR	NR	N: 26 (15)	N: 19 (53)	NR	No.
Ragazzi,2010[14]	Follow-up visits	Practice 3	NR	NR	NR	NR	N: 10 (20)	N: 21 (71)	NR	No.
Ragazzi,2010[14]	Self-management education	Practice 1	NR	NR	Yes	No	N: 17 (47)	N: 24 (79)	NR	No.
Ragazzi,2010[14]	Self-management education	Practice 2	NR	NR	Yes	No	N: 26 (23)	N: 19 (47)	NR	No.
Ragazzi,2010[14]	Self-management education	Practice 3	NR	NR	Yes	No	N: 10 (10)	N: 21 (86)	NR	No.
Rance,20	Prescription	Arm B-	NR	NR	NR	NR	N: 41	N: 41	NR	No.

Author, Year	Health Care Process Outcomes	Arm	Definition of Scale	Range of Scale	Were outcomes measured over a period of at least 12 months?	Is there enough information to determine seasonality?	Measurement at Baseline n (%) mean SD	Measurement at end of treatment n (%) mean SD	Measurement at last follow-up n (%) mean SD	Were outcomes adjusted?
11[55]	s for controller medicine	Decision support					n with outcomes: 28	n with outcomes: 38		
Richman, 2000[29]	Environmental control practice recommendations	Feedback	"environmental screening"	0-100	No	No	N: NR n with outcomes: NR n with events: NR (21)	N: NR n with outcomes: NR n with events: NR (70)	NR	No.
Richman, 2000[29]	Prescription of peak flow meter	Feedback	"peak flow meter"	0-100	No	No	N: NR n with events: NR (18)	N: NR n with events: NR (40)	NR	No.
Richman, 2000[29]	Prescriptions for controller medicine	Feedback	"inhaled anti-inflammatory"	0-100	No	No	N: NR n with events: NR (45)	N: NR n with outcomes: NR n with events: NR (63)	NR	No.
Richman, 2000[29]	Self-management education	Feedback	"basic education"	0-100	No	No	N: NR n with events: NR (30)	N: NR n with events: NR (70)	NR	No.
Richman, 2000[29]	Self-management education	Feedback	"referral for comprehensive education"	0-100	No	No	N: NR n with events: NR (13)	N: NR n with events: NR (34)	NR	No.
Ruoff, 2002[30]	Environmental control practice recommendations	Arm A- Before flow sheet	NR	NR	NR	NR	NR	NR	(27.37)	No.
Ruoff, 2002[30]	Environmental control practice recommendations	Arm B- After implementation of the flow sheet	NR	NR	NR	NR	NR	NR	,(78.95)	No.
Ruoff, 2002[30]	Prescription	Arm A-	Yearly PFT	NR	NR	NR	NR	NR	N: 122 (8.08)	No.

Author, Year	Health Care Process Outcomes	Arm	Definition of Scale	Range of Scale	Were outcomes measured over a period of at least 12 months?	Is there enough information to determine seasonality?	Measurement at Baseline n (%) mean SD	Measurement at end of treatment r (%) mean SD	Measurement at last follow-up n (%) mean SD	Were outcomes adjusted?
2[30]	of peak flow meter	Before the flow sheet								
Ruoff,200 2[30]	Prescription of peak flow meter	Arm B- After implement ation of the flow sheet	Yearly PFT	NR	NR	NR	NR	NR	N: 122 (84.21)	No.
Ruoff,200 2[30]	Self-manageme nt education	Arm A- Before the flow sheet	Inhaler technique education	NR	NR	NR	NR	NR	N: 122 (7.07)	No.
Ruoff,200 2[30]	Self-manageme nt education	Arm B- After implement ation of the flow sheet	Inhaler technique education	NR	NR	NR	NR	NR	N: 122 (78.95)	No.
Ruoff,200 2[30]	Self-manageme nt education	Arm A- Before the flow sheet	Flow meter education	NR	No	No	NR	NR	N: 122 (7.07)	No.
Ruoff,200 2[30]	Self-manageme nt education	Arm B- After implement ation of the flow sheet	Flow meter education	NR	No	No	NR	NR	N: 122 (63.13)	No.
Saini,2004 22	Documenta tion of level of asthma control/sev erity	Arm A- Control 1	Perceived control over asthma	11-55	No	No	N: 22 Mean:36.7 SD:9.5	NR	N: 22 Mean:36.7 SD:9.5	No.
Saini,2004 22	Documenta tion of level of asthma control/sev	Arm B- Control 1	Perceived control over asthma	11-55	No	No	N: 28, Mean:39.2 SD:5.8	NR	N: 28 Mean:39.2 SD:5.8	No.

E-155

Author, Year	Health Care Process Outcomes	Arm	Definition of Scale	Range of Scale	Were outcomes measured over a period of at least 12 months?	Is there enough information to determine seasonality?	Measurement at Baseline n (%) mean SD	Measurement at end of treatment n (%) mean SD	Measurement at last follow-up n (%) mean SD	Were outcomes adjusted?
	erity									
Saini,2004[22]	Documentation of level of asthma control/severity	Arm C- Education	Perceived control over asthma	11-55	No	No	N: 52 Mean:39.4 SD:5.1	NR	N: 39 Mean:42.5 SD:5.2	No.
Schneider, 2008[17]	Asthma action plans (emergency plans)	Arm A- Traditional quality circle	Emergency plan in place	Binary yes/no	Yes	NR	N: NR n with outcomes: 62 n with events: 4 (6.1)	NR	N: 62 n with outcomes: 62 n with events: 7 (10.6)	No.
Schneider, 2008[17]	Asthma action plans (emergency plans)	Arm B- Benchmark quality circle	Emergency plan in place	Binary yes/no	Yes	NR	N: NR n with outcomes: 113 n with events: 8 (6.7)	NR	N: 113 n with outcomes: 113 n with events: 17 (14.3)	No.
Schneider, 2008[17]	Prescription of peak flow meter	Arm A- Traditional quality circle	peak flow use at home	Yes/No	Yes	Follow up questionnaire was sent one year later	N: NR n with outcomes: 62 n with events: 16 (24.2)	NR	N: 62 n with outcomes: 62 n with events: 20 (30.3)	No.
Schneider, 2008[17]	Prescription of peak flow meter	Arm B- Benchmark quality circle	peak flow use at home	Yes/No	Yes	Follow up questionnaire was sent one year later	N: NR n with outcomes: 113 n with events: 27 (22.7)	NR	N: 113 n with outcomes: 113 n with events: 27 (22.7)	No.
Schneider, 2008[17]	Self-management education	Arm A- Traditional quality circle	receipt/non-receipt	binary	Yes	NR	N: NR n with outcomes: 62 n with events: 20 (30.3)	NR	N: 62 n with outcomes: 62 n with events: 20 (30.3)	No.
Schneider, 2008[17]	Self-management education	Arm B- Benchmark quality circle	receipt/non-receipt	binary	Yes	NR	N: NR n with outcomes: 113 n with events: 37 (31.1)	NR	N: 113 n with outcomes: 113 n with events: 39 (32.8)	No.
Shah,201	Asthma	Arm A-	NR	NR	No	No	N: 56	N: 47	NR	No.

Author, Year	Health Care Process Outcomes	Arm	Definition of Scale	Range of Scale	Were outcomes measured over a period of at least 12 months?	Is there enough information to determine seasonality?	Measurement at Baseline n (%) mean SD	Measurement at end of treatment n (%) mean SD	Measurement at last follow-up n (%) mean SD	Were outcomes adjusted?
1[15]	action plans	Control					n with outcomes: 25 (45)	n with outcomes: 25 (53)		
Shah,201 1[15]	Asthma action plans	Arm B-Interventio n	NR	NR	No	No	N: 66 n with outcomes: 30 (45)	N: 55 n with outcomes: 42 (76)	NR	No.
Shapiro,2 011[23]	Documenta tion of level of asthma control/sev erity	SBHC	Documentatio n during any visit	NR	No	No	N: 200 (25.5)	N: 200 (77.5)	NR	No.
Shapiro,2 011[23]	Documenta tion of level of asthma control/sev erity	NYCHP	Documentatio n during any visit	NR	No	No	N: 197 (11.7)	N: 249 (85.1)	NR	No.
Shiffman,2 000[24]	Documenta tion of level of asthma control/sev erity	Arm A-Pre	assessment of PEFR	0-1.0	No	Each interval (pre and post) was under one year	N: 91 n with outcomes: 81 Mean:0.86	NR	NR	No.
Shiffman,2 000[24]	Documenta tion of level of asthma control/sev erity	Arm B-Post	assessment of PEFR	0-1.0	No	Each interval (pre and post) was under one year	N: 74 n with outcomes: 73 Mean:0.94	NR	NR	No.
Shiffman,2 000[24]	Documenta tion of level of asthma control/sev erity	Arm A-Pre	Oxygen saturation measured	0-1	No	No. Each interval, pre and post, was under one year.	N: 91 n with outcomes: 81 Mean:0.29	NR	NR	No.
Shiffman,2 000[24]	Documenta tion of level of asthma control/sev erity	Arm B-Post	Oxygen saturation measured	0-1	No	No. Each interval, pre and post, was under one year.	N: 74 n with outcomes: 73 Mean:0.56	NR	NR	No.

Author, Year	Health Care Process Outcomes	Arm	Definition of Scale	Range of Scale	Were outcomes measured over a period of at least 12 months?	Is there enough information to determine seasonality?	Measurement at Baseline n (%) mean SD	Measurement at end of treatment n (%) mean SD	Measurement at last follow-up n (%) mean SD	Were outcomes adjusted?
Shiffman, 2000[24]	Prescriptions for controller medicine	Arm A-Pre	Prescription of systemic corticosteroid	0-1	No	No. Each interval (pre and post) was under a year	N: 91 n with outcomes: 81 Mean:0.43	NR	NR	No.
Shiffman, 2000[24]	Prescriptions for controller medicine	Arm B-Post	Prescription of systemic corticosteroid	0-1	No	No. Each interval (pre and post) was under a year	N: 74 n with outcomes: 73 Mean:0.57	NR	NR	No.
Smeele, 1999[31]	Environmental control practice recommendations	Arm A-Control	Advice on house dust mite eradication	NR	NR	NR	N: 17 n with events: 17 (21)	N: 17 n with events: 17 (25)	NR	No.
Smeele, 1999[31]	Environmental control practice recommendations	Arm B-Education	Advice or house dust mite eradication	NR	NR	NR	N: 16 n with outcomes: 16 (17)	N: 16 n with outcomes: 16 (15)	NR	No.
Smeele, 1999[31]	Prescriptions for controller medicine	Arm A-Control	Exacerbation: prescription of Oral steroids	NR	NR	NR	N: 17 n with outcomes: 15 n with events: 15 (29)	N: 15 n with outcomes: 15 n with events: 15 (33)	NR	No.
Smeele, 1999[31]	Prescriptions for controller medicine	Arm B-Education	Exacerbation: prescription of Oral steroids	NR	NR	NR	N: 17 n with outcomes: 17 (21)	N: 15 n with outcomes: 15 (34)	NR	No.
Smeele, 1999[31]	Prescriptions for controller medicine	Arm A-Control	Exacerbations: Prescription of Inhaled steroids	NR	NR	NR	N: 17 n with outcomes: 15 n with events: 15 (51)	N: 15 n with outcomes: 15 n with events: 15 (50)	NR	No.
Smeele, 1999[31]	Prescriptions for controller medicine	Arm B-Education	Exacerbations: Prescription of Inhaled steroids	NR	NR	NR	N: 17 n with outcomes: 17 (52)	N: 15 n with outcomes: 15 (65)	NR	No.

E-158

Author, Year	Health Care Process Outcomes	Arm	Definition of Scale	Range of Scale	Were outcomes measured over a period of at least 12 months?	Is there enough information to determine seasonality?	Measurement at Baseline n (%) mean SD	Measurement at end of treatment n (%) mean SD	Measurement at last follow-up n (%) mean SD	Were outcomes adjusted?
Smeele, 1999[31]	Self-management education	Arm A-Control	Written patient education	NR	NR	NR	N: 17 n with outcomes: 17 n with events: 17 (21)	N: 17 n with outcomes: 17 n with events: 17 (25)	NR	No.
Smeele, 1999[31]	Self-management education	Arm B-Education	Written patient education	NR	NR	NR	N: 17 n with outcomes: 16 (26)	N: 17 n with outcomes: 16, (29)	NR	No.
Smeele, 1999[31]	Self-management education	Arm A-Control	Patient education inhalation instruction materials	NR	Yes	No	N: 17 n with events: 11	N: 7 n with events: 13	N: 13	No.
Smeele, 1999[31]	Self-management education	Arm B-Education	Patient education inhalation instruction materials	NR	Yes	No	N: 17 n with outcomes: 16 (15)	N: 6 n with outcomes: 16 (17)	N: 17	No.
Smeele, 1999[31]	Self-management education	Arm A-Control	Peakflow measurement	NR	NR	NR	N: 17 n with outcomes: 17 n with events: 9	N: 17 n with outcomes: 17 n with events: 11	NR	No.
Smeele, 1999[31]	Self-management education	Arm B-Education	Peakflow measurement	NR	NR	NR	N: 17 n with events: 12,	N: 17 n with events: 17	NR	No.
Sondergaard, 2002[56]	Prescriptions for controller medicine	Arm A-Control (Feedback)	incidence of initiation of inhaled steroids among repeat users of beta2 agonists	NR	Yes	NR	NR	NR	N: 751 n with outcomes: 751 n with events: 140 (NR) incidence rate (IR): 0.018 CI (0.015,	Yes. Using survival analysis. Also variance taking into account clustering.

Author, Year	Health Care Process Outcomes	Arm	Definition of Scale	Range of Scale	Were outcomes measured over a period of at least 12 months?	Is there enough information to determine seasonality?	Measurement at Baseline n (%) mean SD	Measurement at end of treatment n (%) mean SD	Measurement at last follow-up n (%) mean SD	Were outcomes adjusted?
									0.021 HR 1.00	
Sondergaard,2002[56]	Prescriptions for controller medicine	Arm A-Control	incidence of initiation of inhaled steroids among first time users of inhaled beta 2 agonists	NR	Yes	NR	NR	NR	N: 1000 n with outcomes: 1000 n with events: 519, (NR) IR 0.060 CI: 0.052, 0.069	Yes. Using survival analysis. Also variance taking into account clustering.
Sondergaard,2002[56]	Prescriptions for controller medicine	Arm A-Control	Change in fraction of asthmatic treated with ICS	NR	Yes	NR	NR	N: NR change in fraction: -0.02 95% CI: -0.05, 0.00	NR	No.
Sondergaard,2002[56]	Prescriptions for controller medicine	Arm A-Control	incidence of initiation of inhaled steroids among repeat users of beta2 agonists	NR	Yes	NR	NR	NR	N: 751 n with outcomes: 751 n with events: 140 (NR) incidence rate (IR): 0.018 CI (0.015, 0.021) HR 1.00	Yes. Using survival analysis. Also variance taking into account clustering.
Sondergaard,2002[56]	Prescriptions for controller medicine	Arm A-Control	incidence of initiation of inhaled steroids among first time users of inhaled beta 2 agonists	NR	Yes	NR	NR	NR	N: 1000 n with outcomes: 1836 n with events: 519 (NR) IR 0.060 CI 0.052, 0.069 HR 1.00	Yes. Using survival analysis. Also variance taking into account clustering.
Sondergaard,2002[56]	Prescriptions for	Arm B-Audit,	Change in fraction of	NR	Yes	NR	NR	N: NR change in	NR	No.

Author, Year	Health Care Process Outcomes	Arm	Definition of Scale	Range of Scale	Were outcomes measured over a period of at least 12 months?	Is there enough information to determine seasonality?	Measurement at Baseline n (%) mean SD	Measurement at end of treatment n (%) mean SD	Measurement at last follow-up n (%) mean SD	Were outcomes adjusted?
	controller medicine	feedback. Individual patient count data	asthmatic treated with ICS					fraction, -0.01, 95% CI -0.04, 0.02		
Sondergaard,2002[56]	Prescriptions for controller medicine	Arm B- Audit, feedback. Individual patient count data	Change in fraction of asthmatic treated with ICS	NR	Yes	NR	NR	N: NR change in fraction, -0.01, 95% CI -0.04, 0.02	NR	No.
Sondergaard,2002[56]	Prescriptions for controller medicine	Arm B- Audit, feedback. Individual patient count data	incidence of initiation of inhaled steroids among repeat users of beta2 agonists	NR	Yes	NR	NR	NR	N: 457 n with outcomes: 457 n with events: 67 (NR) IR: 0.013 CI: 0.011, 0.017 HR: 0.77 CI: 0.59, 1.01	Yes. Using survival analysis. Also variance taking into account clustering.
Sondergaard,2002[56]	Prescriptions for controller medicine	Arm B- Audit, feedback. Individual patient count data	incidence of initiation of inhaled steroids among first time users of inhaled beta 2 agonists	NR	Yes	NR	NR	NR	N: 1000 n with outcomes: 1000 n with events: 305 (NR) IR: 0.064 CI: 0.054, 0.076 HR: 1.08 CI: 0.90, 1.30	Yes. Using survival analysis. Also variance taking into account clustering.
Sondergaard,2002[56]	Prescriptions for controller medicine	Arm C- Audit, feedback. Aggregate data feedback	incidence of initiation of inhaled steroids among repeat users of beta2 agonists	NR	Yes	NR	NR	NR	N: 442 n with outcomes: 442 n with events: 67 (NR) IR: 0.014 CI: 0.011, 0.018 HR: 0.79	Yes. Using survival analysis. Also variance taking into account

Author, Year	Health Care Process Outcomes	Arm	Definition of Scale	Range of Scale	Were outcomes measured over a period of at least 12 months?	Is there enough information to determine seasonality?	Measurement at Baseline n (%) mean SD	Measurement at end of treatment n (%) mean SD	Measurement at last follow-up n (%) mean SD	Were outcomes adjusted?
									CI: 0.59, 1.07	clustering.
Sonderga ard, 2002[56]	Prescription s for controller medicine	Arm C-Audit, feedback. Aggregate data feedback	incidence of initiation of inhaled steroids among first time users of inhaled beta 2 agonists	NR	Yes	NR	NR	NR	N: 868 n with outcomes: 868 n with events: 229 (NR) IR: 0.054 CI 0.045, 0.066; HR: 0.92 CI 0.75, 1.13	-1Using survival analysis. Also variance taking into account clustering.
Sonderga ard, 2002[56]	Prescription s for controller medicine	Arm C-Audit, feedback. Aggregate data feedback	Change in fraction of asthmatic treated with ICS	NR	Yes	NR	NR	N: NR 0.01 95% CI: -0.03, 0.05	NR	No.
Suh, 2001[7]	Prescription s for controller medicine	Intermitten t	"number of uses of short acting controller"	NR	No	Yes. Same period	N: 5665 Mean:0.78 SD:0.89	N: 566 Mean:1.13 SD:1.74	NR	No.
Suh, 2001[7]	Prescription s for controller medicine	Persistent	"number of uses of short acting controller"	NR	No	Yes. Same period	N: 1050 Mean:5.1 SD:4.51	N: 1050 Mean:4.4 SD:4.86	NR	No.
Suh, 2001[7]	Prescription s for controller medicine	Intermitten t	"long acting controller meds per patient"	NR	No	Yes. Same time period	N: 566 n with outcomes: 566 Mean:0.4 SD:0.67	N: 566, n with outcomes: 566 Mean:0.77, SD:1 .67	NR	No.
Suh, 2001[7]	Prescription s for controller medicine	Persistent	"long acting controller meds per patient"	NR	No	Yes. Same time period	N: 1050 n with outcomes: 1050 Mean:4.04 SD:4.81	N: 1050 n with outcomes: 1050 Mean:3.75 SD:5.12	NR	No.
Suh, 2001[7]	Prescription s for	Intermitten t	no of prescriptions	NR	No	Yes. Same time period	N: 566 n with	N: 566 n with	NR	No.

E-162

Author, Year	Health Care Process Outcomes	Arm	Definition of Scale	Range of Scale	Were outcomes measured over a period of at least 12 months?	Is there enough information to determine seasonality?	Measurement at Baseline n (%) mean SD	Measurement at end of treatment n (%) mean SD	Measurement at last follow-up n (%) mean SD	Were outcomes adjusted?
	controller medicine		for inhaled corticosteroids				outcomes: 566 total number 135	outcomes: 566 total scripts 276		
Suh, 2001[5][7]	Prescriptions for controller medicine	Persistent	no of prescriptions for inhaled corticosteroids	NR	No	Yes. Same time period	N: 1050 n with outcomes: 1050 n with events: 2255 (23.5), number of scripts 2255	N: 1050 n with outcomes: 1050 n with events: 2012 (23.4), number of scripts 2012	NR	No.
Suh, 2001[5][7]	Prescriptions for controller medicine	Intermittent	number of leukotriene inhibitor prescriptions	NR	No	Yes. Same time period	N: 566 n with outcomes: 566 n with events: NR,(NR), total 7	N: 566 n with outcomes: 566 n with events: NR,(NR), total 37	NR	No.
Suh, 2001[5][7]	Prescriptions for controller medicine	Persistent	number of leukotriene inhibitor prescriptions	NR	No	Yes. Same time period	N: 1050 n with outcomes: 1050 n with events: 217 (2.3), total 217	N: 1050 n with ou comes: 1050 n with events: 527 (6.2), total 527	NR	No.
Sulaiman, 2010[16]	Asthma action plans	Arm A-Control (ENT education)	NR	NR	No	NR	N: 99 n with outcomes: 31 (31.3)	N: 100 n with outcomes: 35 (35)	NR	No.
Sulaiman, 2010[16]	Asthma action plans	Arm B-Asthma education and guidelines	NR	NR	No	NR	N: 120 n with outcomes: 37 (30.8)	N: 123 n with outcomes: 44 (35.8)	NR	No.
Sulaiman, 2010[16]	Asthma action plans	Arm C-Guidelines only	NR	NR	No	NR	N: 103 n with outcomes: 35 (34)	N: 105 n with outcomes: 40 (38.1)	NR	No.
Veninga, 1999[58]	Prescriptions for	Netherlands control	Proportion of patients on	NR	Yes	"To control for seasonal	N: 12 (58)	NR	(56)	Yes. Weighted

Author, Year	Health Care Process Outcomes	Arm	Definition of Scale	Range of Scale	Were outcomes measured over a period of at least 12 months?	Is there enough information to determine seasonality?	Measurement at Baseline n (%) mean SD	Measurement at end of treatment n (%) mean SD	Measurement at last follow-up n (%) mean SD	Were outcomes adjusted?
	controller medicine	arm	inhaled cortico-steroids (continued in ID2)			influences on asthma treatment, outcome data of a comparable period were collected after the intervention (between sept 1995 and aug 1997)."				mean proportions per group of doctors calculated with multilevel model.
Veninga,1 999[58]	Prescriptions for controller medicine	Netherlands intervention arm	Proportion of patients on inhaled cortico-steroids (continued in ID2)	NR	Yes	"To control for seasonal influences on asthma treatment, outcome data of a comparable period were collected after the intervention (between sept 1995 and aug 1997)."	N: 12 (58)	NR	(63)	Yes. Weighted mean proportions per group of doctors calculated with multilevel model.
Veninga,1 999[58]	Prescriptions for controller medicine	Sweden control arm	Proportion of patients on inhaled cortico-steroids (continued in ID2)	NR	Yes	"To control for seasonal influences on asthma treatment, outcome data of a comparable period were	N: 18 (46)	NR	(50)	Yes. Weighted mean proportions per group of doctors calculated with

Author, Year	Health Care Process Outcomes	Arm	Definition of Scale	Range of Scale	Were outcomes measured over a period of at least 12 months?	Is there enough information to determine seasonality?	Measurement at Baseline n (%) mean SD	Measurement at end of treatment n (%) mean SD	Measurement at last follow-up n (%) mean SD	Were outcomes adjusted?
						collected after the intervention (between sept 1995 and aug 1997)."				multilevel model.
Veninga,1 999[58]	Prescriptions for controller medicine	Sweden intervention arm	Proportion of patients on inhaled cortico-steroids (continued in ID2)	NR	Yes	"To control for seasonal influences on asthma treatment, outcome data of a comparable period were collected after the intervention (between sept 1995 and aug 1997)."	N: 18 (47)	NR	(53)	Yes. Weighted mean proportions per group of doctors calculated with multilevel model
Veninga,1 999[58]	Proportion of patients on inhaled cortico-steroids	Norway control	Proportion of patients on inhaled cortico-steroids (same outcome as ID1)	NR	Yes	"To control for seasonal influences on asthma treatment, outcome data of a comparable period were collected after the intervention (between Sept 1995 and Aug 1997)."	N: 16 (46)	NR	(50)	Yes. Weighted mean proportions per group of doctors calculated with multilevel model.
Veninga,1	Proportion	Norway	Proportion of	NR	Yes	"To control for	N: 16	NR	(54)	Yes.

Author, Year	Health Care Process Outcomes	Arm	Definition of Scale	Range of Scale	Were outcomes measured over a period of at least 12 months?	Is there enough information to determine seasonality?	Measurement at Baseline n (%) mean SD	Measurement at end of treatment n (%) mean SD	Measurement at last follow-up n (%) mean SD	Were outcomes adjusted?
999[58]	of patients on inhaled cortico-steroids	intervention	patients on inhaled cortico-steroids (same outcome as ID1)			seasonal influences on asthma treatment, outcome data of a comparable period were collected after the intervention (between sept 1995 and aug 1997)."	(47)			Weighted mean proportions per group of doctors calculated with multilevel model.
Veninga,1 999[58]	Proportion of patients on inhaled cortico-steroids	Slovakia control	Proportion of patients on inhaled cortico-steroids (same outcome as ID1)	NR	Yes	"To control for seasonal influences on asthma treatment, outcome data of a comparable period were collected after the intervention (between sept 1995 and aug 1997)."	N: 10 (41)	NR	(47)	Yes. Weighted mean proportions per group of doctors calculated with multilevel model.
Veninga,1 999[58]	Proportion of patients on inhaled cortico-steroids	Slovakia intervention	Proportion of patients on inhaled cortico-steroids (same outcome as ID1)	NR	Yes	"To control for seasonal influences on asthma treatment, outcome data of a comparable	N: 10 (38)	NR	(50)	Yes. Weighted mean proportions per group of doctors calculated

Author, Year	Health Care Process Outcomes	Arm	Definition of Scale	Range of Scale	Were outcomes measured over a period of at least 12 months?	Is there enough information to determine seasonality?	Measurement at Baseline n (%) mean SD	Measurement at end of treatment n (%) mean SD	Measurement at last follow-up n (%) mean SD	Were outcomes adjusted?
						period were collected after the intervention (between sept 1995 and aug 1997)."				with multilevel model.
Veninga,2000[59]	Prescriptions for controller medicine	Arm A-UTI	Proportion of patients receiving inhaled corticosteroids of all defined asthma patients	0-100	No	Yes. Both data collection periods were from June to Nov (in 1995 and then 1996)	N: NR n with outcomes: NR n with events: NR (0.58)	NR	N: NR n with outcomes: NR n with events: NR (0.56)	Separate article describing analytic approach suggests data were adjusted.
Veninga,2000[59]	Prescriptions for controller medicine	Arm B-Asthma	Proportion of patients receiving inhaled corticosteroids of all defined asthma patients	0-100	No	Yes. Both data collection periods were from June to Nov (in 1995 and then 1996)	N: NR n with outcomes: NR n with events: NR (0.58)	NR	N: NR n with outcomes: NR n with events: NR (0.63)	Separate article describing analytic approach suggests data were adjusted.
Yawn,2010[25]	Documentation of level of asthma control/severity	Education and Feedback	activity modification due to asthma	NR	NR	NR	N: 840 (29)	N: 851 (58)	NR	No.
Yawn,2010[25]	Documentation of level of asthma control/severity	Education and Feedback	Symptom frequency	NR	NR	NR	N: 840 (30)	N: 851 (62)	NR	No.
Yawn,2010[25]	Documentation of level	Education and	nighttime symptom	NR	NR	NR	N: 840 (25)	N: 851 (63)	NR	No.

Author, Year	Health Care Process Outcomes	Arm	Definition of Scale	Range of Scale	Were outcomes measured over a period of at least 12 months?	Is there enough information to determine seasonality?	Measurement at Baseline n (%) mean SD	Measurement at end of treatment n (%) mean SD	Measurement at last follow-up n (%) mean SD	Were outcomes adjusted?
	of asthma control/severity	Feedback	frequency							
Yawn, 2010[25]	Follow-up visits	Education and Feedback	NR	NR	NR	NR	N: 840 (4)	N: 850 (21)	NR	No.
Yawn, 2010[25]	Prescriptions for controller medicine	Education and Feedback	daily ant-inflammatory medication	NR	NR	NR	N: 840 (24)	N: 851 (73)	NR	No.
Yawn, 2010[25]	Self-management education	Education and Feedback	NR	NR	Unable to determine	No	N: 840 (8)	N: 851 (54)	NR	No.

ENT = ear nose throat; ER = Emergency Room; GP = General Practitioner; HCSD = Health Care Services Division; HPQOL = Health Profile Quality of Life;ICS = Inhaled Corticosteroids; NR = Not Reported; NYCHP = New York Children's Health Project;PLE = Peer Leader Education; QOL = Quality of Life;SBHC = South Bronx Health Center; SP = Suburban Practice;TOM = Therapeutic Outcomes Monitoring; UP = Urban Practice; UTI = Urinary Tract Infection

References

1. Bender BG, Dickinson P, Rankin A, Wamboldt FS, Zittleman L, Westfall JM. J Am Board Fam Med: The Colorado Asthma Toolkit Program: a practice coaching intervention from the High Plains Research Network. 2011; 24:240-8.

2. Clark, N. M Gong M. Schork M. et al. Impact of education for physicians on patient outcomes. Pediatrics 1998; 101(5):831-6.

3. Daniels EC, Bacon J, Denisio S et al.. Asthma: Translation squared: improving asthma care for high-disparity populations through a safety net practice-based research network. 2005; 42:499-505.

4. Frankowski BL, Keating K, Rexroad A et al. J Sch Health: Community collaboration: concurrent physician and school nurse education and cooperation increases the use of asthma action plans. 2006; 76:303-6.

5. Glasgow NJ, Ponsonby AL, Yates R, Beilby J, Dugdale P. BMJ: Proactive asthma care in childhood: general practice based randomised controlled trial. 2003; 327:659.

6. Halterman JS, Fisher S, Conn KM et al. Archives of Pediatrics & Adolescent Medicine: Improved preventive care for asthma: a randomized trial of clinician prompting in pediatric offices. 2006; 42:499-505.

160:1018-25.

7. Homer CJ, Forbes P, Horvitz L, Peterson LE, Wypij D, Heinrich P. Archives of Pediatrics and Adolescent Medicine: Impact of a quality improvement program on care and outcomes for children with asthma. 2005; 159:464-9.

8. Horswell R, Butler MK, Kaiser M et al. Dis Manag: Disease management programs for the underserved. 2008; 11:145-52.

9. Liaw ST, Sulaiman ND, Barton CA et al. BMC Fam Pract: An interactive workshop plus locally adapted guidelines can improve general practitioners asthma management and knowledge: a cluster randomised trial in the Australian setting. 2008; 9:22.

10. Mangione-Smith R, Schonlau M, Chan KS et al. Ambulatory Pediatrics: Measuring the effectiveness of a collaborative for quality improvement in pediatric asthma care: Does implementing the chronic care model improve processes and outcomes of care? 2005; 5:75-82.

11. McCowan C, Neville RG, Ricketts IW, Warner FC, Hoskins G, Thomas GE. Medical Informatics and the Internet in Medicine: Lessons from a randomized controlled trial designed to evaluate computer decision support software to improve the management of asthma. 2001; 26:191-201.

12. Newton WP, Lefebvre A, Donahue KE, Bacon T, Dobson A. J Contin Educ Health Prof: Infrastructure for large-scale quality-improvement projects: early lessons from North Carolina Improving Performance in Practice. 2010; 30:106-13.

13. Patel PH, Welsh C, Foggs MB. Dis Manag: Improved asthma outcomes using a coordinated care approach in a large medical group. 2004; 7:102-11.

14. Ragazzi H, Keller A, Ehrensberger R, Irani AM. J Urban Health: Evaluation of a practice-based intervention to improve the management of pediatric asthma. 2011; 88 Suppl 1:38-48.

15. Shah S, Sawyer SM, Toelle BG et al. Med J Aust: Improving paediatric asthma outcomes in primary health care: a randomised controlled trial. 2011; 195:405-9.

16. Sulaiman ND, Barton CA, Liaw ST et al. Fam Pract: Do small group workshops and locally adapted guidelines improve asthma patients' health outcomes? A cluster randomized controlled trial. 2010; 27:246-54.

17. Schneider A, Wensing M, Hessecker K, Quinzler R, Kaufmamm-Kolle P, Szecsenyi J. J Eval Clin Pract: Impact of quality circles for improvement of asthma care: results of a randomized controlled trial. 2008; 14:185-90.

18. Armour C, Bosnic-Anticevich S, Brillant M et al. Thorax: Pharmacy Asthma Care Program (PACP) improves outcomes for patients in the community. 2007; 62:496-502.

19. Ables AZ, Godenick MT, Lipsitz SR. Family Medicine: Improving family practice residents' compliance with asthma practice guidelines. 2002; 34:23-8.

20. Davis AM, Cannon M, Ables AZ, Bendyk H. Family Medicine: Using the electronic medical record to improve asthma severity documentation and treatment among family medicine residents. 2010; 42:334-7.

21. Fox P, Porter PG, Lob SH, Boer JH, Rocha DA, Adelson JW. Pediatrics: Improving asthma-related health outcomes among low-income, multiethnic, school-aged children: Results of a demonstration project that combined continuous quality improvement and community health worker strategies. 2007; 120:e902-e911.

22. Saini B, Krass I, Armour C. Annals of Pharmacotherapy: Development, implementation, and evaluation of a community pharmacy-based asthma care model. 2004; 38:1954-60.

23. Shapiro A, Gracy D, Quinones W, Applebaum J, Sarmiento A. Arch Pediatr Adolesc Med: Putting guidelines into practice: improving

24. Shiffman RN, Freudigman M, Brandt CA, Liaw Y, Navedo DD. Pediatrics: A guideline implementation system using handheld computers for office management of asthma: effects on adherence and patient outcomes. 2000; 105:767-73.

25. Yawn BP, Bertram S, Wollan P. Journal of Asthma and Allergy: Introduction of asthma APGAR tools improve asthma management in primary care practices. 2008; 1-10

26. Baker R, Fraser RC, Stone M, Lambert P, Stevenson K, Shiels C. Br J Gen Pract: Randomised controlled trial of the impact of guidelines, prioritized review criteria and feedback on implementation of recommendations for angina and asthma. 2003; 53:284-91.

27. Eccles M, McColl E, Steen N et al. BMJ: Effect of computerised evidence based guidelines on management of asthma and angina in adults in primary care: cluster randomised controlled trial. 2002; 325:941.

28. Fairall L, Bachmann MO, Zwarenstein M et al. Trop Med Int Health: Cost-effectiveness of educational outreach to primary care nurses to increase tuberculosis case detection and improve respiratory care: economic evaluation alongside a randomised trial. 2010; 15:277-86.

29. Richman MJ, Poltawsky JS. Stud Health Technol Inform: Partnership for excellence in asthma care: evidence-based disease management. 2000; 76:107-21.

30. Ruoff G. Family Medicine: Effects of flow sheet implementation on physician performance in the management of asthmatic patients. 2002; 34:514-7.

31. Smeele IJ, Grol RP, van Schayck CP, van den Bosch WJ, van den Hoogen HJ, Muris JW. Qual Health Care: Can small group education and peer review improve care for patients with asthma/chronic obstructive pulmonary disease? 1999; 3:92-8.

32. Feder G, Griffiths C, Highton C, Eldridge S, Spence M, Southgate L. British Medical Journal: Do clinical guidelines introduced with practice based education improve care of asthmatic and diabetic patients? A randomised controlled trial in general practices in east London. 1995; 311:1473-8.

33. Finkelstein JA, Lozano P, Fuhlbrigge AL et al. Health Serv Res: Practice-level effects of interventions to improve asthma care in primary care settings: the Pediatric Asthma Care Patient Outcomes Research Team. 2005; 40:1737-57.

34. Kattan M, Crain EF, Steinbach S et al. Pediatrics: A randomized clinical trial of clinician feedback to improve quality of care for inner-city children with asthma. 2006; 117:e1095-103.

35. Bryce FP, Neville RG, Crombie IK, Clark RA, McKenzie P. British Medical Journal: Controlled trial of an audit facilitator in diagnosis and treatment of childhood asthma in general practice. 1995; 310:838-42.

36. Coleman CI, Reddy P, Laster-Bradley NM, Dorval S, Munagala B, White CM. Ann Pharmacother: Effect of practitioner education on adherence to asthma treatment guidelines. 2003; 37:956-61.

37. Gorton TA, Cranford CO, Golden WE, Walls RC, Pawelak JE. Arch Fam Med: Primary care physicians' response to dissemination of practice guidelines. 1995; 4:135-42.

38. Bell LM, Grundmeier R, Localio R et al. Pediatrics: Electronic health record-based decision support to improve asthma care: a cluster-randomized trial. 2010; 125:e770-7.

39. Cho SH, Jeong JW, Park HW et al. J Asthma: Effectiveness of a computer-assisted asthma management program on physician adherence to guidelines. 2010; 47:680-6.

40. Cloutier MM, Wakefield DB, Carlisle PS, Bailit HL, Hall CB. Arch Pediatr Adolesc Med: The effect of Easy Breathing on asthma management and knowledge. 2002; 156:1045-51.

documentation of pediatric asthma management using a decision-making tool. 2011; 165:412-8.

41. Cloutier MM, Grosse SD, Wakefield DB, Nurmagambetov TA, Brown CM. American Journal of Managed Care: The economic impact of an urban asthma management program. 2009; 15:345-51.

42. Cowie RL, Underwood MF, Mack S. Can Respir J: The impact of asthma management guideline dissemination on the control of asthma in the community. 2001; 8 Suppl A:41A-5A.

43. Davis RS, Bukstein DA, Luskin AT, Kailin JA, Goodenow G. Ann Allergy Asthma Immunol: Changing physician prescribing patterns through problem-based learning: an interactive, teleconference case-based education program and review of problem-based learning. 2004; 93:237-42.

44. de Vries TW, van den Berg PB, Duiverman EJ, de Jong-van den Berg LT. Arch Dis Child: Effect of a minimal pharmacy intervention on improvement of adherence to asthma guidelines. 2010; 95:302-4.

45. Hagmolen of ten Have W, van den Berg NJ, van der Palen J, van Aalderen WM, Bindels PJ. Prim Care Respir J: Implementation of an asthma guideline for the management of childhood asthma in general practice: a randomised controlled trial. 2008; 17:90-6.

46. Halterman JS, McConnochie KM, Conn KM et al. Archives of Pediatrics and Adolescent Medicine: A randomized trial of primary care provider prompting to enhance preventive asthma therapy. 2005; 159:422-7.

47. Herborg H, Soendergaard B, Jorgensen T et al. J Am Pharm Assoc (Wash): Improving drug therapy for patients with asthma-part 2: Use of antiasthma medications. 2001; 41:551-9.

48. Hoskins G, Neville RG, Smith B, Clark RA. Health Bull (Edinb): Does participation in distance learning and audit improve the care of patients with acute asthma attacks? The General Practitioners in Asthma Group. 1997; 55:150-5.

49. Lesho EP, Myers CP, Ott M, Winslow C, Brown JE. Mil Med: Do clinical practice guidelines improve processes or outcomes in primary care? 2005; 170:243-6.

50. Lundborg CS, Wahlstrom R, Oke T, Tomson G, Diwan VK. J Clin Epidemiol: Influencing prescribing for urinary tract infection and asthma in primary care in Sweden: a randomized controlled trial of an interactive educational intervention. 1999; 52:801-12.

51. Mahi-Taright S, Belhocine M, Ait-Khaled N. Int J Tuberc Lung Dis: Can we improve the management of chronic obstructive respiratory disease? The example of asthma in adults. 2004; 8:873-81.

52. Martens JD, Winkens RA, van der Weijden T, de Bruyn D, Severens JL. BMC Health Serv Res: Does a joint development and dissemination of multidisciplinary guidelines improve prescribing behaviour: a pre/post study with concurrent control group and a randomised trial. 2006; 6:145.

53. Martens JD, van der Weijden T, Severens JL et al. Int J Med Inform: The effect of computer reminders on GPs' prescribing behaviour: a cluster-randomised trial. 2007; 76 Suppl 3:S403-16.

54. Mitchell EA, Didsbury PB, Kruithof N et al. Acta Paediatr: A randomized controlled trial of an asthma clinical pathway for children in general practice 2005; 94:226-33.

55. Rance K, OLaughlen M, Tng S. J Pediatr Health Care: Improving asthma care for African American children by increasing national asthma guideline adherence. 2011; 25:235-49.

56. Sondergaard J, Andersen M, Vach K, Kragstrup J, Maclure M, Gram LF. Eur J Clin Pharmacol: Detailed postal feedback about prescribing to asthma patients combined with a guideline statement showed no impact: a randomised controlled trial. 2002; 58:127-32.

57. Suh DC, Shin SK, Okpara I, Voytovich RM, Zimmerman A. Am J Manag Care: Impact of a targeted asthma intervention program on treatment costs in patients with asthma. 2001; 7:897-906.

58. Veninga CCM, Lagerlv P, Wahlstrom R et al. American Journal of Respiratory and Critical Care Medicine: Evaluating an educational intervention to improve the treatment of asthma in four european countries. 1999; 160 :1254-62.

E-171

59.	Veninga CCM, Denig P, Zwaagstra R, Haaijer-Ruskamp FM. Journal of Clinical Epidemiology: Improving drug treatment in general practice. 2000; 53:762-72.

Evidence Table 7. Mean difference between groups- Clinical outcomes

Author, Year	Clinical Outcome	Arm	Comparison Arm	Total N in Arm A	Total N in Comparison Arm	Total N in both arms	Definition of Scale	Range of Scale	Time	Statistical comparison (OR, RR, RD, HR P value 95% CI)
Armour,2007[12]	Quality of Life	Arm A: Control	Arm B: Pharmacy Asthma Care Program (PACP)	186	160	346	Asthma related quality of life questionnaire (mean change from baseline)	NR	NR	-0.23 p-value:0.05 95%CI:-0.46,0.00
Armour,2007[12]	Lung function tests	Arm A: Control	Arm B: Pharmacy Asthma Care Program (PACP)	135	122	257	FEV1(% predicted)	NR	NR	Risk diff: -1.81 p-value: 0.14
Armour,2007[12]	Lung function tests	Arm A: Control	Arm B: Pharmacy Asthma Care Program (PACP)	135	122	257	FEV1/FVC (% predicted)	NR	NR	Risk diff: 0.41 p-value: 0.71 95% CI: -1.76,2.57
Armour,2007[12]	Patient perceptions	Arm A: Control	Arm B: Pharmacy Asthma Care Program (PACP)	176	153	329	Perceived control of asthma questionnaire	11-55		Risk diff: -1.39 p-value: <0.01 95% CI: -2.44,-0.35
Baker,2003[17]	Patient perceptions	Arm A: Guidelines only	NR	NR	NR	NR	patients are satisfied that everything possible was done to treat asthma	NR	NR	p-value: 0.83 Generalized Wald tests
Baker,2003[17]	Patient perceptions	Arm A: Guidelines only	NR	NR	NR	NR	patients are satisfied with explanations given by the doctor about asthma	NR	NR	p-value: 0.75 Generalized Wald tests
Baker,2003[17]	Symptom Score	Arm A: Guidelines only	NR	NR	NR	NR	mean symptom score	NR	NR	p-value: 0.02 Generalized Wald tests
Bell,2009[13]	Lung function tests	Arm A: UP Control	Arm B: Up intervention	NR	NR	NR	Spirometry performed	NR	NR	P-value: 0.04

E-173

Study	Outcome	Arm A	Arm B				Measure			Result
Bryce,1995[1]	Emergency department visits	Arm A: Control	Arm B: Reminders and Tools	1563	1585	NR	No of patients attending: Accident and emergency departments	NR	NR	Risk ratio: 0.42 95%CI: 0.09 to 1.94
Bryce,1995[1]	hospitalizations	Arm A: Control	Arm B: Reminders and Tools	1563	1585	NR	No of patients admitted	NR	NR	Risk ratio: 0.53 95%CI: 0.22,1.26
Cabana, 2006[2]	Emergency department visits	Arm A: Control	Arm B: Physician Asthma Care Education (PACE)	368	363	731	Mean # visits per year	NR	NR	p-value:<0.05
Cabana, 2006[2]	Hospitalizations	Arm A: Control	Arm B: Physician Asthma Care Education (PACE)	368	363	731	Mean # hospitalizations	NR	NR	p-value:>0.05
Cabana, 2006[2]	Symptom days	Arm A: Control	Arm B: Physician Asthma Care Education (PACE)	368	363	731	Mean # days	NR	NR	p-value: <0.05
Cabana, 2006[2]	Urgent doctor visits	Arm A: Control	Arm B: Physician Asthma Care Education (PACE)	368	363	731	Mean # days	NR	NR	p-value: >0.05
Clark,1998[3]	Emergency department visits	Arm A	NR	NR	NR	NR	NR	NR	NR	p-value: ns
Clark,1998[3]	hospitalizations	Arm A	Arm B: Education	NR	NR	NR	NR	NR	NR	p-value: ns
Coleman, 2003[4]	Emergency department visits	Arm A: Patient specific information: Prescribers with patients on 'high dose'	Arm B: Patient specific information: Prescribers with patients on 'low dose'	510	135	645	NR	NR	6	p-value: 0.372 Unit: months mean difference; Pre intervention: p=0.357 mean difference between groups post intervention Post Intervention: p=0.372
Glasgow,	Emergency	Arm A	Arm B:	71	95	NR	Attended emergency	NR	NR	Odds ratio: 0.4

Study	Outcome	Arm A	Arm B				Measure			Results
2003[5]	department visits		Decision support				department 1-3 times in past 12 months	NR	NR	p-value: 0.06 95% CI: 0.2,1.04
Glasgow, 2003[5]	Missed days of school	Arm A	Arm B: Decision support	71	95	NR	Did not miss any school days with wheezing or asthma in past 12 months†	NR	NR	Odds ratio: 0.8 p-value: 0.3 95% CI: 0.5,1.2
Halterman, 2005[6]	Emergency department visits	Arm A:Control (standard practice)	Arm B: Decision support	77	73	150	NR	NR	NR	p-value: 0.25
Halterman, 2005[6]	Hospitalizations	Arm A:Control (standard practice)	Arm B: Decision support	77	73	150	NR	NR	NR	p-value: 0.62 95%
Holton, 2011[14]	Lung function tests	Arm A: Control (standard practice)	Arm B: Spirometry training	119	171	290	Post-bronchodilator FEV_1/FVC ratio (mean)	NR	12	Risk difference: -0.01 95%CI: -0.03,0.02 Unit: months "mean difference"
Holton, 2011[14]	Lung function tests	Arm A: Control (standard practice)	Arm B: Spirometry training	153	225	NR	Patients who had spirometry performed in the previous 6 months	NR	12	Risk ratio: 0.91, 95%CI: 0.37,2.28
Holton, 2011[14]	Lung function tests	Arm A: Control (standard practice)	Arm B: Spirometry training	119	171	290	Post-bronchodilator FEV_1/FVC ratio (mean)	NR	12	Risk difference: -0.01 95%CI: -0.03,0.02 Unit: months "mean difference"
Holton, 2011[14]	Lung function tests	Arm A: Control (standard practice)	Arm B: Spirometry training	153	225	NR	Patients who had spirometry performed in the previous 6 months	NR	12	Risk ratio: 0.91, 95%CI: 0.37,2.28, Unit: months

Study	Outcome	Arm A		Arm B		Outcome description	Range	Months	Results
Holton,20 11[14]	Missed days of work	Arm A: Control (standard practice)	129	Arm B: Spirometry training	194	days off work due to asthma ("at least 1 day in the last 4 weeks")	NR	12	Risk ratio: 1.52 95%CI: 0.91,2.54 Unit: months "rate ratio"
Holton,20 11[14]	Missed days of work	Arm A: Control (standard practice)	129	Arm B: Spirometry training	194	days off work due to asthma ("at least 1 day in the last 4 weeks")	NR	12	Risk ratio: 1.52 95%CI: 0.91,2.54 Unit: months "rate ratio"
Holton,20 11[14]	Patient perceptions	Arm A: Control (standard practice)	129	Arm B: Spirometry training	194	Patient rating of acceptability of spirometry (mean; max 10)	0-10	12	Risk difference: -0.1, 95%CI: -0.55,0.34, Unit: months "mean difference"
Holton,20 11[14]	Patient perceptions	Arm A: Control (standard practice)	129	Arm B: Spirometry training	194	Patient rating of usefulness of spirometry (mean; max 10)	0-10	12	Risk difference: 0.14, 95%CI: -0.39,0.68, Unit: months "mean difference"
Holton,20 11[14]	Quality of Life	Arm A: Control (standard practice)	129	Arm B: Spirometry training	194	Asthma Quality of Life-TOTAL SCORE	NR	12	Risk difference: -0.23 95%CI: -0.44,-0.01, Unit: months "mean difference"
Holton,20 11[14]	Symptom Days	Arm A: Control (standard practice)	129	Arm B: Spirometry training	194	exacerbations (at least 1 in the last 4 weeks)	NR	12	Risk ratio: 1.09 95%CI: 0.85,1.41 Unit: months "rate ratio"
Holton,20 11[14]	Symptom Days	Arm A: Control (standard practice)	129	Arm B: Spirometry training	194	asthma on waking (at least 1 night in the last 4 weeks)	NR	12	Risk ratio: 1.21 95%CI: 0.79,1.85 Unit: months "rate ratio"

Study	Outcome	Arm A	Arm B				Measure			Result
Holton,2011[14]	Symptom Days	Arm A: Control (standard practice)	Arm B: Spirometry training	129	194	323	nocturnal asthma (at least 1 night in the last 4 weeks)	NR	12	Risk ratio: 0.98 95%CI: 0.63, 1.51 Unit: months "rate ratio"
Kattan,2006[15]	Missed days of school	Arm A: Control (standard practice)	Arm B: Decision support	463	466	929	Mean # days per two weeks	NR	NR	p-value: 0.38
Kattan,2006[15]	Symptom days	Arm A: Control (standard practice)	Arm B: Decision support	463	466	929	Mean # per two weeks	NR	NR	p-value: 0.54
McCowan,2001[7]	Emergency department visits	Arm A: Control (standard practice)	Arm B: Decision support	330	147	NR	Accident and emergency	NR	NR	Odds ratio: 0, 95%CI: (0,9.16)
McCowan,2001[7]	Hospitalizations	Arm A: Control (standard practice)	Arm B: Decision support	330	147	NR	Admissions	NR	NR	Odds ratio: 0, 95%CI: (0,3.44)
McCowan,2001[7]	Rescue use of short-acting B2 agonists	Arm A: Control (standard practice)	Arm B: Decision support	330	147	NR	Received emergency nebulisations	NR	NR	Odds ratio: 0.13, 95%CI: (0.01,0.91)
Mitchell,2005[8]	Emergency department visits	Arm A: Control	Arm B: Decisioon support	NR	NR	104501	# of attendance per person week x10^5	NR	NR	p-value:0.3
Mitchell,2005[8]	Hospitalizations	Arm A: Control	Arm B: Decisioon support	NR	NR	104501	# of admissions per person week x 10^5	NR	NR	p-value: 0.7
Premaratne,1999[1]	Quality of Life	Arm A: Control	Arm B: Education	NR	NR	NR	Mean square root quality of life	NR	NR	Risk difference: - 0.003

Study	Outcome	Arm A	Arm B			Outcome measure			Results
9									p-value: 0.96 95%CI: -0.121,0.115
Renzi,2006[9]	Emergency department visits	Arm A: Group 4 (Standard practice)	Arm B (Group 1: Education), C (Group 2: Education) and D (Group 3: Education)	222	1390	NR	NR	NR	p-value: 0.009
Renzi,2006[9]	Hospitalizations	Arm A: Group 4 (Standard practice)	Arm B (Group 1: Education), C (Group 2: Education) and D (Group 3: Education)	222	1390	NR	NR	NR	p-value: 0.09
Ruoff,2002[10]	Emergency department visits	Arm A: Before the Flow Sheet	After implementation of the Flow Sheet	122	122	Emergency room visits	NR	NR	p-value: <0.0001
Ruoff,2002[10]	Hospitalizations	Arm A: Before the Flow Sheet	After implementation of the Flow Sheet	122	122	Hospitalizations	NR	NR	p-value: <0.0001
Ruoff,2002[10]	Missed days of work	Arm A: Before the Flow Sheet	After implementation of the Flow Sheet	122	122	Days of school/work missed	NR	NR	p-value: <0.0001
Smeele,1999[18]	Prescriptions for controller medicine	Arm A- Control	Arm B- Education	15	30	Exacerbations: Prescription of inhaled steroids	NR	NR	Risk difference: 14 p-value: 0.1 95%CI: -4% to32%
Smeele,1999[18]	Self-management education	Arm A- Control	Arm B- Education	17	33	Advise on house dust mite	NR	NR	Risk difference p-value: 0.1 95%CI: -16%to 2%
Weinberger,2002[11]	Emergency department visits	Arm A: Usual Care Control Group	Arm C: Education, Feedback, pay-for-performance	246	602	Hospital or emergency department visit in past month (admission)	NR	12	Odds ratio: 1.08 95%CI: 0.93,1.2
Weinberger,2002[11]	Emergency department visits	Arm B: Peak Flow Meter Monitoring Control	Arm C: Education, Feedback, pay-for-performance	296	652	Hospital or emergency department visit in past month (admission)	NR	12	Odds ratio 2.16 95%CI: 1.76,2.6

References

1. Bryce FP, Neville RG, Crombie IK, Clark RA, McKenzie P. British Medical Journal: Controlled trial of an audit facilitator in diagnosis and treatment of childhood asthma in general practice. 1995; 310:838-42.

2. Cabana MD, Slish KK, Evans D *et al.* Pediatrics: Impact of physician asthma care education on patient outcomes. 2006; 117:2149-57.

3. Clark N, Gong M, Schork M, et al . Impact of education for physicians on patient outcomes. Pediatrics 1998; 101(5):831-6.

4. Coleman CI, Reddy P, Laster-Bradley NM, Dorval S, Munagala B, White CM. Ann Pharmacother: Effect of practitioner education on adherence to asthma treatment guidelines. 2003; 37:956-61.

5. Glasgow NJ, Ponsonby AL, Yates R, Beilby J, Dugdale P. BMJ: Proactive asthma care in childhood: general practice based randomised controlled trial. 2003; 327:659.

6. Halterman JS, McConnochie KM, Conn KM *et al.* Archives of Pediatrics and Adolescent Medicine: A randomized trial of primary care provider prompting to enhance preventive asthma therapy. 2005; 159:422-7.

7. McCowan C, Neville RG, Ricketts IW, Warner FC, Hoskins G, Thomas GE. Medical Informatics and the Internet in Medicine: Lessons from a randomized controlled trial designed to evaluate computer decision support software to improve the management of

asthma. 2001; 26:191-201.

8. Mitchell EA, Didsbury PB, Kruithof N *et al.* Acta Paediatr: A randomized controlled trial of an asthma clinical pathway for children in general practice. 2005; 94:226-33.

9. Renzi PM, Ghezzo H, Goulet S, Dorval E, Thivierge RL. Can Respir J: Paper stamp checklist tool enhances asthma guidelines knowledge and implementation by primary care physicians. 2006; 13:193-7.

10. Ruoff G. Family Medicine: Effects of flow sheet implementation on physician performance in the management of asthmatic patients. 2002; 34:514-7.

11. Weinberger M , Murray MD, Marrero DG *et al.* Journal of the American Medical Association: Effectiveness of pharmacist care for patients with reactive airways disease: A randomized controlled trial. 2002; 288:1594-602.

12. Armour C, Bosnic-Anticevich S, Brillant M *et al.* Thorax: Pharmacy Asthma Care Program (PACP) improves outcomes for patients in the community. 2007; 62:496-502.

13. Bell LM, Grundmeier R, Localio R *et al.* Pediatrics: Electronic health record-based decision support to improve asthma care: a cluster-randomized trial. 2010; 125:e770-7.

14. Holton C, Crockett A, Nelson M *et al.* International Journal for

FEV = Forced Expiratory Volume; FVC = Forced Vital Capacity: NR = Not Reported;

	Group				

and peer review improve care for patients with asthma/chronic obstructive pulmonary disease? 1999; 8:92-8.

19. Premaratne UN, Sterne JA, Marks GB, Webb JR, Azima H, Burney PG. BMJ: Clustered randomised trial of an intervention to improve the management of asthma: Greenwich asthma study. 1999; 318:1251-5.

20. Lob SH, Boer JH, Porter PG, et al. Promoting Best-Care Practices in Childhood Asthma: Quality Improvement in Community Health Centers. Pediatrics 2011;128;20; Originally Published Online June 13, 2011; DOI: 10.1542/Peds.2010-1962.

21. Fox P, Porter PG, Lob SH, et al. Pediatrics: Improving asthma-related health outcomes among low-income, multiethnic, school-aged children: Results of a demonstration project that combined continuous quality improvement and community health worker strategies2007; 120e902-e911

Quality in Health Care: Does spirometry training in general practice improve quality and outcomes of asthma care? 2011; 23:545-53.

15. Kattan M, Crain EF, Steinbach S et al. Pediatrics: A randomized clinical trial of clinician feedback to improve quality of care for inner-city children with asthma. 2006; 117:e1095-103.

16. Mangione-Smith R, Schonlau M, Chan KS et al. Ambulatory Pediatrics: Measuring the effectiveness of a collaborative for quality improvement in pediatric asthma care: Does implementing the chronic care model improve process and outcomes of care? 2005; 5:75-82.

17. Baker R, Fraser RC, Stone M, Lambert P, Stevenson K, Shiels C. Br J Gen Pract: Randomised controlled trial of the impact of guidelines, prioritized review criteria and feedback on implementation of recommendations for angina and asthma. 2003; 53:284-91.

18. Smeele IJ, Grol RP, van Schayck CP, van den Bosch WJ, van den Hoogen HJ, Muris JW. Qual Health Care: Can small group education

Evidence Table 8. Mean difference between groups- Healthcare process outcomes

Author, Year	Healthcare Process Outcomes	Arm	Comparison Arm	Total N in Arm A	Total N in Comparison Arm	Total N in both Arms	Definition of Scale	Time	Statistical comparison (OR, RR, RD, HR P value 95% CI)
Baker,2003[12]	Self-management education	Arm A- Guidelines only	NR	NR	NR	NR	patient's inhaler technique has been checked and recorded	NR	p-value: 0.56 Generalized Wald tests
Baker,2003[12]	Environmental control practice recommendations	Arm A- Guidelines only	NR	NR	NR	NR	patients have been advised to avoid passive smoking	NR	p-value: 0.72 Generalized Wald tests
Baker,2003[12]	Environmental control practice recommendations	Arm A- Guidelines only	NR	NR	NR	NR	patient's current smoking status has been established and recorded (past 12 months)	NR	p-value: 0.74 Generalized Wald tests
Baker,2003[12]	Prescriptins for controller medicines	Arm A- Guidelines only	NR	NR	NR	NR	Patients have been treated with cheapest inhaled corticosteroid	NR	P-value: 0.044 Generalized Wald tests
Bell,2009[7]	Prescriptions for controller medicine	Arm A-UP control	Arm B-UP intervention	1328	1205	NR	Controller medication prescribed	NR	p-value: 0.006
Bryce,1995[10]	Prescriptions for controller medicine	Arm A- Control	Arm B- Physician Asthma Care Education (PACE)	1563	1585	NR	Bronchodilators Inhaled	NR	Risk ratio: 1.16 95%CI: 0.93,1.45
Bryce,1995[10]	Prescriptions for controller medicine	Arm A- Control	Arm B- Physician Asthma Care Education (PACE)	1563	1585	NR	Bronchodilators Oral	NR	Risk ratio: 1.43 95%CI: 1.06,1.94
Bryce,1995[10]	Prescriptions for controller medicine	Arm A- Control	Arm B- Physician Asthma Care Education (PACE)	1563	1585	NR	Prophylactic agents Cromoglycae	NR	Risk ratio: 1.52 95%CI: 1.02,2.25
Bryce,1995[10]	Prescriptions for controller medicine	Arm A- Control	Arm B- Physician Asthma Care Education (PACE)	1563	1585	NR	Prophylactic agents: Inhaled steroids	NR	Risk ratio: 1.02 95%CI: 0.71,1.47

E-181

Author, Year	Healthcare Process Outcomes	Arm	Comparison Arm	Total N in Arm A	Total N in Comparison Arm	Total N in both Arms	Definition of Scale	Time	Statistical comparison (OR, RR, RD, HR P value 95% CI)
Bryce, 1995[10]	Prescriptions for controller medicine	Arm A-Control	Arm B-Physician Asthma Care Education (PACE)	1563	1585	NR	Peak flow meters	NR	Risk ratio: 1.99 95%CI: 0.86,4.60
Clark,1998[5]	Follow-up visits	Arm A-Control	Arm B-Education	NR	NR	NR	Visits/patient	NR	p-value: .018
Clark,1998[5]	Asthma action plans	Arm A-Control	Arm B-Education	NR	NR	NR	NR	NR	Odds ratio: 1.74 p-value: .03
Clark,1998[5]	Follow-up visits	Arm A-Control	Arm B-Education	NR	NR	NR	Scheduled	NR	p-value: .005
Clark,1998[5]	Follow-up visits	Arm A-Control	Arm B-Education	NR	NR	NR	After an episode of symptoms	NR	p-value: .005
Cloutier M.M.,2012[21]	Asthma action plan	Arm A-Control	Arm B-Physician-directed intervention	34	36	70	NR	NR	No difference in use or creation of asthma action plan.
Cloutier M.M.,2012[21]	Prescription of controller medicine	Arm A-Control	Arm B-Physician-directed intervention	34	36	70	NR	NR	No difference in anti-inflammatory use.
Coleman, 2003[13]	Prescription of peak flow meter	Arm A-Patient specific information: Prescribers with patients on 'high dose'	Arm B: Patient specific information: Prescribers with patients cn 'low dose'	510	135	645	NR	6	p-value: 0.607 Unit: months
Daniels,2005[19]	Asthma action plan	Arm A-Control (standard practice)	Arm B-Education	136079	90555	222634	z	NR	Z=0.17
Daniels,20	Prescriptions for	Arm A-	Arm B-	136079	90555	222634	Z	NR	Z=0.006*

Author, Year	Healthcare Process Outcomes	Arm	Comparison Arm	Total N in Arm A	Total N in Comparison Arm	Total N in both Arms	Definition of Scale	Time	Statistical comparison (OR, RR, RD, HR P value 95% CI)
05[19]	peak flow meter	Control (standard practice)	Education						
Daniels,2005[19]	NR	Arm A- Control (standard practice)	Arm B- Education	136079	90555	222634	Z	NR	Z=0.30
Daniels,2005[19]	Prescriptions for medicine	Arm A- Control (standard practice)	Arm B- Education	136079	90555	222634	Z	NR	Z=0.63
Daniels,2005[19]	Follow-up visits	Arm A- Control (standard practice)	Arm B- Education	136079	90555	222634	Z	NR	Z=0.24
Glasgow,2003[16]	Asthma action plans	Arm A	Arm B- Decision support	73	71	NR	Have a written asthma action plan	NR	Odds ratio: 2.2 p-value: 0.01 95% CI: 1.2,4.1
Glasgow,2003[16]	Prescriptions for controller medicine	Arm A	Arm B- Decision support	71	95	NR	Uses nebuliser	NR	Odds ratio: 0.5 p-value: 0.09 95%CI: 0.2,1.1
Halterman,2005[3]	Prescriptions for controller medicine	Arm A- Control (standard practice)	Arm B	77	73	150	NR	NR	p-value: 0.57
Halterman,2005[3]	Prescriptions for controller medicine	Arm A- Control (standard practice)	Arm B	77	73	150	NR	NR	Odds ratio: 0.78 p-value: 0.62
Halterman,2006[2]	Asthma action plans	Arm A- Control (standard practice)	Arm B	114	112	226	NR	NR	Odds ratio: 4 p-value: <0.001 95%CI: 2.1,7.8
Halterman,2006[2]	Prescriptions for controller medicine	Arm A- Control (standard	Arm B	114	112	226	NR	NR	Odds ratio: 1.6 p-value: 0.12 95%CI: 0.9,3.0

Author, Year	Healthcare Process Outcomes	Arm	Comparison Arm	Total N in Arm A	Total N in Comparison Arm	Total N in both Arms	Definition of Scale	Time	Statistical comparison (OR, RR, RD, HR P value 95% CI)
		practice)							
Holton,2011[4]	Asthma action plans	Arm A- Control	Arm B- Spirometry training	153	225	378	Written asthma action plan prepared or revised in the previous 6 months	12	Unit: months
Hoskins,1997[1]	Prescriptions for controller medicine	Arm A- Before intervention	Arm B- Education and feedback	272	268	NR	NR	NR	Odds ratio: 0.8 95%CI: 0.64,0.99
Hoskins,1997[1]	Prescriptions for controller medicine	Arm A- Before intervention	Arm B- Education and feedback	563	506	NR	NR	NR	Odds ratio: 0.83 95%CI: 0.65,1.06
Hoskins,1997[1]	Prescriptions for controller medicine	Arm A- Before intervention	Arm B- Education and feedback	402	382	NR	NR	NR	Odds ratio 0.7995 95%CI: 0.64,0.98
Kattan,2006[18]	Follow-up visits	Arm A- Control (standard practice)	Arm B- Decision support	463	466	929	# of visits per year	NR	P-value: 0.14
Mangione-Smith,2005[8]	Asthma action plans	Arm A- Control (standard practice)	Arm B- Learning collaborative	348	153	NR	All patients should have a written action plan in the medical record that is based on changes in symptoms or peak flow measurements	NR	Risk difference: 33 p-value: <0.0001
Mangione-Smith,2005[8]	Self-management education	Arm A- Control (standard practice)	Arm B- Learning collaborative	348	153	NR	Patients should be educated in self-management of asthma	NR	Risk difference: 21 p-value: <0.0001
Mangione-Smith,2005[8]	Follow up visits	Arm A - Intervention	Arm A - Control	348	153		Patients whose asthma medications are changed during one visit should have a follow up visit within 6 weeks		Risk difference: -4, p-value: 0.64
Mangione-	Follow up visits	Arm A -	Arm A -	348	153	NR	Patients with asthma		Risk difference: 15, p-

E-184

Author, Year	Healthcare Process Outcomes	Arm	Comparison Arm	Total N in Arm A	Total N in Comparison Arm	Total N in both Arms	Definition of Scale	Time	Statistical comparison (OR, RR, RD, HR P value 95% CI)
Smith,2005[8]		Intervention	Control				should have at least two routine follow up visits annually		value: 0.004
McGowan, 2001[11]	Prescription of peak flow meter	Arm A- Control (standard practice)	Arm B- Decision support	330	147	NR	Issued peak flow meter	NR	Odds ratio: 1.52, 95%CI: (0.58–4.01)
Mitchell,2005[20]	Prescriptions for controller medicine	Arm A- Control (standard practice)	Arm B- Decision support	NR	NR	104501	% decrease in # of inhaled corticosteroids	NR	p-value: 0.4
Mitchell,2005[20]	Prescriptions for controller medicine	Arm A- Control (standard practice)	Arm B- Decision support	NR	NR	104501	% decrease in the # of inhalers relievers prescribed	NR	Other:0.2
Mitchell,2005[20]	Prescriptions for controller medicine	Arm A- Control (standard practice)	Arm B- Decision support	NR	NR	104501	% decrease in oral relievers prescribed	NR	p-value: <0.001
Mitchell,2005[20]	Prescriptions for controller medicine	Arm A- Control (standard practice)	Arm B- Decision support	NR	NR	104501	% decrease in Rx's for reliever dry powder	NR	p-value:0.3
Mitchell,2005[20]	Prescriptions for controller medicine	Arm A- Control (standard practice)	Arm B- Decision support	NR	NR	104501	% decrease of # Rx's for mast cell stabilizers	NR	p-value:0.5
Mitchell,2005[20]	Prescriptions for controller medicine	Arm A- Control (standard practice)	Arm B- Decision support	NR	NR	104501	% decrease in # of Rx's for the theophylline group of drugs	NR	p-value:0.3
Premaratne,1999[15]	Prescriptions for controller medicine	Arm A- Control	Arm B- Education	870	627	NR	Possession of steroid inhaler	NR	Odds ratio: 1.07 95%CI: 0.87-1.31
Premaratne,1999[15]	Prescriptions for controller medicine	Arm A- Control	Arm B- Education	880	623	NR	Possession of peak flow meter	NR	Odds ratio: 0.78 95%CI: 0.49-1.24
Premaratn	Prescriptions for	Arm A-	Arm B-	869	628	NR	Explanation of appropriate	NR	Odds ratio: 0.81

Author, Year	Healthcare Process Outcomes	Arm	Comparison Arm	Total N in Arm A	Total N in Comparison Arm	Total N in both Arms	Definition of Scale	Time	Statistical comparison (OR, RR, RD, HR P value 95% CI)
e, 1999[15]	controller medicine	Control	Education				actions if asthma symptoms worsen		95%CI: 0.64-1.01
Ruoff, 2002[6]	Self-management education	Arm A-Before the flow sheet	Arm B-After implementation of the flow sheet	122	122	NR	Flow meter education	NR	p-value: <.0001
Ruoff, 2002[6]	Self-management education	Arm A-Before the flow sheet	Arm B-After implementation of the flow sheet	122	122	NR	Inhaler technique education	NR	p-value: <.0001
Ruoff, 2002[6]	Prescription of peak flow meter	Arm A-Before the flow sheet	Arm B-After implementation of the flow sheet	122	122	NR	Yearly PFT	NR	p-value: <0.0001
Smeele, 1999[14]	Self-management education	Arm B-Control	Arm B-Education	17	17	34	patient education inhalation instruction materials	NR	p-value: 0.4
Smeele, 1999[14]	Self-management education	Arm A-Control	Arm B-Education	17	16	33	Advise on house dust mite	NR	Risk difference p-value: 0.1 95%CI: -16%to 2%
Smeele, 1999[14]	Self-management education	Arm A-Control	Arm B-Education	17	16	33	Written patient education	NR	Risk difference: -1 p-value: 0.8 95%CI: -13%; -11%
Smeele, 1999[14]	Prescriptions for controller medicine	Arm A-Control	Arm B-Education	15	15	30	Exacerbations: prescription of Oral steroids	NR	Risk difference: 5 p-value: 0.7 95%CI: -19%-28%
Smeele, 1999[14]	Prescriptions for controller medicine	Arm A-Control	Arm B-Education	15	15	30	Exacerbations: Prescription of inhaled steroids	NR	Risk difference: 14 p-value: 0.1 95%CI: -4% to32%
Veninga, 1999[7]	Prescriptions for controller medicine	Arm A-Netherlands	NR	12	12	24	Proportion of patients on inhaled cortico-steroids	NR	1.27, p-value: <0.05 effect size
Veninga, 1999[7]	Prescriptions for controller medicine	Arm A-Netherlands	NR	18	18	36	Proportion of patients on inhaled cortico-steroids	NR	0.33 p-value: >=0.05 effect size
Veninga, 1999[7]	Prescriptions for controller medicine	Arm A-Netherlands	NR	16	16	32	Proportion of patients on inhaled cortico-steroids	NR	0.51 p-value: >=0.05 effect

E-186

Author, Year	Healthcare Process Outcomes	Arm	Comparison Arm	Total N in Arm A	Total N in Comparison Arm	Total N in both Arms	Definition of Scale	Time	Statistical comparison (OR, RR, RD, HR P value 95% CI)
									size
Weinberger, 2002[9]	medication compliance	Arm A-Netherlands	Arm C-Norway	246	356	602	% not compliant	12	Odds ratio: 1.09 95%CI: 0.80,1.49

NR = Not Reported; OR = odds ratio; PFT = Pulmonary Function Test; RR = Relative risk

References

1. Hoskins G, Neville RG, Smith B, Clark RA. Health Bull (Edinb): Does participation in distance learning and audit improve the care of patients with acute asthma attacks? The General Practitioners in Asthma Group. 1997; 55:150-5.

2. Halterman JS, Fisher S, Conn KM *et al*. Archives of Pediatrics & Adolescent Medicine: Improved preventive care for asthma: a randomized trial of clinician prompting in pediatric offices. 2006; 160:1018-25.

3. Halterman JS, McConnochie KM, Conn KM *et al*. Archives of Pediatrics and Adolescent Medicine: A randomized trial of primary care provider prompting to enhance preventive asthma therapy. 2005; 159:422-7.

4. Holton C, Crockett A, Nelson M *et al*. International Journal for Quality in Health Care: Does spirometry training in general practice improve quality and outcomes of asthma care? 2011; 23:545-53.

5. Clark Gong M. Schork M. et al.. Impact of education for physicians on patient outcomes. Pediatrics 1998; 101(5):831-6.

6. Ruoff G. Family Medicine: Effects of flow sheet implementation on physician performance in the management of asthmatic patients. 2002; 34:514-7.

7. Veninga CCM, Lagerlv P, Wahlstrom R *et al*. American Journal of Respiratory and Critical Care Medicine: Evaluating an educational intervention to improve the treatment of asthma in four european countries. 1999; 160 :1254-62.

8. Mangione-Smith R, Schonlau M, Chan KS *et al*. Ambulatory Pediatrics: Measuring the effectiveness of a collaborative for quality improvement in pediatric asthma care: Does implementing the chronic care model improve processes and outcomes of care? 2005; 5:75-82.

9. Weinberger M, Murray MD, Marrero DG *et al*. Journal of the American Medical Association: Effectiveness of pharmacist care for patients with reactive airways disease: A randomized controlled trial. 2002; 288:1594-602.

10. Bryce FP, Neville RG, Crombie IK, Clark RA, McKenzie P. British Medical Journal: Controlled trial of an audit facilitator in diagnosis and treatment of childhood asthma in general practice. 1995; 310:838-42.

11. McCowan C, Neville RG, Ricketts IW, Warner FC, Hoskins G,

Thomas GE. Medical Informatics and the Internet in Medicine: Lessons from a randomized controlled trial designed to evaluate computer decision support software to improve the management of asthma. 2001; 26:191-201.

12. Baker R, Fraser RC, Stone M, Lambert P, Stevenson K, Shiels C. Br J Gen Pract: Randomised controlled trial of the impact of guidelines, prioritized review criteria and feedback on implementation of recommendations for angina and asthma. 2003; 53:284-91.

13. Coleman CI, Reddy P, Laster-Bradley NM, Dorval S, Munagala B, White CM. Ann Pharmacother: Effect of practitioner education on adherence to asthma treatment guidelines. 2003; 37:956-61.

14. Smeele IJ, Grol RP, van Schayck CP, van den Bosch WJ, van den Hoogen HJ, Muris JW. Qual Health Care: Can small group education and peer review improve care for patients with asthma/chronic obstructive pulmonary disease? 1999; 8:92-8.

15. Premaratne UN, Sterne JA, Marks GB, Webb JR, Azima H, Burney PG. BMJ: Clustered randomised trial of an intervention to improve the management of asthma: Greenwich asthma study. 1999; 318:1251-5.

16. Glasgow NJ, Ponsonby AL, Yates R, Beilby J, Dugdale P. BMJ: Proactive asthma care in childhood: general practice based randomised controlled trial. 2003; 327:659.

17. Bell LM, Grundmeier R, Localio R et al. Pediatrics: Electronic health record-based decision support to improve asthma care: a cluster-randomized trial. 2010; 125:e770-7.

18. Kattan M, Crain EF, Steinbach S et al. Pediatrics: A randomized clinical trial of clinician feedback to improve quality of care for inner-city children with asthma. 2006; 117:e1095-103.

19. Daniels EC, Bacon J, Denisio S et al. J Asthma: Translation squared:

improving asthma care for high-disparity populations through a safety net practice-based research network. 2005; 42:499-505.

20. Mitchell EA, Didsbury PB, Kruithof N et al. Acta Paediatr: A randomized controlled trial of an asthma clinical pathway for children in general practice. 2005; 94:226-33.

21. Cloutier MM, Tennen H, Wakefield DB, et al. Improving clinician self-efficacy does not increase asthma guideline use by primary care clinicians. Acad. Pediatr. 2012; 12(4):312-318; ISSN: 1876-2859. 1876-2867.

Evidence Table 9. Mean difference within groups- Clinical outcomes

Author, Year	Arm, N	Clinical Outcome	Definition of Scale	Range of Scale	End of treatment Mean difference • SD • 95% CI • P-value	Last Follow-up Mean difference • SD • 95% CI • P-value	Additional Comments
Baker,2003[15]	Arm A: Guidelines only	Patient perceptions	Patients are satisfied with explanations given by the doctor about asthma	NR	NR	NR	Generalized Wald tests were used to calculate P-values for differences between the interventions after adjustment
Baker,2003[15]	Arm B: Guidelines with audit criteria	Patient perceptions	Patients are satisfied with explanations given by the doctor about asthma	NR	NR	NR	Generalized Wald tests were used to calculate P-values for differences between the interventions after adjustment
Baker,2003[15]	Arm C: Guidelines with audit criteria and feedback	Patient perceptions	Patients are satisfied with explanations given by the doctor about asthma	NR	NR	NR	Generalized Wald tests were used to calculate P-values for differences between the interventions after adjustment
Baker,2003[15]	Arm B: Guidelines with audit criteria	Patient perceptions		NR	NR	NR	NR
Baker,2003[15]	Arm C: Guidelines with audit criteria and feedback	Patient perceptions	NR	NR	NR	NR	NR
Blackstien-Hirsch,2000[16]	Education, 11	Quality of Life	NR	NR	Time: 6 Mean diff: 1.8	Time: 6 Mean diff: 1.8	quality of life activity subscale (ages 7-9 years); SE 0.30; P-
Blackstien-Hirsch,2000[16]	Education, 11	Quality of Life	NR	NR	Time: 6 Mean diff: 0.9	Time: 6 Mean diff: 0.9	quality of life symptoms subscale (ages 7-9 years); SE=0.31 P-
Blackstien-Hirsch,2000[16]	Education, 123	Quality of Life	NR	NR	Time: 6 Mean diff: 0.42 p-value: <0.001	Time: 6 Mean diff: 0.42 p-value: <0.001	quality of life symptoms subscore, ages 10+ years; SE= 0.10
Blackstien-Hirsch,2000[16]	Education, 123	Quality of Life	NR	NR	Time: 6 Mean diff: 0.4 p-value: <0.001	Time: 6 Mean diff: 0.4 p-value: <0.001	quality of life emotions subscore, ages 10+; SE =0.10

E-189

Author, Year	Arm, N	Clinical Outcome	Definition of Scale	Range of Scale	End of treatment Mean difference • SD • 95% CI • P-value	Last Follow-up Mean difference • SD • 95% CI • P-value	Additional Comments
Blackstien-Hirsch,2000[16]	Education, 11	Quality of Life	NR	NR	Time: 6 Mean diff. 1.23	Time: 6 Mean diff. 1.23	quality of life emotions subscale (ages 7-9 years) SE=0.40 P-
Blackstien-Hirsch,2000[16]	Education, 123	Quality of Life	NR	NR	Time: 6 Mean diff. 0.12 p-value: 0.20	Time: 6 Mean diff. 0.12 p-value: 0.20	quality of life, environment, ages 10+; SE=0.10
Blackstien-Hirsch,2000[16]	Education, 123	Quality of Life	NR	NR	Time: 6 Mean diff. 0.28 p-value: 0.001	Time: 6 Mean diff. 0.28 p-value: 0.001	quality of life activity subscale, ages 10+; SE 0.08
Blackstien-Hirsch,2000[16]	Education, 11	Quality of Life	NR	NR	Time: 6 Mean diff. 1.19	Time: 6 Mean diff. 1.19	quality of life overall subscale (ages 7-9 years) SE=1.19 P-
Blackstien-Hirsch,2000[16]	Education, 123	Quality of Life	NR	NR	Time: 6 Mean diff. 0.33 p-value: <0.001	Time: 6 Mean diff. 0.33 p-value: <0.001	quality of life subscale, overall (ages 10+); SE=0.08
Cabana,2006[1]	Arm A-Control (standard practice), 368	Emergency department visits	Mean # ED visits per year	NR	NR	Time: 12 Mean diff. -0.3	Mean # ED visits per year
Cabana,2006[1]	Arm B-Physician Asthma Care Education (PACE), 363	Emergency department visits	Mean # ED visits per year	NR	NR	Time: 12 Mean diff. -0.55	Mean # ED visits per year
Cabana,2006[1]	Arm C-	Emergency department visits	Mean # ED visits per year	NR	NR	NR	Mean # ED visits per year
Cabana,2006[1]	Arm A-Control (standard practice), 368	Hospitalizations	mean # per year	NR	NR	Time: 12 Mean diff. -0.06	*OUTCOME: Mean hospitalizations for asthma per year.
Cabana,2006[1]	Arm B-Physician Asthma Care Education (PACE),, 363	Hospitalizations	mean # per year	NR	NR	Time: 12 Mean diff. -0.06	*OUTCOME: Mean hospitalizations for asthma per year.
Cabana,2006[1]	Arm C-	Hospitalizations	mean # per year	NR	NR	NR	*OUTCOME: Mean hospitalizations for asthma per year.
Cabana,2006[1]	Arm A-Control	Symptom Days	Change in # of days	NR	NR	Time: 12	OUTCOME: Change in

Author, Year	Arm, N	Clinical Outcome	Definition of Scale	Range of Scale	End of treatment Mean difference • SD • 95% CI • P-value	Last Follow-up Mean difference • SD • 95% CI • P-value	Additional Comments
	(standard practice), 368					Mean diff: -8.5	number of days for which activity was limited by asthma
Cabana,2006[1]	Arm B- Physician Asthma Care Education (PACE),, 363	Symptom Days	Change in # of days	NR	NR	Time: 12 Mean diff: -15.6 SD diff: NR 95%CI: NR p-value: NR	OUTCOME: Change in number of days for which activity was limited by asthma
Cabana,2006[1]	Arm C-	Symptom Days	Change in # of days	NR	NR	NR	OUTCOME: Change in number of days for which activity was limited by asthma
Cabana,2006[1]	Arm A-Control (standard practice), 368	urgent doctor visits	Change in Mean # visits per year	NR	NR	Time: 12 Mean diff: -0.9	OUTCOME: Mean # urgent asthma office visits per year
Cabana,2006[1]	Arm B- Intervention, 363	urgent doctor visits	Change in Mean # visits per year	NR	NR	Time: 12 Mean diff: -1.07	OUTCOME: Mean # urgent asthma office visits per year
Cabana,2006[1]	Arm C-	urgent doctor visits	Change in Mean # visits per year	NR	NR	NR	OUTCOME: Mean # urgent asthma office visits per year
Cloutier, 2005[3]	Arm B-Decision support: intermittent asthma	Emergency department visits	ED visit/child/year	NR	Time: NR 95%CI: 0.799,1.049 p-value: 0.82 Adjusted RR- 0.915	NR	NR
Cloutier, 2005[3]	Arm C-Decision support: persistent asthma, 1799	Emergency department visits	ED visit/child/year	NR	Time: NR 95%CI: 0.776,0.999 p-value: 0.05 Adjusted RR- 0.880	NR	NR
Cloutier, 2005[3]	Arm B- Decision support: intermittent asthma	Hospitalizations	NR	NR	Time: NR 95%CI: 0.453,1.350 p-value: 0.38 Adjusted RR- 0.782	NR	NR
Cloutier, 2005[3]	Arm C-Decision support: persistent asthma, 1799	Hospitalizations	NR	NR	Time: NR 95%CI: 0.454,0.932 p-value: 0.02 Adjusted RR- 0.651	NR	NR
Cloutier, 2009[2]	Decision support	Emergency department visits	NR	NR	p-value: < 0.01 27% decrease	p-value: <0.01 27% decrease	Number of Emergency Department visits per

Author, Year	Arm, N	Clinical Outcome	Definition of Scale	Range of Scale	End of treatment Mean difference • SD • 95% CI • P-value	Last Follow-up Mean difference • SD • 95% CI • P-value	Additional Comments
							100 children per 12 months eligibility. "other" refers to the percentage decrease in overall hospitalization after the Easy Breathing intervention versus pre intervention.
Cloutier, 2009[2]	Decision support	Hospitalizations	NR	NR	p-value: <0.006 35% decrease	p-value: <0.006 35% decrease	Number of hospital visits per 100 children per 12 months eligibility. "other" refers to the percentage decrease in overall hospitalization after the Easy Breathing intervention versus pre intervention.
Finkelstein, 2005[4]	Arm A-Control (standard practice), 1531	Emergency department visits	Unadjusted mean absolute change from baseline	NR	Time: 12 Mean diff: NR	Time: 24 Mean diff: -0.01 95%CI: -0.04, 0.02	1(+) ED/hospitalization
Finkelstein, 2005[4]	Arm B-PLE Intervention, 2003	Emergency department visits	Unadjusted mean absolute change from baseline	NR	Time: 12 Mean diff: NR	Time: 24 Mean diff: -0.01 95%CI: -0.05, 0.03	1(+) ED/hospitalization
Finkelstein, 2005[4]	Arm C-Planned care intervention, 1635	Emergency department visits	Unadjusted mean absolute change from baseline	NR	Time: 12 Mean diff: NR	Time: 24	1(+) ED/hospitalization
Hagmolen, 2008[11]	Arm A-Guidelines only, 98	Lung function tests	PEF variability	NR	NR	Time: 12 Mean diff: -1.3 p-value: 0.05	NR
Hagmolen, 2008[11]	Arm B-Education and guidelines, 133	Lung function tests	PEF variability	NR	NR	Time: 12 Mean diff: -1.7 p-value: <0.001	NR
Hagmolen, 2008[11]	Arm C-Education, guidelines, and individualized	Lung function tests	PEF variability	NR	NR	Time: 12 Mean diff: -1.6 p-value: 0.001	NR

Author, Year	Arm, N	Clinical Outcome	Definition of Scale	Range of Scale	End of treatment Mean difference • SD • 95% CI • P-value	Last Follow-up Mean difference • SD • 95% CI • P-value	Additional Comments
	treatment advice, 131						
Hagmolen,2008[11]	Arm A- Guidelines only, 98	Lung function tests	FEV1 % predicted	0-100	NR	Time: 12 Mean diff: 0.1	NR
Hagmolen,2008[11]	Arm B- Education and guidelines, 133	Lung function tests	FEV1 % predicted	0-100	NR	Time: 12 Mean diff: -1	NR
Hagmolen,2008[11]	Arm C- Education, guidelines, and treatment advice, 131	Lung function tests	FEV1 % predicted	0-100	NR	Time: 12 Mean diff: 0.2	NR
Hagmolen,2008[11]	Arm A- Guidelines only, 58	Symptom Days	Number of symptom free days	0-14	Time: 12 Mean diff: 1.5 p-value: <0.05	NR	P values are less than the stated number (won't allow symbols).
Hagmolen,2008[11]	Arm B- Education and guidelines, 133	Symptom Days	Number of symptom free days	0-14	Time: 12 Mean diff: 1.3 p-value: 0.05	NR	P values are less than the stated number (won't allow symbols).
Hagmolen,2008[11]	Arm C- Education, guidelines, and individual treatment advice, 131	Symptom Days	Number of symptom free days	0-14	Time: 12 Mean diff: 1.9 SD diff: NR 95%CI: NR p-value: 0.001	NR	P values are less than the stated number (won't allow symbols).
Hagmolen,2008[11]	Arm A- Guidelines only, 98	Symptom Score	Total symptom score	0-18	NR	Time: 12 Mean diff: -0.6 p-value: <0.05	The frequency of asthma-related symptoms, cough, wheeze, and shortness of breath were scored twice daily. 0=no complaints 1=once a day 2=more than daily 3= whole daily in a two week diary. P value is < 0.05, won't allow symbols
Hagmolen,2008[11]	Arm B- Education and	Symptom Score	Total symptom score	0-18	NR	Time: 12 Mean diff: -0.3	The frequency of asthma-related

Author, Year	Arm, N	Clinical Outcome	Definition of Scale	Range of Scale	End of treatment Mean difference • SD • 95% CI • P-value	Last Follow-up Mean difference • SD • 95% CI • P-value	Additional Comments
	guidelines, 133						symptoms, cough, wheeze, and shortness of breath were scored twice daily. 0=no complaints 1=once a day 2=more than daily 3= whole daily in a two week diary. P value is < 0.05, won't allow symbols
Hagmolen, 2008[11]	Arm C- Education, guidelines, and individualized treatment advice, 131	Symptom Score	Total symptom score	0-18	NR	Time: 12 Mean diff: -0.5 p-value: 0.05	The frequency of asthma-related symptoms, cough, wheeze, and shortness of breath were scored twice daily. 0=no complaints 1=once a day 2=more than daily 3= whole daily in a two week diary. P value is < 0.05, won't allow symbols
Hagmolen, 2008[11]	Arm A- Guidelines only, 98	Symptom Score	Nocturnal symptom score	NR	NR	Time: 12 Mean diff: -0.24 p-value: <0.05	NR
Hagmolen, 2008[11]	Arm B- Education and guidelines, 133	Symptom Score	Nocturnal symptom score	NR	NR	Time: 12 Mean diff: -0.7	NR
Hagmolen, 2008[11]	Arm C- Education, guidelines, and individualized treatment advice, 131	Symptom Score	Nocturnal symptom score	NR	NR	Time: 12 Mean diff: -0.15 p-value: <0.05	NR
Lesho, 2005[5]	Decision Support	Emergency department visits	NR	NR	Time: NR Mean diff: 0.65 p-value: <0.001	NR	NR
Lesho, 2005[5]	Decision Support, 582	Hospitalizations	NR	NR	Time: NR Mean diff: 0.6	NR	NR

E-194

Author, Year	Arm, N	Clinical Outcome	Definition of Scale	Range of Scale	End of treatment Mean difference • SD • 95% CI • P-value	Last Follow-up Mean difference • SD • 95% CI • P-value	Additional Comments
					p-value: <0.001		
Lesho,2005[5]	Decision support, 334	Lung function tests	NR	NR	Time: NR Mean diff: 0.07 p-value: 0.15	NR	Result reported only for those with persistent asthma
Lesho,2005[5]	Decision Support,334	NR	NR	NR	Time: NR Mean diff: 0.02 p-value: 0.78	NR	Result reported only for those with persistent asthma
Lesho,2005[5]	Decision Support	Rescue use of short-acting B2 agonists	NR	NR	NR Mean diff: 0.54 p-value: <0.001	NR	NR
Lozano,2004[17]	Arm A-Control (standard practice)	Symptom Days	NR	NR	NR	NR	NR
Lozano,2004[17]	Arm B-Peer leader education, 226	Symptom Days	NR	NR	Time: 24 Mean diff: -14.8 95%CI: -22.4,-7.28	NR	NR
Lozano,2004[17]	Arm C-Chronic care model, 213	Symptom Days	NR	NR	Time: 24 Mean diff: -13.3 95%CI: -24.7,-2.1	NR	NR
Mitchell,2005[6]	Arm A-Control (standard practice)	Emergency department visits	Percent decrease in the number of attendances at Children's ED per person week x 10^ 5 (95% confidence intervals)	NR	Time: 9 Mean diff: NR SD diff: 9.99E+02 30%	NR	Percent decrease in the number of attendances at Children's ED per person week x 10^ 5 (95% confidence intervals)
Mitchell,2005[6]	Arm B-Decision support	Emergency department visits	Percent decrease in the number of attendances at Children's ED per person week x 10^ 5 (95% confidence intervals)	NR	Time: 9 Mean diff: NR 25% decrease	NR	Percent decrease in the number of attendances at Children's ED per person week x 10^ 5 (95% confidence intervals)
Mitchell,2005[6]	Arm A-Control (standard practice)	Hospitalizations	Percent decrease in the number of admissions per person week x 10^ 5 (95% confidence intervals)	NR	Time: 9 33% decrease	NR	% decrease in the number of admissions per person week x 10^ 5 (95% confidence intervals)

Author, Year	Arm, N	Clinical Outcome	Definition of Scale	Range of Scale	End of treatment Mean difference • SD • 95% CI • P-value	Last Follow-up Mean difference • SD • 95% CI • P-value	Additional Comments
Mitchell, 2005[6]	Arm B-Decision support	Hospitalizations	Percent decrease in the number of admissions per person week x 10^5 (95% confidence intervals)	NR	Time: 9 40% decrease	NR	% decrease in the number of admissions per person week x 10^5 (95% confidence intervals)
Mitchell, 2005[6]	Arm C-	Hospitalizations	Percent decrease in the number of admissions per person week x 10^5 (95% confidence intervals)	NR	NR	NR	% decrease in the number of admissions per person week x 10^5 (95% confidence intervals)
O'Laughlen, 2008[12]	MSAGR group, 24	Lung function tests	FEV1	NR	NR	NR	p = 0.01 : p value for test of trends
O'Laughlen, 2008[12]	MSAGR group,24	Quality of Life	Physical health of child	NR	NR	NR	p < 0.01 difference between base line and las follow up
O'Laughlen, 2008[12]	MSAGR, 24	Quality of Life	Activity of child1	NR	NR	NR	p = 0.78: difference between baseline and last follow up
O'Laughlen, 2008[12]	MSAGR, 24	Quality of Life	Activity of family	NR	NR	NR	p = 0.01; diff btw baseline and last follow up
O'Laughlen, 2008[12]	MSAGR, 24	Quality of Life	Emotional health of child	NR	NR	NR	p = 0.06; diff btw baseline and last follow up
O'Laughlen, 2008[12]	MSAGR, 24	Quality of Life	Emotional health of family	NR	NR	NR	p = 0.13; diff btw baseline and last follow up
Patel, 2004[7]	Organizational Change, 427	Emergency department visits	Visits/1000 population		Time: 13 Mean diff.: -0.41 p-value: <0.001	NR	NR
Patel, 2004[7]	Organizational change, 427	Hospitalizations	Hospitalization/1000 population	NR	Time: 13 Mean diff.: -0.54 p-value: <0.001	NR	NR
Saini, 2004[13]	Arm C- Education	NR	NR	NR	NR	p-value: <0.001	NR
Shapiro, 2011[9]	SBHC, 200	Hospitalizations	NR	NR	Time: 12 p-value: <0.001	NR	NR

E-196

Author, Year	Arm, N	Clinical Outcome	Definition of Scale	Range of Scale	End of treatment Mean difference • SD • 95% CI • P-value	Last Follow-up Mean difference • SD • 95% CI • P-value	Additional Comments
Shapiro, 2011[9]	NYCHP, 249	Hospitalizations	NR	NR	Time: 12 p-value: <0.001	NR	NR
Suh, 2001[8]	Arm A-intermittent, 566	Emergency department visits	mean number of ED visits per patient	NR	Time: 9 Intermittent Mean diff: 0.06 95% CI: 0.04,0.09 p-value: 0.001	NR	P for intermittent and persistent less than value in cell
Suh, 2001[8]	Arm B-persistent, 1050	Emergency department visits	mean number of ED visits per patient	NR	Time: 9 Persistent Mean diff: -0.11 95%CI: -0.14, -0.08 p-value: 0.001	NR	P for intermittent and persistent less than value in cell
Suh, 2001[8]	Arm A-intermittent, 566	Hospitalizations	number of hospitalizations per patient	NR	Time: 9 Mean diff: 0.02 95%CI: 0.12,0.03 p-value: 0.001	NR	
Suh, 2001[8]	Arm B-persistent, 1050	Hospitalizations	number of hospitalizations per patient	NR	Time: 9 Mean diff: -0.03 SD diff: NR 95%CI: -0.05,0.02, p-value: 0.003	NR	NR
To, 2008[10]	PCAPP Intervention, 1014	Hospitalizations	NR	NR	NR	Time: 12 95%CI: 0.32–2.03 p-value: p>0.05 OR: 0.80	Hospitalizations in last 6 months (dichotomous outcome).
To, 2008[10]	PCAPP Intervention, 463	Missed days of school	NR	NR	NR	Time: 12 95%CI: 0.25–0.54 OR: 0.37	Lost days of school among children (dichotomous outcome).
To, 2008[10]	PCAPP Intervention, 551	Missed days of work	NR	NR	NR	Time: 12 95%CI: 0.34,0.71 0.49	OUTCOME: Missed days of work among adults (dichotomous outcome).
To, 2008[10]	PCAPP Intervention, 1014	Symptom Days	NR	NR	NR	Time: 12 95%CI: 0.27,0.42 OR: 0.34	OUTCOME: Any uncontrolled daytime symptoms (dichotomous outcome)
To, 2008[10]	PCAPP Intervention, 1014	Symptom Days	NR	NR	NR	Time: 12 95%CI: 0.23,0.37 OR: 0.29	OUTCOME: Any uncontrolled nighttime symptoms

Author, Year	Arm, N	Clinical Outcome	Definition of Scale	Range of Scale	End of treatment Mean difference • SD • 95% CI • P-value	Last Follow-up Mean difference • SD • 95% CI • P-value	Additional Comments
							(dichotomous outcome).
To,2008[10]	PCAPP Intervention, 1014	urgent doctor visits	NR	NR	NR	Time: 12 95%CI: 0.32,0.62 p-value: p<0.0001 OR: 0.45	Any urgent or walk-in clinic visits in last 6 months (dichotomous outcome).

AAP = Asthma Action Plan; CME = Continuing medical education; CLIQ = Clinical Inquiry: DM = Diabetes mellitus; ED = Emergency department; EMR = Electronic Medical Records; ENT = ear nose throat; HCSD = Health Care Services Division; HMO = Health maintenance organization ; ICS = Inhaled Corticosteroids; MD = Medical Doctor; MSAGR = Multicolored, Simplified, Asthma Guideline Reminder; NAEPP = National Asthma Education and Prevention Program; NR = Not reported; NYCHP = New York Children's Health Project; PCAPP = Primary Care Asthma Pilot Project; PDSA = Plan-do-study-act; PEFR = Peak Exploratory Flow Rate; PLE = Peer Leader Education; PPO-FFS = Preferred provider organization – Fee for service; SBHC = South Bronx Health Center; SF = Short-Form ; UP =Urban Practice; SP = Suburban Practice; UTI = Urinary tract infection;

References

1. Cabana MD, Slish KK, Evans D *et al.* Pediatrics: Impact of physician asthma care education on patient outcomes. 2006; 117:2149-57.

2. Cloutier MM, Grosse SD, Wakefield EB, Nurmagambetov TA, Brown CM. American Journal of Managed Care: The economic impact of an urban asthma management program. 2009; 15:345-51.

3. Cloutier MM, Hall CB, Wakefield DB, Bailit H. J Pediatr: Use of asthma guidelines by primary care providers to reduce hospitalizations and emergency department visits in poor, minority, urban children. 2005; 146:591-7.

4. Finkelstein JA, Lozano P, Fuhlbrigge AL *et al.* Health Serv Res: Practice-level effects of interventions to improve asthma care in primary care settings: the Pediatric Asthma Care Patient Outcomes Research Team. 2005; 40:1737-57.

5. Lesho EP, Myers CP, Ott M, Winslow C, Brown JE. Mil Med: Do

6. Mitchell EA, Didsbury PB, Kruithof N *et al.* Acta Paediatr: A randomized controlled trial of an asthma clinical pathway for children in general practice. 2005; 94:226-33.

7. Patel PH, Welsh C, Foggs MB. Dis Manag: Improved asthma outcomes using a coordinated care approach in a large medical group. 2004; 7:102-11.

8. Suh DC, Shin SK, Okpara I, Voytovich RM, Zimmerman A. Am J Manag Care: Impact of a targeted asthma intervention program on treatment costs in patients with asthma. 2001; 7:897-906.

9. Shapiro A, Gracy D, Quinones W, Applebaum J, Sarmiento A. Arch Pediatr Adolesc Med: Putting guidelines into practice: improving documentation of pediatric asthma management using a decision-

clinical practice guidelines improve processes or outcomes in primary care? 2005; 170:243-6.

making tool. 2011; 165:412-8.

10. To T, Cicutto L, Degani N, McLimont S, Beyene J. Med Care: Can a community evidence-based asthma care program improve clinical outcomes?: a longitudinal study. 2008; 46:1257-66.

11. Hagmolen of ten Have W, van den Berg NJ, van der Palen J, van Aalderen WM, Bindels PJ. Prim Care Respir J: Implementation of an asthma guideline for the management of childhood asthma in general practice: a randomised controlled trial. 2008; 17:90-6.

12. O'Laughlen MC, Hollen PJ, Rakes G, Ting S. Pediatric Asthma, Allergy and Immunology: Improving pediatric asthma by the MSAGR algorithm: A multicolored, simplified, asthma guideline reminder. 2008; 21:119-27.

13. Saini B, Krass I, Armour C. Annals of Pharmacotherapy: Development, implementation, and evaluation of a community pharmacy-based asthma care model. 2004; 38:1954-60.

14. Mangione-Smith R, Schonlau M, Chan KS et al. Ambulatory Pediatrics: Measuring the effectiveness of a collaborative for quality improvement in pediatric asthma care: Does implementing the chronic care model improve processes and outcomes of care? 2005; 5:75-82.

15. Baker R, Fraser RC, Stone M, Lambert P, Stevenson K, Shiels C. Br J Gen Pract: Randomised controlled trial of the impact of guidelines, prioritized review criteria and feedback on implementation of recommendations for angina and asthma. 2003; 53:284-91.

16. Blackstien-Hirsch P, Anderson G, Cicutto L, McIvor A, Norton P. Journal of Asthma: Implementing continuing education strategies for family physicians to enhance asthma patients' quality of life. 2000; 37:247-57.

17. Lozano P, Finkelstein JA, Carey VJ et al. Arch Pediatr Adolesc Med: A multisite randomized trial of the effects of physician education and organizational change in chronic-asthma care: health outcomes of the Pediatric Asthma Care Patient Outcomes Research Team II Study. 2004; 158:875-83.

Evidence Table 10. Mean difference within groups- Healthcare process outcomes

Author, Year	Arm, N	Health Care Process Outcome	Definition of Scale	Range of Scale	End of treatment Mean difference • SD • 95% CI • P-value	Last Follow-up Mean difference • SD • 95% CI • P-value	Additional Comments
Ables,2002[6]	Education and Reminders,175	Documentation of level of asthma control/severity	NR	NR	Time: 18 p-value: <0.0001	NR	NR
Bender,201 1[1]	Arm B- Education, Coaching, Toolkit, NR	Asthma action plans	NR	NR	NR	NR	P-value= <0.0001
Bender,201 1[1]	Arm B- Education, Coaching, Toolkit, NR	Prescriptions for controller medicine	NR	NR	NR	NR	P-value= <0.0001
Cho,2010[13]	Decision support, 96	Prescriptions for controller medicine	NR	NR	Time: 3	NR	Mean difference= +86% P value= <0.001
Cloutier,20 05[14]	Arm B- Decision support: intermitten t asthma, NR	Prescriptions for controller medicine	NR	NR	95%CI: 1.7984 - 3.614 p-value:<0.001 Adjusted RR- 2.539	NR	NR
Cloutier,20 05[14]	Arm C- Decision support: persistent asthma, 1799	Prescriptions for controller medicine	NR	NR	95%CI: 1.031 - 1.295 p-value:0.01 Adjusted RR- 1.155	NR	NR
Daniels,200 5[2]	Arm A- Control (standard practice), 136,079	Asthma action plans	Percent increase	NR	NR	-6%	Percent increase from baseline to follow-up between intervention and control groups (compliance from chart audit)

E-200

Author, Year	Arm, N	Health Care Process Outcome	Definition of Scale	Range of Scale	End of treatment Mean difference • SD • 95% CI • P-value	Last Follow-up Mean difference • SD • 95% CI • P-value	Additional Comments
Daniels,200 5[2]	Arm B-Education, 90555	Asthma action plans	Percent increase	NR	-0.07%	NR	Percent Increase from baseline to follow-up between intervention and control groups (compliance from chart audit)
Daniels,200 5[2]	Arm A-Control (standard practice), 136079	Follow-up visits	% increase from baseline	NR	NR	+11%	Percent increase from baseline to follow-up b/w intervention and control groups (compliance from chart audit)
Daniels,200 5[2]	Arm B-Education, 90,555	Follow-up visits	% increase from baseline	NR	NR	+28%	Percent increase from baseline to follow-up b/w intervention and control groups (compliance from chart audit)
Daniels,200 5[2]	Arm A-Control (standard practice), 136,079	Prescription of peak flow meter	% increase	NR	NR	+0.04%	Percent increase from baseline to follow-up b/w intervention and control groups (compliance from chart audit)
Daniels,200 5[2]	Arm B-Education, 90,555	Prescription of peak flow meter	% increase	NR	NR	+11%	Percent increase from baseline to follow-up b/w intervention and control groups (compliance from chart audit)
Daniels,200 5[2]	Arm A-Control (standard practice), 136,079	Prescriptions for controller medicine	% increase from baseline	NR	NR	+9%	Percent increase from baseline to follow-up b/w intervention and control groups (compliance from chart audit)
Daniels,200 5[2]	Arm B-Education, 90,555	Prescriptions for controller medicine	% increase from baseline	NR	NR	+19%	Percent increase from baseline to follow-up b/w intervention and control groups (compliance from chart audit)
Daniels,200 5[2]	Arm A-Control	Self-management	% increase from baseline	NR	NR	+3%	Percent increase from baseline to follow-up b/w

Author, Year	Arm, N	Health Care Process Outcome	Definition of Scale	Range of Scale	End of treatment Mean difference • SD • 95% CI • P-value	Last Follow-up Mean difference • SD • 95% CI • P-value	Additional Comments
	(standard practice), 136079	education					intervention and control groups (compliance from chart audit)
Daniels,200 5[2]	Arm B- Education, 90,555	Self- management education	% increase from baseline	NR	NR	+19%	Percent increase from baseline to follow-up b/w intervention and control groups (compliance from chart audit)
Davis,2004 [15]	Arm A- Guidelines only, 30	Prescriptions for controller medicine	ICS prescriptions/m onth	NR	Mean diff: 9.99E+02	NR	NR
Davis,2004 [15]	Arm B- Education and toolkit, 20	Prescriptions for controller medicine	ICS prescriptions/m onth	NR	Time: 6 p-value: <0.001	NR	NR
Davis,2010 [7]	Decision Support, 180	Documentation of level of asthma control/severity	NR	NR	Time: 180 p-value: 0.0013	NR	NR
Davis,2010 [7]	Decision support, 180	Prescriptions for controller medicine	NR	NR	Time: 18 p-value: 0.017	NR	NR
Finkelstein, 2005[11]	Arm A- Control (standard practice), 1531	Prescriptions for controller medicine	Mean absolute change from baseline Proportional to each practice	NR	Time: 12 Mean diff: NR 95%CI: NR	Time: 24 Mean diff: 0.07 95%CI: -0.01, 0.15	Among all patients with asthma, 1(+) asthma controller dispensed.
Finkelstein, 2005[11]	Arm B- PLE Interventio n, 2003	Prescriptions for controller medicine	Mean absolute change from baseline Proportional to each practice	NR	Time: 12 Mean diff: NR	Time: 24 Mean diff: 0.16 95%CI: 0.08, 0.24	Among all patients with asthma, 1(+) asthma controller dispensed.
Finkelstein, 2005[11]	Arm C- Planned Care Interventio n, 1635	Prescriptions for controller medicine	Mean absolute change from baseline proportional to each practice	NR	Time: 12 Mean diff: NR	Time: 24 Mean diff: 0.13 95%CI: 0.07, 0.19	Among all patients with asthma, 1(+) asthma controller dispensed.
Finkelstein,	Arm A-	Prescriptions for	Mean absolute	NR	Time: 12	Time: 24	Among all patients with

E-202

Author, Year	Arm, N	Health Care Process Outcome	Definition of Scale	Range of Scale	End of treatment Mean difference • SD • 95% CI • P-value	Last Follow-up Mean difference • SD • 95% CI • P-value	Additional Comments
2005[11]	Control (standard practice) 1531	controller medicine	change from baseline proportional to each practice		Mean diff: NR	Mean diff: 0.04 95%CI: -0.02, 0.10	asthma, 3(+) asthma controller dispensed.
Finkelstein, 2005[11]	Arm B-PLE Intervention, 2003	Prescriptions for controller medicine	Mean absolute change from baseline proportional to each practice	NR	Time: 12 Mean diff: NR	Time: 24 Mean diff: 0.08 95%CI: 0.02, 0.14	Among all patients with asthma, 3(+) asthma controller dispensed.
Finkelstein, 2005[11]	Arm C-Planned care intervention, 1635	Prescriptions for controller medicine	Mean absolute change from baseline proportional to each practice	NR	Time: 12 Mean diff: NR	Time: 24 Mean diff: 0.1 95%CI: 0.06, 0.14	Among all patients with asthma, 3(+) asthma controller dispensed.
Finkelstein, 2005[11]	Arm A-Control (standard practice), 1531	Prescriptions for controller medicine	Mean absolute change from baseline proportional to each practice	NR	Time: 12 Mean diff: NR	Time: 24 Mean diff: 0.1 95%CI: 0.00, 0.20	Among all patients with asthma, 1(+) inhaled corticosteroid.
Finkelstein, 2005[11]	Arm B-PLE Intervention, 2003	Prescriptions for controller medicine	Mean absolute change from baseline proportional to each practice	NR	Time: 12 Mean diff: NR	Time: 24 Mean diff: 0.18 95%CI: 0.10, 0.26	Among all patients with asthma, 1(+) inhaled corticosteroid.
Finkelstein, 2005[11]	Arm C-Planned care intervention, 1635	Prescriptions for controller medicine	Mean absolute change from baseline proportional to each practice	NR	Time: 12 Mean diff: NR	Time: 24 Mean diff: 0.17 95%CI: 0.11, 0.23	Among all patients with asthma, 1(+) inhaled corticosteroid.
Finkelstein, 2005[11]	Arm A-Control (standard practice), 1531	Prescriptions for controller medicine	Mean absolute change from baseline proportional to each practice	NR	Time: 12 Mean diff: NR	Time: 24 Mean diff: 0.03 95%CI: -0.03, 0.09	Among all patients with asthma, 3(+) inhaled corticosteroid.
Finkelstein, 2005[11]	Arm B-PLE Intervention, 2003	Prescriptions for controller medicine	Mean absolute change from baseline proportional to	NR	Time: 12 Mean diff: NR	Time: 24 Mean diff: 0.09 95%CI: 0.03, 0.15	Among all patients with asthma, 3(+) inhaled corticosteroid.

Author, Year	Arm, N	Health Care Process Outcome	Definition of Scale	Range of Scale	End of treatment Mean difference • SD • 95% CI • P-value	Last Follow-up Mean difference • SD • 95% CI • P-value	Additional Comments
			each practice				
Finkelstein, 2005[11]	Arm C-Planned care interventio n, 1635	Prescriptions for controller medicine	Mean absolute change from baseline proportional to each practice	NR	Time: 12 Mean diff: NR	Time: 24 Mean diff: 0.09 95%CI: 0.07,0.11	Among all patients with asthma, 3(+) inhaled corticosteroid.
Finkelstein, 2005[11]	Arm A-Control (standard practice), 1531	Prescriptions for controller medicine	Mean absolute change from baseline proportional to each practice	NR	Time: 12 Mean diff: NR	Time: 24 Mean diff: 0.02 95%CI: -0.01, 0.05	Among all patients with asthma, 1(+) oral steroid dispensed.
Finkelstein, 2005[11]	Arm B-PLE Interventio n, 2003	Prescriptions for controller medicine	Mean absolute change from baseline proportional to each practice	NR	Time: 12 Mean diff: NR	Time: 24 Mean diff: 0.05 95%CI: 0.00,0.10	Among all patients with asthma, 1(+) oral steroid dispensed.
Finkelstein, 2005[11]	Arm C-Planned care interventio n, 1635	Prescriptions for controller medicine	Mean absolute change from baseline proportional to each practice	NR	Time: 12 Mean diff: NR	Time: 24 Mean diff: 0.04 95%CI: 0.00, 0.08	Among all patients with asthma, 1(+) oral steroid dispensed.
Finkelstein, 2005[11iii]	Arm A-Control (standard practice), 1531	Follow-up visits	Unadjusted mean absolute change from baseline	NR	Time: 12 Mean diff: NR	Time: 24 Mean diff: -0.01 95%CI: -0.23,0.14	Ambulatory visits
Finkelstein, 2005[11iii]	Arm B-PLE Interventio n, 2003	Follow-up visits	Unadjusted mean absolute change from baseline	NR	Time: 12 Mean diff: NR	Time: 24 Mean diff: 0.17 95%CI: -0.01, 0.35	Ambulatory visits
Gorton, 199 5[12]	Arm A-Control compariso n site, 19	Prescription of peak flow meter	NR	NR	NR	Mean diff: -0.05 SD diff: 1.08	*p<0.05 for site A and p<0.01 for Site b.
Lesho,2005[16]	Decision Support, 334	Prescriptions for controller medicine	NR	NR	Mean diff: 0.02 p-value: 0.78	NR	Result reported only for those with persistent asthma
Lesho,2005	Decision	Self-	NR	NR	Mean diff: 0.28	NR	Result reported only for

E-204

Author, Year	Arm, N	Health Care Process Outcome	Definition of Scale	Range of Scale	End of treatment Mean difference • SD • 95% CI • P-value	Last Follow-up Mean difference • SD • 95% CI • P-value	Additional Comments
[16]	Support, 334	management education			p-value: <0.001		those with persistent asthma
Mangione-Smith, 2005[3]	Arm A-Control (standard practice), 385	Asthma action plans	All patients should have a written action plan in the medical record that is based on changes in symptoms or peak flow measurement	NR	NR	Mean diff: 1	NR
Mangione-Smith, 2005[3]	Arm B-Learning collaborative, 126	Asthma action plans	All patients should have a written action plan in the medical record that is based on changes in symptoms or peak flow measurement	NR	NR	Mean diff: 34	NR
Mangione-Smith, 2005[3]	Arm A-Control (standard practice), 385	Follow-up visits	Patients whose asthma medications are changed during one visit have a follow-up visit within 6 weeks	NR	NR	Mean diff: 3	NR
Mangione-Smith, 2005[3]	Arm B-Learning collaborative, 126	Follow-up visits	Patients whose asthma medications are changed during one visit have a follow-up visit within 6 weeks	NR	NR	Mean diff: 0	NR
Mangione-Smith, 2005	Arm A-Control	Self-management	NR	NR	NR	Mean diff: -8	NR

Author, Year	Arm, N	Health Care Process Outcome	Definition of Scale	Range of Scale	End of treatment Mean difference • SD • 95% CI • P-value	Last Follow-up Mean difference • SD • 95% CI • P-value	Additional Comments
[3]	(standard practice) 385	education					
Mangione-Smith,2005 [3]	Arm B-Learning collaborative, 126	Self-management education	NR	NR	NR	Mean diff: 16	NR
Mangione-Smith, 2005[21]	Arm A-Control	Followup visits	Patients with asthma shoul have at least two routine planned followup visits for asthma annually.	NR	NR	Mean diff: 4	NR
Mangione-Smith, 2005[21]	Arm B-Learning collaborative	Followup visits	Patients with asthma shoul have at least two routine planned followup visits for asthma annually.	Nr	NR	Mean diff: -12	NR
Mitchell,20 05[17]	Arm A-Control (standard practice)	Prescriptions for controller medicine	% decrease in the number of inhalers prescribed	NR	Time: 9 Mean diff: NR SD diff: 9.99E+02 95%CI: NR p-value: NR 13.3% decrease	NR	NR
Mitchell,20 05[17]	Arm B-Decision support	Prescriptions for controller medicine	% decrease in the number of inhalers prescribed	NR	Time: 9 Mean diff: NR 6.7% decrease	NR	% decrease in the number of inhalers prescribed
Mitchell,20 05[17]	Arm A-Control (standard practice)	Prescriptions for controller medicine	Percent decrease in # of inhaled corticosteroids inhalers	NR	Time: 9 Mean diff: NR SD diff: 9.99E+02 3.5% decrease	NR	Percent decrease in # of inhaled corticosteroids inhalers prescribed.

Author, Year	Arm, N	Health Care Process Outcome	Definition of Scale	Range of Scale	End of treatment Mean difference • SD • 95% CI • P-value	Last Follow-up Mean difference • SE • 95% CI • P-value	Additional Comments
Mitchell, 2005[17]	Arm B- Decision support	Prescriptions for controller medicine	prescribed. Percent decrease in # of inhaled corticosteroids inhalers prescribed.	NR	Time: 9 Mean diff. NR SD diff. NR 95%CI: NR p-value: NR 3.6% decrease	NR	Percent decrease in # of inhaled corticosteroids inhalers prescribed.
Mitchell, 2005[17]	Arm A- Control (standard practice)	Prescriptions for controller medicine	% decrease in Rx's for mast cell stabilizers	NR	Time: 9 Mean diff. NR SD diff. 9.99E+02 44.9% decrease	NR	% decrease in Rx's for mast cell stabilizers
Mitchell, 2005[17]	Arm B- Decision support, NR	Prescriptions for controller medicine	% decrease in Rx's for mast cell stabilizers	NR	Time: 9 Mean diff. NR 38.5% decrease	NR	% decrease in Rx's for mast cell stabilizers
Mitchell, 2005[17]	Arm A- Control (standard practice)	Prescriptions for controller medicine	% decrease in theophylline group of drugs	NR	Time: 9 Mean diff. NR SD diff. 9.99E+02 83.3% decrease	NR	% decrease in Rx's for theophylline group of drugs
Mitchell, 2005[17]	Arm B- Decision support, NR	Prescriptions for controller medicine	% decrease in theophylline group of drugs	NR	Time: 9 Mean diff. NR 31.0% decrease	NR	% decrease in Rx's for theophylline group of drugs
Mitchell, 2005[17]	Arm A- Control (standard practice), NR	Prescriptions for controller medicine	Percent decrease in # of inhaled corticosteroids inhalers prescribed.	NR	Time: 9 Mean diff. NR SD diff. 9.99E+02 3.5% decrease	NR	Percent decrease in # of inhaled corticosteroids inhalers prescribed.
Mitchell, 2005[17]	Arm B- Decision support	Prescriptions for controller medicine	Percent decrease in # of inhaled corticosteroids inhalers prescribed.	NR	Time: 9 Mean diff. NR 3.6% decrease	NR	Percent decrease in # of inhaled corticosteroids inhalers prescribed.
Mitchell, 2005[17]	Arm A- Control (standard	Prescriptions for controller medicine	% decrease in Rx of oral relievers	NR	Time: 9 Mean diff. NR SD diff. 9.99E+02	NR	% decrease in Rx of oral relievers

Author, Year	Arm, N	Health Care Process Outcome	Definition of Scale	Range of Scale	End of treatment Mean difference • SD • 95% CI • P-value	Last Follow-up Mean difference • SD • 95% CI • P-value	Additional Comments
	practice), NR				28.6% decrease		
Mitchell, 2005[17]	Arm B- Decision support	Prescriptions for controller medicine	% decrease in Rx of oral relievers	NR	Time: 9 Mean diff: NR 28.6%	NR	% decrease in Rx of oral relievers
Mitchell, 2005[17]	Arm A- Control (standard practice), NR	Prescriptions for controller medicine	% decrease in Rxs for reliever dry powder devices (in under 5's)	NR	Time: 9 Mean diff: NR SD diff: 9.99E+02 8.2% decrease	NR	% decrease in Rxs for reliever dry powder devices (in under 5's)
Mitchell, 2005[17]	Arm B- Decision support	Prescriptions for controller medicine	% decrease in Rxs for reliever dry powder devices (in under 5's)	NR	Time: 9 Mean diff: NR 23.9% decrease	NR	% decrease in Rxs for reliever dry powder devices (in under 5's)
Patel, 2004[4]	Organizational Change, 427	Asthma action plans	NR	NR	Time: 13 95%CI: 1.8,-4.1 p-value: <0.001 OR= 2.72	NR	NR
Patel, 2004[4]	Organizational Change, 427	Self-management education	NR	NR	Time: 13 95%CI: 1.4,2.7 p-value: <0.001 OR= 1.89	NR	NR
Saini, 2004[8]	Arm C- Education, 39	Documentation of level of asthma control/severity	Perceived control over asthma	11-55	NR	p-value: 0.04	NR
Shapiro, 2011[9]	SBHC, 200	Documentation of level of asthma control/severity	NR	NR	Time: 12 p-value: <0.01	NR	NR
Shapiro, 2011[9]	NYCHP, 249	Documentation of level of asthma control/severity	NR	NR	Time: 12 p-value: <0.001	NR	NR
Smeele, 1999[19]	Arm A- Control (standard	Prescriptions for controller medicine	Exacerbations: Prescription of oral steroids	NR	Mean diff: 0.04 95%CI: -11%,19% p-value: 0.7	NR	NR

Author, Year	Arm, N	Health Care Process Outcome	Definition of Scale	Range of Scale	End of treatment Mean difference • SD • 95% CI • P-value	Last Follow-up Mean difference • SD • 95% CI • P-value	Additional Comments
	practice), 15						
Smeele, 1999[19]	Arm A-Control (standard practice), 17	Prescriptions for controller medicine	Exacerbations: Prescription of inhaled steroids	NR	Mean diff: -0.01 95%CI: -13%, 14% p-value: 0.9	NR	NR
Smeele, 1999[19]	Arm B-Education, 17	Prescriptions for controller medicine	Exacerbations: Prescription of inhaled steroids	NR	Mean diff: 0.13 95%CI: -1%, 27% p-value: 0.08	NR	NR
Smeele, 1999[19]	Arm A-control group	Self-management education	Patient education inhalation instruction materials	NR	change in number of GP=2	NR	NR
Smeele, 1999[19]	Arm B-Education, 17	Self-management education	Patient education inhalation instruction materials	NR	Change in number of GP =+2	NR	NR
Smeele, 1999[19]	Arm A-Control, 17	Self-management education	Advise on house dust mite	NR	Mean diff: 0.04 95%CI: -2%, 10% p-value: 0.2	NR	NR
Smeele, 1999[19]	Arm B-Intervention, 16	Self-management education	Advise on house dust mite	NR	Mean diff: -0.02 95%CI: -6%, 2% p-value: 0.3	NR	NR
Smeele, 1999[19]	Arm A-Control (standard practice), 17	Self-management education	Written patient education	NR	Mean diff: 0.07 95%CI: -1%, 15% p-value: 0.1	NR	NR
Smeele, 1999[19]	Arm B-Education, 16	Self-management education	Written patient education	NR	Mean diff: 0.03 95%CI: -7%, 13% p-value: 0.6	NR	NR
Suh, 2001[10]	Arm A-intermittent, 566	Environmental control practice recommendations	number of prescriptions of long term controller meds	NR	Time: 9 Mean diff: 0.37 SD diff: NR 95%CI: 0.25, 0.47	NR	Mean difference by bootstrap method used to determine the confidence interval was

E-209

Author, Year	Arm, N	Health Care Process Outcome	Definition of Scale	Range of Scale	End of treatment Mean difference • SD • 95% CI • P-value	Last Follow-up Mean difference • SD • 95% CI • P-value	Additional Comments
			per patient		p-value: 0.001		0.37 for intermittent and -0.29 for persistent group. P is less than value in cell for intermittent group.
Suh, 2001[10]	Arm A-intermittent, 566	Prescriptions for controller medicine	"short acting controller"	NR	Time: 9 Mean diff: 0.36 95%CI: 0.23,0.48 p-value: 0.001	NR	p-values less than value in cell — short acting = short acting beta agonist, but not clear in study.
To, 2008[5]	PCAPP Intervention, 1014	Asthma action plans	NR	NR	NR	Time: 12 95%CI: 1.88,3.07 p-value: <0.0001 OR: 2.41	Dichotomous outcome: Have you been given a personal asthma self-management plan or action plan?
Yawn, 2010[20]	Education and Feedback 851	Self-management education	NR	NR	Time: 9 Mean diff: 5.75 p-value: <0.0001	NR	NR

GP = General Practitioner; NR = Not Reported; OR = odds ratio; PCAPP = Primary Care Asthma Pilot Project; PLE = Peer Leader Education; SBHC = South Bronx Health; SD = standard deviation

References

1. Bender BG, Dickinson P, Rankin A, Wamboldt FS, Zittleman L, Westfall JM. J Am Board Fam Med: The Colorado Asthma Toolkit Program: a practice coaching intervention from the High Plains Research Network. 2011; 24:240-8.

2. Daniels EC, Bacon J, Denisio S *et al.* J Asthma: Translation squared: improving asthma care for high-disparity populations through a safety net practice-based research network. 2005; 42:499-505.

3. Mangione-Smith R, Schonlau M, Chan KS *et al.* Ambulatory Pediatrics: Measuring the effectiveness of a collaborative for quality improvement in pediatric asthma care: Does implementing the chronic care model improve processes and outcomes of care? 2005; 5:75-82.

4. Patel PH, Welsh C, Foggs MB. Dis Manag: Improved asthma outcomes using a coordinated care approach in a large medical group. 2004; 7:102-11.

5. To T, Cicutto L, Degani N, McLimont S, Beyene J. Med Care: Can a community evidence-based asthma care program improve clinical outcomes?: a longitudinal study. 2008; 46:1257-66.

6. Ables AZ, Godenick MT, Lipsitz SR. Family Medicine: Improving

family practice residents' compliance with asthma practice guidelines. 2002; 34:23-8.

7. Davis AM, Cannon M, Ables AZ, Bendyk H. Family Medicine: Using the electronic medical record to improve asthma severity documentation and treatment among family medicine residents. 2010; 42:334-7.

8. Saini B, Krass I, Armour C. Annals of Pharmacotherapy: Development, implementation, and evaluation of a community pharmacy-based asthma care model. 2004; 38:1954-60.

9. Shapiro A, Gracy D, Quinones W, Applebaum J, Sarmiento A. Arch Pediatr Adolesc Med: Putting guidelines into practice: improving documentation of pediatric asthma management using a decision-making tool. 2011; 165:412-8.

10. Suh DC, Shin SK, Okpara I, Voytovich RM, Zimmerman A. Am J Manag Care: Impact of a targeted asthma intervention program on treatment costs in patients with asthma. 2001; 7:897-906.

11. Finkelstein JA, Lozano P, Fuhlbrigge AL et al. Health Serv Res: Practice-level effects of interventions to improve asthma care in primary care settings: the Pediatric Asthma Care Patient Outcomes Research Team. 2005; 40:1737-57.

12. Gorton TA, Cranford CO, Golden WE, Walls RC, Pawelak JE. Arch Fam Med: Primary care physicians' response to dissemination of practice guidelines. 1995; 4:135-42.

13. Cho SH, Jeong JW, Park HW et al. J Asthma: Effectiveness of a computer-assisted asthma management program on physician adherence to guidelines. 2010; 47:680-6.

14. Cloutier MM, Hall CB, Wakefield DB, Bailit H. J Pediatr: Use of asthma guidelines by primary care providers to reduce hospitalizations and emergency department visits in poor, minority, urban children. 2005; 146:591-7.

15. Davis RS, Bukstein DA, Luskin AT, Kailin JA, Goodenow G. Ann Allergy Asthma Immunol: Changing physician prescribing patterns through problem-based learning: an interactive, teleconference case-based education program and review of problem-based learning. 2004; 93:237-42.

16. Lesho EP, Myers CP, Ott M, Winslow C, Brown JE. Mil Med: Do clinical practice guidelines improve processes or outcomes in primary care? 2005; 170:243-6.

17. Mitchell EA, Didsbury PB, Kruithof N et al. Acta Paediatr: A randomized controlled trial of an asthma clinical pathway for children in general practice. 2005; 94:226-33.

18. Premaratne UN, Sterne JA, Marks GB, Webb JR, Azima H, Burney PG. BMJ: Clustered randomised trial of an intervention to improve the management of asthma: Greenwich asthma study. 1999; 318:1251-5.

19. Smeele IJ, Grol RP, van Schayck CP, van den Bosch WJ, van den Hoogen HJ, Muris JW. Qual Health Care: Can small group education and peer review improve care for patients with asthma/chronic obstructive pulmonary disease? 1999; 8:92-8.

20. Yawn BP, Bertram S, Wollan P. Journal of Asthma and Allergy: Introduction of asthma APGAR tools improve asthma management in primary care practices. 2008; 1-10.

21. Mangione-Smith R, Schonlau M, Chan KS, et al. Ambulatory Pediatrics: Measuring the effectiveness of a collaborative for quality improvement in pediatric asthma care: Does implementing the chronic care model improve processes and outcomes of care? 2005; 575-82.

Evidence Table 11. Risk of bias

	Randomized Control Studies									
Author, year	Random sequence generation	Allocation concealment	Blinding of Participants	Blinding of Investigators	Blinding of healthcare process outcome assessment	Blinding of clinical outcome assessment	Incomplete healthcare process outcome data	Incomplete clinical outcome data	Selective reporting	Other bias
Shah S., 2011[50]	Low Risk	Low Risk	Low Risk	Low Risk	Unclear Risk	Unclear Risk	Unclear Risk	Unclear Risk	Unclear Risk	N/A
Shapiro A., 2011[51]	High Risk	High Risk	High Risk	High Risk	Low Risk	Unclear Risk	Low Risk	Unclear Risk	Low Risk	N/A
Fairall L., 2010[19]	Low Risk	Low Risk	High Risk	Unclear Risk	Low Risk	N/A	Unclear Risk	N/A	Unclear Risk	Unclear Risk
De Vries, 2010[17]	High Risk	High Risk	High Risk	Unclear Risk	Low Risk	N/A	Unclear Risk	N/A	Low Risk	N/A
Liaw ST, 2008[33]	Low Risk	Unclear Risk	Unclear Risk	High Risk	Low Risk	N/A	Unclear Risk	N/A	High Risk	N/A
Hagmolen, W., 2008[24]	Unclear Risk	Unclear Risk	Low Risk	Unclear Risk	Unclear Risk	Unclear Risk	Low Risk	Low Risk	Low Risk	Low Risk
Hagmolen, W., 2008[24]	Unclear Risk	Unclear Risk	Low Risk	Low Risk	High Risk	High Risk	Low Risk	Low Risk	Low Risk	Low Risk
Schneider A., 2008[49]	Unclear Risk	Unclear Risk	Unclear Risk	Unclear Risk	Unclear Risk	Unclear Risk	Low Risk	Low Risk	Low Risk	Low Risk
Martens J.D., 2007[38]	Unclear Risk	Unclear Risk	Low Risk	Unclear Risk	Low Risk	Low Risk	High Risk	High Risk	Low Risk	High Risk
Renzi PM 2006[45]	Unclear Risk	Unclear Risk	High Risk	High Risk	High Risk	High Risk	N/A		Low Risk	

Randomized Control Studies

Author, year	Random sequence generation	Allocation concealment	Blinding of Participants	Blinding of Investigators	Blinding of healthcare process outcome assessment	Blinding of clinical outcome assessment	Incomplete healthcare process outcome data	Incomplete clinical outcome data	Selective reporting	Other bias
Shah S, 2011[50]	Low Risk	Low Risk	Low Risk	Low Risk	Unclear Risk	Unclear Risk	Unclear Risk	Unclear Risk	Unclear Risk	N/A
Shapiro A., 2011[51]	High Risk	High Risk	High Risk	High Risk	Low Risk	Unclear Risk	Low Risk	Unclear Risk	Low Risk	N/A
Fairall L., 2010[19]	Low Risk	Low Risk	High Risk	Unclear Risk	Low Risk	N/A	Unclear Risk	N/A	Unclear Risk	Unclear Risk
De Vries, 2010[17]	High Risk	High Risk	High Risk	Unclear Risk	Low Risk	N/A	Unclear Risk	N/A	Low Risk	N/A
Liaw ST, 2008[33]	Low Risk	Unclear Risk	Unclear Risk	High Risk	Low Risk	N/A	Unclear Risk	N/A	High Risk	N/A
Cabana MD, 2006[7]	Low Risk	High Risk	High Risk	High Risk	High Risk	High Risk	Low Risk	Low Risk	Low Risk	N/A
Kattan M, 2006[31]	Low Risk	Low Risk	High Risk	High Risk	Unclear Risk	Unclear Risk	Low Risk	Low Risk	Low Risk	N/A
Finkelstein J. A., 2005[21]	Low Risk	Unclear Risk	High Risk	Low Risk	Low Risk	Low Risk	Low Risk	Low Risk	Low Risk	N/A
Daniels E. C., 2005[14]	Low Risk	Unclear Risk	High Risk	Unclear Risk	Unclear Risk	N/A	Low Risk	N/A	Low Risk	N/A
Mitchell E.A.,2005[40]	Low Risk	Unclear Risk	High Risk	High Risk	High Risk	High Risk	Low Risk	Low Risk	Low Risk	N/A
Lozano P, 2004[34]	Unclear Risk	High Risk	High Risk	High Risk	Unclear Risk	Low Risk	High Risk	High Risk	Low Risk	Low Risk
Baker R., 2003[2]	Low Risk	Low Risk	High Risk	Unclear Risk	Low Risk	Low Risk	High Risk	High Risk	Unclear Risk	N/A

Randomized Control Studies

Author, year	Random sequence generation	Allocation concealment	Blinding of Participants	Blinding of Investigators	Blinding of healthcare process outcome assessment	Blinding of clinical outcome assessment	Incomplete healthcare process outcome data	Incomplete clinical outcome data	Selective reporting	Other bias
Shah S., 2011[50]	Low Risk	Low Risk	Low Risk	Low Risk	Unclear Risk	Unclear Risk	Unclear Risk	Unclear Risk	Unclear Risk	N/A
Shapiro A., 2011[51]	High Risk	High Risk	High Risk	High Risk	Low Risk	Unclear Risk	Low Risk	Unclear Risk	Low Risk	N/A
Fairall L., 2010[19]	Low Risk	Low Risk	High Risk	Unclear Risk	Low Risk	N/A	Unclear Risk	N/A	Unclear Risk	Unclear Risk
De Vries, 2010[17]	High Risk	High Risk	High Risk	Unclear Risk	Low Risk	N/A	Unclear Risk	N/A	Low Risk	N/A
Liaw ST, 2008[33]	Low Risk	Unclear Risk	Unclear Risk	High Risk	Low Risk	N/A	Unclear Risk	N/A	High Risk	N/A
Eccles M, 2002[18]	Low Risk	Unclear Risk	High Risk	Unclear Risk	Low Risk	Unclear Risk	Low Risk	High Risk	High Risk	Low Risk
Sondergaard J., 2002[54]	Unclear Risk	Unclear Risk	High Risk	Unclear Risk	Low Risk		Low Risk		Low Risk	Low Risk
Herborg H., 2001[27]	High Risk	High Risk	Low Risk	High Risk	Low Risk	Low Risk	High Risk	High Risk	High Risk	Low Risk
Smeele I. J., 1999[53]	Low Risk	Unclear Risk	Unclear Risk	Unclear Risk	Unclear Risk	Unclear Risk	Low Risk	Unclear Risk	Unclear Risk	Low Risk
Lundborg C. S., 1999[35]	High Risk	High Risk	Unclear Risk	Unclear Risk	Low Risk	Low Risk	High Risk	High Risk	High Risk	Low Risk
Premaratne U. N., 1999[43]	Low Risk	High Risk	Unclear Risk	Unclear Risk	Unclear Risk	Low Risk	Low Risk	High Risk	Low Risk	Low Risk

Randomized Control Studies										
Author, year	Random sequence generation	Allocation concealment	Blinding of Participants	Blinding of Investigators	Blinding of healthcare process outcome assessment	Blinding of clinical outcome assessment	Incomplete healthcare process outcome data	Incomplete clinical outcome data	Selective reporting	Other bias
Shah S., 2011[50]	Low Risk	Low Risk	Low Risk	Low Risk	Unclear Risk	Unclear Risk	Unclear Risk	Unclear Risk	Unclear Risk	N/A
Shapiro A., 2011[51]	High Risk	High Risk	High Risk	High Risk	Low Risk	Unclear Risk	Low Risk	Unclear Risk	Low Risk	N/A
Fairall L., 2010[19]	Low Risk	Low Risk	High Risk	Unclear Risk	Low Risk	N/A	Unclear Risk	N/A	Unclear Risk	Unclear Risk
De Vries, 2010[17]	High Risk	High Risk	High Risk	Unclear Risk	Low Risk	N/A	Unclear Risk	N/A	Low Risk	N/A
Liaw ST, 2008[33]	Low Risk	Unclear Risk	Unclear Risk	High Risk	Low Risk	N/A	Unclear Risk	N/A	High Risk	N/A
Gorton TA, 1995[23]	High Risk	High Risk	High Risk	Unclear Risk	Unclear Risk	Unclear Risk	High Risk	High Risk	Low Risk	High Risk
Halterman J.S., 2006[25]	Low Risk	Low Risk	High Risk	N/A	Low Risk	Low Risk	Low Risk	N/A	Low Risk	N/A
Halterman JS, 2005[26]	Low Risk	Unclear Risk	High Risk	Unclear Risk	Low Risk	Low Risk	Low Risk	Low Risk	Unclear Risk	Low Risk
Holton C., 2011[28]	Unclear Risk	Low Risk	High Risk	Unclear Risk	Unclear Risk	Unclear Risk	Low Risk	Unclear Risk	High Risk	High Risk
Veninga CCM, 2000[59]	Unclear Risk	Unclear Risk	High Risk	High Risk	Low Risk	Unclear Risk	Unclear Risk	Unclear Risk	Low Risk	Low Risk

Randomized Control Studies

Author, year	Random sequence generation	Allocation concealment	Blinding of Participants	Blinding of Investigators	Blinding of healthcare process outcome assessment	Blinding of clinical outcome assessment	Incomplete healthcare process outcome data	Incomplete clinical outcome data	Selective reporting	Other bias
Shah S., 2011[50]	Low Risk	Low Risk	Low Risk	Low Risk	Unclear Risk	Unclear Risk	Unclear Risk	Unclear Risk	Unclear Risk	N/A
Shapiro A., 2011[51]	High Risk	High Risk	High Risk	High Risk	Low Risk	Unclear Risk	Low Risk	Unclear Risk	Low Risk	N/A
Fairall L., 2010[19]	Low Risk	Low Risk	High Risk	Unclear Risk	Low Risk	N/A	Unclear Risk	N/A	Unclear Risk	Unclear Risk
De Vries, 2010[17]	High Risk	High Risk	High Risk	Unclear Risk	Low Risk	N/A	Unclear Risk	N/A	Low Risk	N/A
Liaw ST, 2008[33]	Low Risk	Unclear Risk	Unclear Risk	High Risk	Low Risk	N/A	Unclear Risk	N/A	High Risk	N/A
Yawn BP, 2008[62]	High Risk	Unclear Risk	High Risk	High Risk	High Risk	N/A	Unclear Risk	N/A	Unclear Risk	Unclear Risk
Yawn BP, 2008[62]	High Risk	Unclear Risk	High Risk	High Risk	High Risk	N/A	Unclear Risk	N/A	Unclear Risk	Unclear Risk
Brown R, 2004[5]	Unclear Risk	High Risk	Unclear Risk	High Risk	Unclear Risk	Unclear Risk	Unclear Risk	Low Risk	Low Risk	N/A
Ruoff G., 2002[47]	Low Risk	Low Risk	Unclear Risk	High Risk	High Risk	Unclear Risk	Unclear Risk	Unclear Risk	Unclear Risk	Low Risk
Davis A.M., 2010[15]	Low Risk		High Risk	High Risk	High Risk	High Risk	Unclear Risk	Unclear Risk	Unclear Risk	Unclear Risk

Randomized Control Studies

Author, year	Random sequence generation	Allocation concealment	Blinding of Participants	Blinding of Investigators	Blinding of healthcare process outcome assessment	Blinding of clinical outcome assessment	Incomplete healthcare process outcome data	Incomplete clinical outcome data	Selective reporting	Other bias
Shah S., 2011[50]	Low Risk	Low Risk	Low Risk	Low Risk	Unclear Risk	Unclear Risk	Unclear Risk	Unclear Risk	Unclear Risk	N/A
Shapiro A., 2011[51]	High Risk	High Risk	High Risk	High Risk	Low Risk	Unclear Risk	Low Risk	Unclear Risk	Low Risk	N/A
Fairall L., 2010[19]	Low Risk	Low Risk	High Risk	Unclear Risk	Low Risk	N/A	Unclear Risk	N/A	Unclear Risk	Unclear Risk
De Vries, 2010[17]	High Risk	High Risk	High Risk	Unclear Risk	Low Risk	N/A	Unclear Risk	N/A	Low Risk	N/A
Liaw ST, 2008[33]	Low Risk	Unclear Risk	Unclear Risk	High Risk	Low Risk	N/A	Unclear Risk	N/A	High Risk	N/A
Veninga CCM, 1999[60]	Unclear Risk	Unclear Risk	Low Risk	High Risk	Low Risk	N/A	Unclear Risk	N/A	Low Risk	N/A
Feder G, 1995[20]	Unclear Risk	High Risk	High Risk	High Risk	High Risk	N/A	Unclear Risk	N/A	Unclear Risk	Unclear Risk
Mangione-Smith R., 2005[37]	High Risk	High Risk	High Risk	High Risk	High Risk	High Risk	Unclear Risk	Unclear Risk	Unclear Risk	N/A
Weinberger M, 2002[61]	Low Risk	Unclear Risk	Low Risk	Low Risk	Low Risk	Low Risk	Low Risk	Low Risk	Low Risk	Low Risk
Saini B, 2004[48]	High Risk	High Risk	High Risk	High Risk	High Risk	High Risk	Low Risk	Low Risk	Unclear Risk	High Risk

	Randomized Control Studies									
Author, year	Random sequence generation	Allocation concealment	Blinding of Participants	Blinding of Investigators	Blinding of healthcare process outcome assessment	Blinding of clinical outcome assessment	Incomplete healthcare process outcome data	Incomplete clinical outcome data	Selective reporting	Other bias
Shah S., 2011[50]	Low Risk	Low Risk	Low Risk	Low Risk	Unclear Risk	Unclear Risk	Unclear Risk	Unclear Risk	Unclear Risk	N/A
Shapiro A., 2011[51]	High Risk	High Risk	High Risk	High Risk	Low Risk	Unclear Risk	Low Risk	Unclear Risk	Low Risk	N/A
Fairall L., 2010[19]	Low Risk	Low Risk	High Risk	Unclear Risk	Low Risk	N/A	Unclear Risk	N/A	Unclear Risk	Unclear Risk
De Vries, 2010[17]	High Risk	High Risk	High Risk	Unclear Risk	Low Risk	N/A	Unclear Risk	N/A	Low Risk	N/A
Liaw ST, 2008[33]	Low Risk	Unclear Risk	Unclear Risk	High Risk	Low Risk	N/A	Unclear Risk	N/A	High Risk	N/A
Saini B, 2004[48]	High Risk	High Risk	High Risk	High Risk	High Risk	High Risk	Low Risk	Low Risk	Unclear Risk	High Risk
Bryce FP, 1995[6]	Low Risk	Unclear Risk	Low Risk	Low Risk	Low Risk	Low Risk	Low Risk	Low Risk	Low Risk	Low Risk
Bryce FP, 1995[6]	Low Risk	Unclear Risk	Low Risk	Low Risk	Low Risk	Low Risk	Low Risk	Low Risk	Low Risk	Low Risk
McCowan C., 2001[39]	Low Risk	Low Risk	Unclear Risk	Unclear Risk	Unclear Risk	Unclear Risk	High Risk	High Risk	Unclear Risk	High Risk
Cloutier MM, 2012[63]	Unclear Risk	Unclear Risk	High Risk	High Risk	Unclear Risk		High Risk		High Risk	

Pre-post studies

Author, year	Random sequence generation	Allocation concealment	Blinding of Participants	Blinding of Investigators	Blinding of healthcare process outcome assessment	Blinding of clinical outcome assessment	Incomplete healthcare process outcome data	Incomplete clinical outcome data	Selective reporting	Other bias	Independent intervention	Intervention unlikely to affect data collection
Rance K., 2011[44]	High Risk	High Risk	High Risk	Unclear Risk	Low Risk	Unclear Risk	Low Risk	Low Risk	Low Risk	Low Risk	Yes	Yes
Bender B. G., 2011[3]	Unclear Risk	Unclear Risk	High Risk	Low Risk	Unclear Risk	High Risk	Unclear Risk	Unclear Risk	Low Risk	Low Risk	Yes	Yes
Cho S. H., 2010[8]	Unclear Risk	Unclear Risk	High Risk	Low Risk	Low Risk	Unclear Risk	Low Risk	Unclear Risk	Low Risk	Low Risk	Yes	Yes
Sulaiman N. D., 2010[56]	Low Risk	Low Risk	High Risk	Low Risk	Low Risk	Low Risk	Low Risk	Low Risk	Low Risk	Low Risk	Yes	Yes
To T., 2008[58]	N/A	N/A	High Risk	High Risk	High Risk	High Risk	Low Risk	Low Risk	Low Risk	N/A	Yes	Yes
Horswell R., 2008[29]	High Risk	High Risk	High Risk	High Risk	Low Risk	Low Risk	Unclear Risk	Unclear Risk	Low Risk	N/A	Yes	Yes
Frankowski B. L., 2006[22]	High Risk	High Risk	High Risk	High Risk	High Risk	Unclear Risk	Low Risk	Unclear Risk	Unclear Risk	N/A	Yes	No
Cloutier M.M., 2005[11]	Unclear Risk	Unclear Risk	High Risk	High Risk	Low Risk	Low Risk	Low Risk	Low Risk	Low Risk	N/A	Yes	No
Lesho EP, 2005[32]	Unclear Risk	Unclear Risk	High Risk	High Risk	High Risk	High Risk	Low Risk	Low Risk	High Risk	N/A	Yes	No
Davis R. S., 2004[16]	Unclear Risk	Unclear Risk	High Risk	High Risk	High Risk	Unclear Risk	Low Risk	Unclear Risk	Low Risk	N/A	Yes	Yes
Mahi-Taright S., 2004[36]	Unclear Risk	Unclear Risk	High Risk	High Risk	Low Risk	Low Risk	Unclear Risk	Unclear Risk	Unclear Risk	N/A	Yes	Yes

E-219

Pre-post studies

Author, year	Random sequence generation	Allocation concealment	Blinding of Participants	Blinding of Investigators	Blinding of healthcare process outcome assessment	Blinding of clinical outcome assessment	Incomplete healthcare process outcome data	Incomplete clinical outcome data	Selective reporting	Other bias	Independent intervention	Intervention unlikely to affect data collection
Patel P. H., 2004 [42]	Unclear Risk	Unclear Risk	High Risk	High Risk	High Risk	High Risk	Low Risk	Low Risk	Low Risk	N/A	Yes	Yes
Coleman C. I., 2003 [13]	Low Risk	Low Risk	Low Risk	Unclear Risk	Low Risk	Low Risk	Low Risk	Low Risk	Low Risk	Low Risk	Yes	No
Cloutier M.M., 2002 [12]	Low Risk	Low Risk	Unclear Risk	Unclear Risk	Low Risk	Low Risk	Unclear Risk	Low Risk	Low Risk	Low Risk	Yes	Yes
Suh D. C., 2001 [55]	Low Risk	Low Risk	Low Risk	Low Risk	Low Risk	Unclear Risk	Unclear Risk	Unclear Risk	Unclear Risk	Low Risk	No	Yes
Richman M. J, 2000 [46]	High Risk	High Risk	Unclear Risk	Unclear Risk	Unclear Risk	Unclear Risk	High Risk	High Risk	Unclear Risk	Low Risk	No	No
Shiffman R.N., 2000 [52]	High Risk	High Risk	High Risk	High Risk	High Risk	High Risk	Unclear Risk	Unclear Risk	Unclear Risk	Low Risk	No	Yes
Hoskins G., 1997 [30]	High Risk	High Risk	Unclear Risk	Unclear Risk	Unclear Risk	Unclear Risk	High Risk	High Risk	Unclear Risk	Low Risk	No	No

Pre-post studies

Author, year	Random sequence generation	Allocation concealment	Blinding of Participants	Blinding of Investigators	Blinding of healthcare process outcome assessment	Blinding of clinical outcome assessment	Incomplete healthcare process outcome data	Incomplete clinical outcome data	Selective reporting	Other bias	Independent intervention	Intervention unlikely to affect data collection
Blackstien-Hirsch P., 2000 [4]	High Risk	High Risk	High Risk	High Risk	High Risk	High Risk	High Risk	High Risk	Unclear Risk	Unclear Risk	Yes	No
Cloutier MM, 2009 [10]	High Risk	High Risk	High Risk	High Risk	Unclear Risk	Unclear Risk	Unclear Risk	Unclear Risk	Low Risk		Yes	Yes
Thyne S.M., 2007 [57]	Unclear Risk	Unclear Risk	High Risk	High Risk	Unclear Risk	Unclear Risk	Unclear Risk	High Risk	Low Risk	Low Risk	Yes	Yes
O'Laughlen MC, 2008 [41]	High Risk	Unclear Risk	High Risk	High Risk	Unclear Risk	High Risk	Unclear Risk	Unclear Risk	Unclear Risk	N/A	Yes	No
Ables AZ, 2002 [1]	Unclear Risk	Unclear Risk	High Risk	High Risk	High Risk	High Risk	Unclear Risk	Unclear Risk	Unclear Risk	N/A	Yes	No

N/A= Not applicable

References

1. Ables AZ, Godenick MT, Lipsitz SR. Family Medicine: Improving family practice residents' compliance with asthma practice guidelines. 2002; 34:23-8.

2. Baker R, Fraser RC, Stone M, Lambert P, Stevenson K, Shiels C. Br J Gen Pract: Randomised controlled trial of the impact of guidelines, prioritized review criteria and feedback on implementation of recommendations for angina and asthma. 2003; 53:284-91.

3. Bender BG, Dickinson P, Rankin A, Wamboldt FS, Zittleman L, Westfall JM. J Am Board Fam Med: The Colorado Asthma Toolkit Program: a practice coaching intervention from the High Plains Research Network. 2011; 24:240-8.

4. Blackstien-Hirsch P, Anderson G, Cicutto L, McIvor A, Norton P. Journal of Asthma: Implementing continuing education strategies for family physicians to enhance asthma patients' quality of life. 2000; 37:247-57.

5. Brown R, Bratton SL, Cabana MD, Kaciroti N, Clark NM. Chest: Physician asthma education program improves outcomes for children of low-income families. 2004; 126:369-74.

6. Bryce FP, Neville RG, Crombie IK, Clark RA, McKenzie P. British Medical Journal: Controlled trial of an audit facilitator in diagnosis and treatment of childhood asthma in general practice. 1995; 310:838-42.

7. Cabana MD, Slish KK, Evans D et al. Pediatrics: Impact of physician asthma care education on patient outcomes. 2006; 117:2149-57.

8. Cho SH, Jeong JW, Park HW et al. J Asthma: Effectiveness of a computer-assisted asthma management program on physician adherence to guidelines. 2010; 47:680-6.

9. Clark NMGMSMeal . Impact of education for physicians on patient outcomes. Pediatrics 1998; 101(5):831-6.

10. Cloutier MM, Grosse SD, Wakefield DB, Nurmagambetov TA, Brown CM. American Journal of Managed Care: The economic impact of an urban asthma management program. 2009; 15:345-51.

11. Cloutier MM, Hall CB, Wakefield DB, Bailit H. J Pediatr: Use of asthma guidelines by primary care providers to reduce hospitalizations and emergency department visits in poor, minority, urban children. 2005; 146:591-7.

12. Cloutier MM, Wakefield DB, Carlisle PS, Bailit HL, Hall CB. Arch Pediatr Adolesc Med: The effect of Easy Breathing on asthma management and knowledge. 2002; 156:1045-51.

13. Coleman CI, Reddy P, Laster-Bradley NM, Dorval S, Munagala B, White CM. Ann Pharmacother: Effect of practitioner education on adherence to asthma treatment guidelines. 2003; 37:956-61.

14. Daniels EC, Bacon J, Denisio S et al. J Asthma: Translation squared: improving asthma care for high-disparity populations through a safety net practice-based research network. 2005; 42:499-505.

15. Davis AM, Cannon M, Ables AZ, Bendyk H. Family Medicine: Using the electronic medical record to improve asthma severity documentation and treatment among family medicine residents. 2010; 42:334-7.

16. Davis RS, Bukstein DA, Luskin AT, Kailin JA, Goodenow G. Ann Allergy Asthma Immunol: Changing physician prescribing patterns through problem-based learning: an interactive, teleconference case-based education program and review of problem-based learning. 2004; 93:237-42.

17. de Vries TW, van den Berg PB, Duiverman EJ, de Jong-van den Berg LT. Arch Dis Child: Effect of a minimal pharmacy intervention on improvement of adherence to asthma guidelines. 2010; 95:302-4.

18. Eccles M, McColl E, Steen N et al. BMJ: Effect of computerised evidence based guidelines on management of asthma and angina in adults in primary care: cluster randomised controlled trial. 2002; 325:941.

19. Fairall L, Bachmann MO, Zwarenstein M et al. Trop Med Int Health: Cost-effectiveness of educational outreach to primary care nurses to increase tuberculosis case detection and improve respiratory care: economic evaluation alongside a randomised trial. 2010; 15:277-86.

20. Feder G, Griffiths C, Highton C, Eldridge S, Spence M, Southgate L. British Medical Journal: Do clinical guidelines introduced with practice based education improve care of asthmatic and diabetic patients? A randomised controlled trial in general practices in east London. 1995; 311:1473-8.

21. Finkelstein JA, Lozano P, Fuhlbrigge AL et al. Health Serv Res: Practice-level effects of interventions to improve asthma care in primary care settings: the Pediatric Asthma Care Patient Outcomes Research Team. 2005; 40:1737-57.

22. Frankowski BL, Keating K, Rexroad A et al. J Sch Health: Community collaboration: concurrent physician and school nurse education and cooperation increases the use of asthma action plans. 2006; 76:303-6.

23. Gorton TA, Cranford CO, Golden WE, Walls RC, Pawelak JE. Arch Fam Med: Primary care physicians' response to dissemination of practice guidelines. 1995; 4:135-42.

24. Hagmolen ten Have W, van den Berg NJ, van der Palen J, van Aalderen WM, Bindels PJ. Prim Care Respir J: Implementation of an asthma guideline for the management of childhood asthma in general practice: a randomised controlled trial. 2008; 17:90-6.

25. Halterman JS , Fisher S, Conn KM et al. Archives of Pediatrics & Adolescent Medicine: Improved preventive care for asthma: a randomized trial of clinician prompting in pediatric offices. 2006; 160:1018-25.

26. Halterman JS , McConnochie KM, Conn KM et al. Archives of Pediatrics and Adolescent Medicine: A randomized trial of primary care provider prompting to enhance preventive asthma therapy. 2005; 159:422-7.

27. Herborg H, Soendergaard B, Jorgensen T et al. J Am Pharm Assoc (Wash): Improving drug therapy for patients with asthma-part 2: Use of antiasthma medications. 2001; 41:551-9.

28. Holton C, Crockett A, Nelson M et al. International Journal for Quality in Health Care: Does spirometry training in general practice improve quality and outcomes of asthma care? 2011; 23:545-53.

29. Horswell R, Butler MK, Kaiser M et al. Dis Manag: Disease management programs for the underserved. 2008; 11:145-52.

30. Hoskins G, Neville RG, Smith B, Clark RA. Health Bull (Edinb): Does participation in distance learning and audit improve the care of patients with acute asthma attacks? The General Practitioners in Asthma Group. 1997; 55:150-5.

31. Kattan M, Crain EF, Steinbach S et al. Pediatrics: A randomized clinical trial of clinician feedback to improve quality of care for inner-city children with asthma. 2006; 117:e1095-103.

32. Lesho EP, Myers CP, Ott M, Winslow C, Brown JE. Mil Med: Do clinical practice guidelines improve processes or outcomes in primary care? 2005; 170:243-6.

33. Liaw ST, Sulaiman ND, Earton CA et al. BMC Fam Pract: An interactive workshop plus locally adapted guidelines can improve general practitioners asthma management and knowledge: a cluster randomised trial in the Australian setting. 2008; 9:22.

34. Lozano P, Finkelstein JA, Carey VJ et al. Arch Pediatr Adolesc Med: A multisite randomized trial of the effects of physician education and organizational change in chronic-asthma care: health outcomes of the Pediatric Asthma Care Patient Outcomes Research Team II Study. 2004; 158:875-83.

35. Lundborg CS, Wahlstrom R, Oke T, Tomson G, Diwan VK. J Clin Epidemiol: Influencing prescribing for urinary tract infection and asthma in primary care in Sweden: a randomized controlled trial of an interactive educational intervention. 1999; 52:801-12.

36. Mahi-Taright S, Belhocine M, Ait-Ehaled N. Int J Tuberc Lung Dis: Can we improve the management of chronic obstructive respiratory disease? The example of asthma in adults. 2004; 8:873-81.

37. Mangione-Smith R, Schonlau M, Chan KS et al. Ambulatory Pediatrics: Measuring the effectiveness of a collaborative for quality improvement in pediatric asthma care: Does implementing the chronic care model improve processes and outcomes of care? 2005; 5:75-82.

38. Martens JD, van der Weijden T, Severens JL et al. Int J Med Inform: The effect of computer reminders on GPs' prescribing behaviour: a cluster-randomised trial. 2007; 76 Suppl 3:S403-16.

39. McCowan C, Neville RG, Ricketts IW, Warner FC, Hoskins G, Thomas GE. Medical Informatics and the Internet in Medicine: Lessons from a randomized controlled trial designed to evaluate computer decision support software to improve the management of asthma. 2001; 26:191-201.

40. Mitchell EA, Didsbury PB, Kruithof N et al. Acta Paediatr: A randomized controlled trial of an asthma clinical pathway for children in general practice. 2005; 94:226-33.

41. OLaughlen MC, Hollen PJ, Rakes G, Ting S. Pediatric Asthma, Allergy and Immunology: Improving pediatric asthma by the MSAGR algorithm: A multicolored, simplified, asthma guideline reminder. 2008; 21:119-27.

42. Patel PH, Welsh C, Foggs MB. Dis Manag: Improved asthma outcomes using a coordinated care approach in a large medical group. 2004; 7:102-11.

43. Premaratne UN, Sterne JA, Marks GB, Webb JR, Azima H, Burney PG. BMJ: Clustered randomised trial of an intervention to improve the management of asthma: Greenwich asthma study. 1999; 318:1251-5.

44. Rance K, OLaughlen M, Ting S. J Pediatr Health Care: Improving asthma care for African American children by increasing national asthma guideline adherence. 2011; 25:235-49.

45. Renzi PM, Ghezzo H, Goulet S, Dorval E, Thivierge RL. Can Respir J: Paper stamp checklist tool enhances asthma guidelines knowledge and implementation by primary care physicians. 2006; 13:193-7.

46. Richman MJ, Poltawsky JS. Stud Health Technol Inform: Partnership for excellence in asthma care: evidence-based disease management. 2000; 76:107-21.

47. Ruoff G. Family Medicine: Effects of flow sheet implementation on physician performance in the management of asthmatic patients. 2002; 34:514-7.

48. Saini B, Krass I, Armour C. Annals of Pharmacotherapy: Development, implementation, and evaluation of a community pharmacy-based asthma care model. 2004; 38:1954-60.

49. Schneider A, Wensing M, Biessecker K, Quinzler R, Kaufmann-Kolle P, Szecsenyi J. J Eval Clin Pract: Impact of quality circles for improvement of asthma care: results of a randomized controlled trial. 2008; 14:185-90.

50. Shah S, Sawyer SM, Toelle BG et al. Med J Aust: Improving paediatric asthma outcomes in primary health care: a randomised controlled trial. 2011; 195:405-9.

51. Shapiro A, Gracy D, Quinones W, Applebaum J, Sarmiento A. Arch Pediatr Adolesc Med: Putting guidelines into practice: improving documentation of pediatric asthma management using a decision-making tool. 2011; 165:412-8.

52. Shiffman RN, Freudigman M, Brandt CA, Liaw Y, Navedo DD. Pediatrics: A guideline implementation system using handheld computers for office management of asthma: effects on adherence and patient outcomes. 2000; 105:767-73.

53. Smeele IJ, Grol RP, van Schayck CP, van den Bosch WJ, van den Hoogen HJ, Muris JW. Qual Health Care: Can small group education and peer review improve care for patients with asthma/chronic obstructive pulmonary disease? 1999; 8:92-8.

54. Sondergaard J, Andersen M, Vach K, Kragstrup J, Maclure M, Gram LF. Eur J Clin Pharmacol: Detailed postal feedback about prescribing to asthma patients combined with a guideline statement showed no impact: a randomised controlled trial. 2002; 58:127-32.

55. Suh DC, Shin SK, Okpara I, Voytovich RM, Zimmerman A. Am J Manag Care: Impact of a targeted asthma intervention program on treatment costs in patients with asthma. 2001; 7:897-906.

56. Sulaiman ND, Barton CA, Liaw ST et al. Fam Pract: Do small group workshops and locally adapted guidelines improve asthma patients' health outcomes? A cluster randomized controlled trial. 2010; 27:246-54.

57. Thyne SM, Marmor AK, Madden N, Herrick G. Paediatric and Perinatal Epidemiology: Comprehensive asthma management for underserved children. 2007; 21:29-34.

58. To T, Cicutto L, Degani N, McLimont S, Beyene J. Med Care: Can a community evidence-based asthma care program improve clinical outcomes?: a longitudinal study. 2008; 46:1257-66.

59. Veninga CCM, Denig P, Zwaagstra R, Haaijer-Ruskamp FM. Journal of Clinical Epidemiology: Improving drug treatment in general practice. 2000; 53:752-72.

60. Veninga CCM, Lagerl++v P, Wahlstr+¦m R et al. American Journal of Respiratory and Critical Care Medicine: Evaluating an educational intervention to improve the treatment of asthma in four european countries. 1999; 160 :1254-62.

61. Weinberger M, Murray MD, Marrero DG et al. Journal of the American Medical Association: Effectiveness of pharmacist care for patients with reactive airways disease: A randomized controlled trial. 2002; 288: 594-602.

62. Yawn BP, Bertram S, Wollan P. Journal of Asthma and Allergy: Introduction of asthma APGAR tools improve asthma management in primary care practices. 2008; 1-10.

63. Cloutier MM, Tennen H, Wakefield DB, Brazil K, Hall CB. Improving clinician self-efficacy does not increase asthma guideline use by primary care clinicians. Acad. Pediatr. 2012; 12(4):312-8.

www.ingramcontent.com/pod-product-compliance
Lightning Source LLC
Chambersburg PA
CBHW081430170526
45166CB00008B/2154